The Mommy MD Guide

to
Your Baby's First Year

Tips That 70 Doctors Who Are Also
Mothers Use During Their Babies' First Year

By Rallie McAllister, MD, MPH
and Jennifer Bright Reich

MOMOSA PUBLISHING

© 2011 by Momosa Publishing LLC

Printed in Hong Kong

Illustrations by Carrie Wendel

Book design by Leanne Coppola

Library of Congress Control Number 2011931922

ISBN 978-0-9844804-2-5

2 4 6 8 10 9 7 5 3 1 paperback

The Mommy MD Guides

Motherhood is a journey.
Mommy MDs are your guides.

MommyMDGuides.com

To my son Staff Sergeant Chad Andrew Millice, USMC
—RM

To Mike, Tyler, and Austin
—JBR

Contents

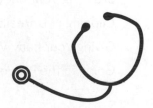

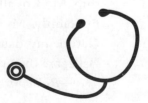

Acknowledgments

Life is full of delightful surprises. Four years ago, I received an e-mail from a journalist who politely inquired if she could interview me for a book she was writing for *Prevention* magazine. The e-mail arrived on an ordinary day in the middle of an ordinary workweek, and the message was short, simple, and straightforward. How could I have known that it would end up changing the course of my life so dramatically? The writer was Jennifer Bright Reich, who has since become my business partner, coauthor, and closest friend. Working with Jennifer to create the Mommy MD Guides books and website hasn't seemed like work at all; it's been more fun and rewarding than I ever could have imagined.

Although Jennifer and I began our venture as a two-woman enterprise, our team has grown to include a number of creative and talented individuals. I'm deeply grateful to Jennifer Goldsmith, Amy Kovalski, Leanne Coppola, Susan Eugster, Carrie Wendel, and Nanette Bendyna for their hard work and dedication to our goal of supporting moms in one of the most important jobs in the world—raising happy and healthy children. I'm also grateful to the physicians who have generously given their time and energy to help us create this book. By sharing the stories of their lives as moms, including their struggles as well as their successes, they help make the exciting and rewarding journey of motherhood a little easier for the rest of us.

I'm thankful to Monica Hess and Kathy Engle for their support of the Mommy MD Guides, and especially for their friendship. Most of all, I'm grateful for the love and encouragement of my family. My husband, Robin; my sons, Chad, Oakley, and Gatlin; my daughter-in-law, Lindsey; and my granddaughter, Bella, are the greatest gifts in my life.

—*Rallie McAllister, MD, MPH*

First and foremost, thank you from the bottom of my heart to Rallie. This book would not have been possible without you, and I will forever be grateful. I'm so lucky to get to work each day with such a dear friend.

Thank you to the dozens of smart, kind doctors who shared their stories and their wisdom with us for this book. Talking with you was both an honor and a delight, and I'm so happy for the opportunity to share your experiences and wisdom with our readers.

Many thanks also to the Mommy MD Guides team. I'm so fortunate to work with such a talented group: editor Amy Kovalski, consultant Jennifer Goldsmith, designer Leanne Coppola, layout designer Susan Eugster, illustrator Carrie Wendel, indexer Nanette Bendyna, and executive assistant Crystal Smith.

I am very grateful to Drew Frantzen, our logo designer, who has helped to establish the very tone and style of our brand.

Thank you to my mentors and friends who have shared their wisdom and advice: Susan Berg, Elly Phillips, Anne Egan, Joey Green, Tim Foster, Maggie Agentis-Ryan, and Buddy Lesavoy.

Most of all, thank you to my family—Mike, Tyler, and Austin Reich and John R. Bright, Mary L. Bright, Robyn Swatsburg, and Judy Beck—for all of your support, encouragement, and love and for making my life so rich, rewarding—and fun.

—*Jennifer Bright Reich*

Introduction

The moment your baby is born is unlike any other. How can a person feel so foreign yet so familiar at the same time? A baby's first year is momentous for the baby, of course, but it's also momentous for the new parents. You'll experience so many firsts, face so many challenges, and enjoy so many celebrations. It's a magical year, filled with wonder, newness, and joy.

To create this book, we spoke with 70 Mommy MD Guides—doctors who are also mothers. Some of these Mommy MD Guides have children who are grown up with babies of their own. They're Grammy MD Guides! Combined, these doctors have centuries of experience as doctors, and they have 160 babies.

These smart, funny, fascinating women opened their hearts and lives to us, sharing their challenges of sleepless nights, sore breasts, and strained relationships. They also fondly reminisced about celebrations such as first smiles, first steps, and first birthdays. These Mommy MD Guides generously shared the wisdom, tips, and tricks that they learned to make it through their babies' first years.

Because doctors so often see the things that can go wrong, they try to do everything as right as they can for their own health and for that of their families. Physicians are a healthier group than the whole. Even though women physicians sometimes will just suffer with things that take time and that affect them alone, caring for their babies is different. Mommy MD Guides combine all of their experience and training as physicians with their wisdom and knowledge as moms to skillfully care for their babies.

The more than 900 tips and stories in this book are presented in the Mommy MD Guides' own words, and each tip is clearly attributed to the doctor who *lived* it. Most of these stories contain kernels of advice. This is what doctors who were new mothers did to make it through their babies' first years. Other stories in this book are just that—true stories. The implied advice is: I made it through this pesky problem, and you can too!

Even though this book is filled with advice from a select group—all Mommy MD Guides—you'll find that they hold vastly differing opinions. Parenting is filled with issues that people feel very strongly about. Should your baby sleep with you or in the next room? Should you breastfeed or bottlefeed? Should you use cloth or disposable diapers? We've presented many different viewpoints—but not with the intent to confuse or to offer conflicting advice. Instead, these diverse voices are presented so that you can choose what's best for you and your family.

As you read this book, keep in mind that every baby is different, and in fact every mom is different. Babies change and grow at different rates. We encourage you to use the index at the end of this book as a resource, in addition to reading month by month.

Welcome to the Mommy MD Guides! Best wishes for a happy, healthy baby's first year!

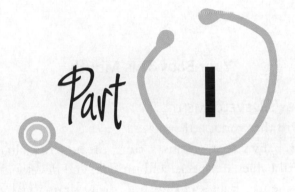

THE FIRST QUARTER

Chapter 1
Birth and 1st Month

Your Baby This Month

YOUR BABY'S DEVELOPMENT

Welcome to the world, little one!

Your baby's first year is a time of amazing change and growth. All babies are special and unique, and development isn't an exact science. Babies change and grow dramatically during their first years, especially in their first few months. Change might well feel like the only constant during your baby's first year.

Perfectly normal—and very common—for newborns is losing up to 10 percent of their weight during their first few days. After that, your baby will likely gain half an ounce a day for his first six months!

If your baby was born with hair, be prepared for him to lose it. This happens when your maternal hormones recede from his body. When your baby's hair regrows, it might be a totally different color and texture. Surprise!

Don't get too attached to your baby's eye color either. Most Caucasian babies are born with blue-gray eyes, and you won't know their permanent color until your baby is around six months old. Most African-American, Hispanic, and Asian babies have dark brown eyes that usually don't change.

A newborn's eyes might appear to be crossed, or they might turn in or out when your baby tries to focus. That's because for the first few weeks, infants don't have good eye muscle control yet.

Perfect vision is 20/20, and your baby's vision is far from that, around 20/400. Right now, your baby can't see very much. He detects patterns and light, and he sees the world in shades of gray. Newborns love to look at faces, and your baby's favorite face to look at is yours.

Baby, can you hear me now? A baby has fully developed hearing at birth, and he recognizes your voice. He probably also recognizes other sounds that he heard while he was in the womb, such as music you played, songs you sang, and stories you read. Your baby might even turn his head in your direction when you talk. Even within your baby's first few weeks, he likely responds to loud noises by blinking, frowning, or startling.

Even though your baby's ears are *functioning* perfectly, they might look a little odd—flattened or misshapen. Your baby's ears will begin to look more normal a week or two after delivery.

Your baby's sense of smell is also fully developed at birth. He recognizes your scent, and he prefers it to all others. Speaking of smell, you probably think that your baby himself has a delicious smell. That's because his apocrine glands, which produce sweat, won't be active until puberty.

At first, your baby's breathing might sound a little noisy. It's because his nose is so tiny that any congestion makes him sound stuffy. Also, your baby might sneeze a lot. That's the only way that he can clear his nose.

At birth, your baby's arm muscles are contracted, and his hands are likely clenched in fists. Your baby's nails might already be long and need to be trimmed. In the weeks ahead, you'll be surprised how quickly they grow.

Because of maternal hormones, both baby boys and baby girls can develop enlarged breasts. They'll return to normal after a month or two. Also, newborns have developed milk ducts that can secrete milk from the nipples. Believe us, and don't press or squeeze on that area, or it can become infected.

Your baby's umbilical cord stump will probably fall off in 10 days to two weeks. Then you'll find out if he has an innie or an outie.

If your baby's genitals are swollen, don't be alarmed. This is normal and common. If your baby boy was circumcised, the tip of his penis will be wrapped in gauze. If your baby is a girl, she might have a bit of mucus-like vaginal discharge and possibly even some bleeding around her fifth or seventh day of life. (Call your doctor if the bleeding lasts for longer than a day.)

When your baby is born, his legs will be curled inward. Babies often sleep like little frogs, with their legs bent at the knees. You might find your baby puts himself into an awkward-looking position. That's because some babies like to return to the positions they were in while in the womb, such as cradling his head upon an arm. As your baby's nervous system matures, his body will straighten, and he'll be in a more relaxed, looser position.

Patches of your baby's skin might peel off in his first few days, which is normal and just fine. Right now his skin might have tiny whiteheads, called millia, especially on his nose and cheeks. They're blocked oil glands caused by your hormones. Those pesky hormones can also cause baby acne, which should disappear on its own in a few weeks.

Babies are born with reflexes that help them to respond to stimuli like light and touch. These reflexes, including grasping, rooting, startling, and sucking, begin soon after birth. They gradually disappear, usually by the time a baby is three to six months old.

In babies' first few weeks, they sleep for an average of 16 out of 24 hours, kind of like cats. Your baby's sleep is divided equally between day and night, and so he probably sleeps around eight hours during the day and around eight hours at night. Unfortunately, that's split into many two- to four-hour periods.

Your baby is already forming memories. In his early months, faces, smells, and voices—especially yours—form the greatest impressions.

Your baby's head will be quite wobbly. His major motor task these first few months is learning head control. Your baby should be able to briefly lift his head when he's lying on his stomach. Babies are curious little creatures, and they're very motivated to lift their heads to see what's going on in their worlds.

Right now, your baby's sole method of communication is to cry. But it won't be long before he can smile and then laugh. When your baby is around a month and a half old, you'll see his first real smile. And it will melt your heart.

TAKING CARE OF YOU

Give your body time to heal from the delivery. Even if you wanted to run a marathon, this isn't the time to do it. It took nine months to get to this point, and it's important to give your body, and your mind, time to regroup. Be kind to yourself!

JUSTIFICATION FOR A CELEBRATION

You can finally hold your baby in your arms!

Meeting Your Baby for the First Time

Your eyes meet, your hearts connect. Finally.

⤳

When my baby was born, I experienced an overpowering, stunned, intoxicating joy. Since the beginning of time, mothers all over the world have been together with their infants in a deeply personal, mind-blowing intimacy. When your baby is born, you join up in your heart with all of these archaic world mothers. It is a gift that life grants to the lucky.

When you meet your baby, your mind is blown in an earth-shattering psychedelic fashion that you have trouble putting into words.

—*Elizabeth Berger, MD, a mom of a 28-year-old son and a 26-year-old daughter, a child psychiatrist, and the author of* Raising Kids with Character, *in New York City*

⤳

I remember the first moment I saw my daughter. I was so surprised. I had thought she would be this delicate little flower I'd need to protect. But when I saw my daughter, she looked at me with an expression that said, *I'm here. I'm in charge. Everything is okay now.*

In that instant, I had such a strong feeling that my daughter was going to be all right. She's rugged. That has continued to be her personality. She dominates the room!

—*Dina Strachan, MD, a mom of a five-year-old daughter, a dermatologist and director of Aglow Dermatology, and an assistant clinical professor in the department of dermatology at Columbia University College of Physicians and Surgeons, in New York City*

⤳

I remember looking at our daughter in the bassinet in the hospital and thinking, *I have no idea what to do with a baby!* Although my husband and I both are physicians, I don't think anything can prepare you for this.

—*Rachel S. Rohde, MD, a mom of a five-month-old daughter, an assistant professor of orthopaedic surgery at the Oakland*

University William Beaumont School of Medicine, and an
orthopaedic upper-extremity surgeon with Michigan Orthopaedic
Institute, P.C., in Southfield, MI

When I met my babies for the first time, I felt very mixed emotions. Here, this person had grown inside of me for nine months. I felt like I should *know* him, yet I was shocked how much I needed to learn about him. I had felt him move inside of me and knew his movement patterns during the day, but now I had to learn new ways that my newborn communicated with me.

—Amy Thompson, MD, a mom of four- and two-year-old
and nine-month-old sons and an ob-gyn at the University of
Cincinnati College of Medicine, in Ohio

My baby was born by C-section. I was in the recovery room for around 45 minutes, so I didn't get to hold or feed her right away. After the doctors were finished closing me up, my husband brought our baby over to me. I was so happy to be able to finally hold her. I'll always remember that my husband commented on how much our baby looked like me because she has cute, chubby cheeks.

—Jennifer Bacani McKenney, MD, a mom of a two month old
daughter and a family physician, in Fredonia, KS

Before my oldest son was born, my father-in-law told me, "Wendy, there's a freight train coming, and there's nothing you can do to stop it." And then it really happens. When you're pregnant, you have all of this excitement and anticipation, and then the baby comes and turns your life upside down. We are all warned, but that's not really helpful at all.

I'll never forget the transformation I felt when my son was born. I felt the most amazing sense of vitality. Here was this new person, and suddenly I had no control over life anymore.

—Wendy Sue Swanson, MD, FAAP, a mom of four- and two-
year-old sons, a board-certified pediatrician, and a blogger for
Seattle Children's Hospital, in Washington

When I was in labor with my youngest daughter, the obstetrician left the room for a few minutes, leaving the midwife in charge. My daughter chose that moment to be born, and the ob was pissed!

When my daughter was born, I grabbed her and put her on my chest. She picked her head up and looked around. It was like she was thinking, *Okay, I'm here now. What's next?* Then she began to nurse. From the very beginning, my daughter had such an ease about her.

—*Nancy Rappaport, MD, a mom of 21- and 16-year-old daughters and an 18-year-old son, an assistant professor of psychiatry at Harvard Medical School, an attending child and adolescent psychiatrist in the Cambridge, MA, public schools, and the author of* In Her Wake: A Child Psychiatrist Explores the Mystery of Her Mother's Suicide

~

When I saw my firstborn for the first time, it was just awesome. She was so beautiful, with gray eyes and perfect features. I have a history of infertility, and it was a long journey to get to see my baby. It was completely unbelievable.

My daughter was born in the afternoon, and we had lots of visitors that afternoon and evening. But that night, after everyone had left, I just held my baby and looked at her for hours, wondering, *How could this beautiful, perfect child be mine?*

—*Sadaf T. Bhutta, MD, a mom of a five-year-old daughter and three-year-old triplets and an assistant professor and the fellowship director of pediatric radiology at the University of Arkansas for Medical Sciences and Arkansas Children's Hospital, both in Little Rock*

~

The moment you meet your baby is one you will never forget. My first pregnancy was the ideal pregnancy, capped off by the ideal delivery. It was just the way that I had planned it: My ob had scheduled an induction so that my husband, who was working in a PhD program in another state, could fly in on a long weekend. When my son was born, he was pink and cute. He was a horrible baby, but for those first few moments, he was perfect!

My second delivery was not so good. In fact, it was about as horrible a delivery as you could possibly imagine. But the moment I held my son in my arms, I forgot all about that. My son was so adorable, even if he was the size of a one-month-old! Ironically, my second son was a wonderful baby, the complete opposite of my first.

—*Carrie Brown, MD, a mom of seven- and five-year-old sons and a general pediatrician who treats medically complex children and specializes in palliative care at Arkansas Children's Hospital, in Little Rock*

My husband and I didn't find out the sex of our babies before they were born, but I somehow knew that I was having a boy first and a girl second. The pregnancies were so different.

When I was pregnant with my son, we had quite a scare. Looking at the ultrasound, the doctors thought that my son's legs were too short, which could have suggested a problem. When my son was born, all I wanted to know was that he looked okay.

"Look at his face," I begged my husband. "Tell me that he's okay." Thank goodness, my son was fine.

My daughter was born a week after my grandfather died. He would have been 90. I remember once he told me, "You need to have a girl because she will never leave you."

When my daughter was born, I looked at her and thought, *She is so beautiful.* I was so very emotional because I felt that my grandfather had sent her to me. That was the other reason I was sure I was having a girl.

When both of my babies were born, I felt so much joy. Their births were the happiest moments of my life.

—*Alanna Kramer, MD, a mom of an eight-year-old son and a six-year-old daughter and a pediatrician with St. Christopher's Hospital for Children, in Philadelphia, PA*

Understanding Newborn Screenings

You might feel sad to have your baby leave your side for a few moments after birth to be weighed, measured, and examined by the doctor and nurses. Or you might feel so busy being cleaned up and adjusting to the new you that you don't mind. Here's what's happening and what to expect.

Your baby will get his very first bath. The nurses will also clean his umbilical cord stump. They'll check his temperature and measure his breathing and heart rate.

Your baby will be given special eye drops to ward off infection, and he'll get a shot of vitamin K to help his blood to clot properly.

When your baby is born, he will be given some of his very first tests, called APGAR. Actually a series of tests, they were developed in 1952 by an anesthesiologist named Virginia Apgar. The tests assign a number between 0 and 2 for each of the following: baby's heart rate, color, breathing, muscle tone, and reflexes. Those numbers are then added up. A total score between 7 and 10 indicates the baby is doing well. Scores below 7 indicate the baby needs special care, and babies with scores below 4 require immediate medical intervention. Your baby will be tested again five minutes after he's born.

Your baby will also be weighed and measured. You might want to have your partner ready with the camera for that! Your baby on the scale, with his weight displayed, makes a really neat photo. His head circumference will also be checked.

At this time, your baby will also receive some very important newborn screenings to check for serious conditions that might not be readily apparent at birth. In most states in the United States, newborn screening is mandatory. Almost all states require testing for more than 30 disorders, but because there is no national standard, the exact screening requirements vary by state. Many of the conditions that babies are screened for are metabolic disorders, which interfere with the way a baby's body uses nutrients to produce energy and maintain healthy tissues and organs. Other disorders screened for can cause problems with the baby's blood or hormones. If you'd like a list of the conditions your baby will be tested for, check with your doctor or the hospital.

From the hustle and bustle of delivering my two sons, I don't have a crystal clear recollection of the screenings of my newborn sons. I do recall the screenings showing no problems, and thus I am blessed.

> —*Amy J. Derick, MD, a mom of two-year-old and nine-month-old sons and a dermatologist in private practice at Derick Dermatology, in Barrington, IL*

My daughter was born by C-section. The nurses took my baby for her screenings while I went to the recovery room. I had anticipated that this would happen, and I asked my husband to please go with our daughter.

"I'll be fine," I assured him.

I was grateful that my husband could go along with our daughter while she had all of her screenings so that she wasn't alone.

> —*Jennifer Bacani McKenney, MD*

The newborn screenings didn't scare me at all because I had studied all about them. I just kept watching to make sure that my babies got all of their screenings. Newborn screenings are very important because they identify certain diseases, metabolic disorders, and blood disorders. If these conditions are detected sooner rather than later, devastating complications might be prevented.

Each state has specific newborn screening requirements. Many screen for hypothyroidism, sickle cell disease, and cystic fibrosis. It's best to check with your doctor or midwife to see what tests are required by your state. Parents should make sure that they have provided the hospital and their child's doctor with accurate contact information so that the hospital and the doctor can get in touch with them easily in case the results of the screening suggest that additional testing is needed.

> —*Leena Shrivastava Dev, MD, a mom of 14- and 10-year-old sons, an assistant professor of medicine at Drexel University College of Medicine, and a general pediatrician, in Philadelphia, PA*

One of the tests performed on newborns is a light reflex test, in which the doctor shines a light into the baby's eyes to determine if there is a symmetrical reflection.

I did this test on my children myself. With my middle child, I couldn't get a normal light reflex. His eyes were never still enough. I took him to a friend of mine who's also a pediatrician, but she thought that his eyes looked fine.

One night, I had a nightmare that my son's eyes grew into insect eyes, and then they cracked! I took my son to see a pediatric ophthalmologist, and she confirmed that he had a condition called nystagmus.

The lesson here is that if you feel something is wrong with your baby, even if indications such as a newborn screening are normal, it's hard to figure out if it's new-parent anxiety or if there is truly something wrong. I think that a good rule of thumb is if you've talked with three doctors, and all of them tell you that something is normal, it probably *is* normal. There's never any harm in getting a second—or even a third—opinion.

—*Amy Baxter, MD, a mom of 13- and 10-year-old sons and an 8-year-old daughter, the CEO of MMJ Labs, and the director of emergency research of Children's Healthcare of Atlanta at Scottish Rite, in Atlanta, GA*

Breastfeeding

It's one of the great ironies of life: Something that should be so simple, so natural, so often isn't.

Among infants born in 2006, the most recent stats available, three-quarters of babies were ever breastfed. Almost half were still breastfeeding at six months old, and almost a quarter were still breastfeeding at their first birthdays.

Studies show many benefits to breastfeeding. Breast milk contains disease-fighting antibodies that can help protect babies from illnesses. Breastfed babies have a lower risk of obesity, diabetes, allergies, and dental cavities. (Look, Ma, no cavities!) Recently, researchers in Australia found that breastfeeding for six months or more was associated with better academic skills, in boys anyway.

For Mom, breastfeeding enhances postpartum weight loss and reduces the risk of developing breast cancer, ovarian cancer, and type 2 diabetes. Moms who breastfeed are likely to miss fewer days of work due to illness than moms who don't breastfeed.

Because breast milk requires no processing, packaging, or shipping, breastfeeding helps protect the environment. From a practical standpoint, breastfeeding saves both time and money. And who couldn't use more of those?

Mommy MD Guides–Recommended Product
Milkin' Cookies

Cheri Wiggins, MD, and Lennox McNeary, MD, had babies about the same age. They had both returned to work and were breast-feeding and trying to find ways to increase their milk supply.

"I had tried taking the herb fenugreek, but I didn't like taking it," says Dr. Wiggins. "I don't like the taste of licorice, so I couldn't drink licorice tea. Dr. McNeary tried a prescription medication called Reglan, but she didn't like the side effects."

Dr. Wiggins and Dr. McNeary decided there had to be some-thing better. They found recipes for lactation cookies but didn't like the taste and wanted to create something healthier. They tinkered with the recipe until they created one that they liked. Thirty-five cookie recipes later, they had a winner.

"We shared them with some other breastfeeding moms at work, who agreed that they really worked!" Dr. Wiggins says.

Milkin' Cookies come in two delicious flavors: oatmeal choco-late chip and cranberry almond oatmeal. Both flavors contain galac-togogues, which can help increase breast milk production. You can buy Milkin' Cookies at **MILKIN-COOKIES.COM**. A two-week supply costs around $21.

Breastfeeding was such a special time. My life was so busy, and I was out of the house a lot, like so many working women. Breastfeeding was a very special opportunity for me to *literally* connect to my child and to veg out. It was so special, and I'll remember it forever.

—*Cathie Lippman, MD, a mom of 30- and 28-year-old sons and a physician who specializes in environmental and preventive medicine at the Lippman Center for Optimal Health, in Beverly Hills, CA*

I loved my Boppy nursing pillow. I used it for breastfeeding. I noticed that as my sons got older, they started to understand that when the Boppy came out, it was time to nurse.

—*Rebecca Reamy, MD, a mom of six- and one-year-old sons and a pediatrician in emergency medicine at Children's Healthcare of Atlanta, in Georgia*

While I was breastfeeding my baby, I settled her on my lap on a Boppy pillow. I found it to be great to help prevent neck, back, shoulder, and arm pain from cradling and leaning.

Also, I bought a mini-fridge and kept it upstairs next to my baby's nursery. It was handy for milk and also snacks for me.

—*Rachel S. Rohde, MD*

When I first started to breastfeed, I was very shy about doing it in public. But in time, I felt more comfortable about it. I simply covered up with a receiving blanket.

—*Charlene Brock, MD, a mom of 28-, 25-, and 23-year-old sons and an 18-year-old daughter and a pediatrician with St. Chris Care at Falls Center, in Philadelphia, PA*

A lot of things that I thought would be hard about having a baby turned out being okay. For example, I really wanted to breastfeed, but I had heard stories about how it was so hard. It wasn't that hard for me, and I think that was partly because I was lucky and partly because I had good help.

Before my daughter was born, I hired a baby nurse to live in my home for my daughter's first three weeks. The nurse was recommended by my ob-gyn. She lived in our spare bedroom, and considering that she lived with us 24 hours a day, the cost wasn't that high.

The nurse got me onto a schedule and helped me to use an electric pump. By the time the nurse left, I was making so much milk that our freezer was packed, and there wasn't any room left for food!

—*Dina Strachan, MD*

All babies are different when it comes to learning to breastfeed, even twins. My twins were born five weeks early, and even though my daughter was premature, she was born knowing exactly how to nurse. On the other hand, it took my son two or three weeks to figure out how to latch on.

The best advice I have about breastfeeding is if a mom really wants to do it, then do it! Although it is a natural process, there is a learning curve for both mom and baby. With careful monitoring of the baby's weight and intake/output, it can be successful and very gratifying. Turn to your pediatrician, lactation consultants, and other moms who've breastfed for help. My twins were exclusively breastfed till they were 12 months old, and then weaned by 15 months. And contrary to popular belief, a working mom can breastfeed successfully, with some planning and support from her employer regarding pumping. As a bonus, ladies, it helps with getting the weight off!

—*Ann Contrucci, MD, a mom of 12-year-old boy-girl twins who works as a pediatric emergency physician, in Atlanta, GA*

My youngest daughter had a lot of difficulty breastfeeding. When she was born, she was 5 pounds, 6 ounces, and she wasn't gaining weight. Within two days of her birth, she weighed just 4 pounds. It seemed like she was latching on okay, and she was pulling and pulling to get the milk, but she was exhausting herself. We weighed her before and after each feeding, and we could tell she was hardly getting any milk.

I took her to see a lactation consultant, and it turned out that my baby didn't have enough strength in her cheeks, like a preemie baby. Based on research done with preemies at Texas Children's Hospital, the lactation consultant recommended that I use breast shields, like the kind used by women with inverted nipples. These helped a lot until my baby got stronger, when she was around two months old. I also pumped after my baby finished nursing to increase my milk production so I could supplement her feedings later if I needed to. Like many women, I had to go back to work six weeks after my baby was born. Increasing my milk production and saving extra milk were very important since I wanted to continue to breastfeed my baby for an entire year and to make sure that she got only breast milk while I was at work.

—*Gabriella Cardone, MD, a mom of five-, three-, and one-year-old daughters and a pediatric emergency physician at Texas Children's Hospital, in Houston*

Breastfeeding can be challenging for some women. You have to mentally prepare yourself that it might not be easy at first. Breastfeeding is a full-time job for the first few weeks at least.

Even after that, it's a huge adjustment to be the primary source of nutrition for a helpless newborn. This is hard if you're used to being on your own and getting out of the house. I had big, fat, healthy 9- and 10-pound babies who were hungry. I felt like I was chained to my recliner for at least their first two months of life. Breastfeeding is a commitment, and you have to be well prepared for that.

Another challenge is that not all moms and babies are good at breastfeeding. I needed three or four visits with a lactation consultant to figure out how to do it. When you're in the hospital, ask to meet the lactation consultant, and get her name and phone number so you can call her when you're at home if you need to. My first baby lost 10 percent of her body weight waiting for my milk to come in and for me to learn how to breastfeed correctly. It's so helpful if you know a lactation consultant you can turn to when you need help and support.

—*Kristin C. Lyle, MD, FAAP, a mom of eight-, six-, and three-year-old daughters, the disaster medical director at Arkansas Children's Hospital, and an assistant professor of pediatrics at the University of Arkansas for Medical Sciences, in Little Rock*

Breastfeeding was a challenge, but I faced it with a sense of humor. Early on, I developed a painful abscess in my breast. I remember that the surgeon didn't believe me. I'm sure she thought that physicians make the worst patients, trying to diagnose ourselves. To placate me, the surgeon aspirated the area, and she was surprised to find that there had indeed been an abscess in my breast. No hard feelings.

Though I got off to a rocky start with breastfeeding the first time, I stuck with it. I think that if you can make it two weeks, you're home free for the most part. For me, the biggest shock was going from a C cup to a G cup. I had to go to a special store to find a brassiere that would accommodate my new physique. Because I wasn't supposed to drive, I called a friend to drive me to the store to get a new bra. She tried very hard not to stare, and she made a joke to make me feel less uncomfortable. She was very supportive and kind. Friends like that are worth their weight in gold.

—*Lesley Burton-Iwinski, MD, a mom of 20- and 18-year-old daughters and a 14-year-old son, a retired family physician, and a parent and teacher educator with Growing Peaceful Families, in Lexington, KY*

I nursed all of my children, and I loved it. But breastfeeding, at least at first, can be difficult. Thankfully, my babies were good at latching on and eating. But one thing I remember from the first few weeks with all of them was that sometimes nursing *hurts*! All of the breastfeeding books I'd read told me that if breastfeeding was painful, something was wrong. For me, though, often the first few minutes of feeding caused what one of my friends called "toe-curling" pain. But I could tell that the baby was latching on well, and after a minute or two, the pain would subside. I had a close friend who had her first baby a few months before mine, and I called her for advice. She had experienced the same thing, and she assured me that it would get better.

So, here's the thing, as indiscreet as it might sound: Your nipples have to get tough. The first few weeks, they're just not used to all of

When to Call Your Doctor

Mastitis is an infection in the breast tissue. It's most common during the first three months of breastfeeding, but it can occur later as well. Women who have sore or cracked nipples are more likely to develop mastitis. If you've had mastitis once, you're more likely to get it again. It's possible that tight-fitting bras can restrict milk flow and contribute to mastitis.

Mastitis develops when bacteria from your skin's surface or your baby's mouth enter your breast through a break in the skin or through the opening to the milk ducts in your nipple.

Signs and symptoms of mastitis are pain, swelling, and redness of the breast, often in a wedge-shaped pattern; feeling exhausted and run-down like you have the flu; chills; and a fever of 101°F or higher.

If you think you have mastitis, call your doctor right away. Mastitis is a serious condition. Your doctor will probably want to see you to confirm the diagnosis. Oral antibiotics are often very effective in treating this condition, but in some cases, intravenous antibiotics are required.

that sucking! And they hurt! But eventually they toughen up, and the pain goes away. I'm so glad that I didn't give up breastfeeding due to this early experience of painful nursing.

—*Lezli Braswell, MD, a mom of a six-year-old daughter and four- and one-year-old sons and a family physician, in Columbus, GA*

Breastfeeding helps babies avoid catching colds, and it also enhances their gastric development. Neurologic benefits and increased IQ have also been well documented.

My time spent nursing my daughter was precious to me. I was disappointed when my breast pump broke while I was on a trip, after my daughter was about six months old. That was the end of nursing for me, but my daughter did just fine.

—*Darlene Gaynor-Krupnick, DO, a mom of five- and two-year-old daughters, a female urologist fellow trained in pelvic reconstruction and neurology, and the inventor of Valera, a USDA-certified organic vaginal lubricant, in northern Virginia*

My milk came in late. For most women, it comes in on day three or four, but mine didn't come in until day five, which meant I didn't get any sleep for two days because my daughter was feeding every two hours.

I got absolutely no help at all from the neonatal nurse, who scolded me for feeding my baby so often. Fortunately, I had an older friend who recognized the problem immediately. She encouraged me to nurse my baby when she was hungry, and she came to stay with me so I could sleep between feedings.

—*Stuart Jeanne Bramhall, MD, a mom of a 30-year-old daughter and a child and adolescent psychiatrist, in New Plymouth, New Zealand*

It's a great idea to find a lactation consultant *before* you have your baby. I hired a consultant to come to my home two days after my daughter and I got home from the hospital, but it would have been so much better to have met with her while I was in the hospital.

Before choosing a lactation consultant, you might want to ask for her views on infant formula. If she says anything along the lines of, "I would *never* use formula; it's the devil," I'd find another lactation consultant.

—*Katja Rowell, MD, a mom of a five-year-old daughter, a family physician, and a childhood feeding specialist with FamilyFeedingDynamics.com, in St. Paul, MN*

I went back to work with my younger daughter when she was about three months old. I was breastfeeding her, and she refused to take a bottle. I tried every single type of bottle I could find, thinking I just needed to find the right one. But with each bottle I tried, my daughter would just look at me like she was thinking, *What are you trying to do to me?* I ended up breastfeeding my daughter before work, running home at lunch to nurse her, and then getting home as quickly as I could after work. And then my daughter flipped her schedule, so she'd nurse every two hours at night—all night long.

—*Cheri Wiggins, MD, a mom of four- and two-year-old daughters, a specialist in physical medicine and rehabilitation at St. Luke's Magic Valley, and a cofounder of the Mommy Doctors Bakery (makers of Milkin' Cookies), in Twin Falls, ID*

Nursing was hard. I have red hair and light skin, and people say that women with fair skin and hair can experience more discomfort breastfeeding. I certainly did!

In the beginning, breastfeeding is a mixed bag of emotions. I remember thinking, *I have to nurse the baby, what a lovely thing.* And at the same time I was thinking, *Oh, no, I have to nurse the baby. It hurts.* I stuck with it, and after about two weeks it felt so much better that I started to experience only the positive side of it.

—*Siobhan Dolan, MD, a mom of 15- and 12-year-old daughters and a 10-year-old son, a consultant to the March of Dimes, and an associate professor of obstetrics and gynecology and women's health at Albert Einstein College of Medicine/Montefiore Medical Center, in Bronx, NY*

When my baby was a few days old, my body started making milk instead of colostrum and my breasts became very engorged. It was painful. One thing that helped to ease the pain was to soak a washcloth in hot water and place it on my breasts. Applying chamomile packs also helped. I just steeped the chamomile tea bags in boiling water, soaked washcloths in the solution, and then placed the washcloths on my breasts.

—*Nancy Rappaport, MD*

I knew that I wanted to breastfeed. I felt very strongly about the benefits of breastfeeding. It had been presented to me as something natural—something that my body would just know how to do. I usually do my homework and prepare for things, but I thought that breastfeeding was just "going to happen."

When my baby was born, the nurses at the hospital were wonderful. But they were under the impression that because I was a doctor, I knew how to breastfeed!

"You don't need a lactation consultant," they said. "You know how to do it."

Not true. It was horrible. Breastfeeding is hard!

My mom hadn't breastfed, so she wasn't able to offer any advice. When I was born, bottlefeeding was a status symbol.

Because I was motivated and determined to breastfeed, I struggled through it. I had a lactation consultant come to my home to help teach me. Breastfeeding got easier with my second baby, and it was easiest of all with my third. By then I had learned to relax and enjoy it.

—*Lisa Dado, MD, a mom of three children, ages 21 to 16, a pediatric anesthesiologist with Valley Anesthesiology Consultants, and a cofounder and CEO of the Center for Human Living, which teaches life skills and martial arts training, in Phoenix, AZ*

I always wanted to try nursing my kids. The importance and benefits of nursing were *seriously* emphasized in medical school! But I found that nursing *did not* come naturally to me.

One of the funniest things I remember was when I had just given birth to my first child, the lactation nurse said that because I was a doctor, I probably knew what to do! No, I don't think so. It's not like we ever had any demonstrations in medical school!

I definitely gave it my all, though, and my daughter latched on well. My milk came in with a vengeance after a couple of days, and my baby seemed permanently attached to me. Things seemed to be going great until about the second week, when my nipples became unbearably sore! It was at this point that I could understand why a lot of new moms give up breastfeeding. I remember speaking to one of my friends, who told me that when she had her first son, the pain of nursing was so intense she would do her Lamaze breathing to get through it!

Another problem for this generation of young mothers is that we do not have anyone from the older generations to help us out. Think about it: Our mothers and grandmothers were actually discouraged from nursing. They were actually told that formula was better than breast milk! My sister-in-law even told me that she thinks nursing is *disgusting!* As mammals, nursing our babies has been a survival advantage for several million years, and in a matter of a few decades, some people have begun to think that you are extreme or weird to even consider it!

I wish that I could offer some advice on how to make things easier, but really I just toughed it out. After a couple of weeks, it got easier, and I never had serious pain with nursing again, not even with my other two babies.

—*Stacey Weiland, MD, a mom of a 12-year-old daughter and 7- and 5-year-old sons and an internist/gastroenterologist, in Denver, CO*

RALLIE'S TIP

I nursed all of my babies, and I loved it! Because I worked full-time when they were young, I needed to pump and store my milk while I was at the hospital. As fate would have it, I worked on the pediatric floor while I was nursing, and the sound of a crying baby or child would cause my milk to let down almost immediately.

I found that the nursing pads I had bought just weren't absorbent

Mommy MD Guides-Recommended Product
Bebe au Lait Nursing Cover

Moms know breastfeeding is 24/7, so it should be comfortable. That's even more important when you're out and about with your baby. Bebe au Lait created a stylish solution—a line of nursing covers that are both functional and fabulous. Bebe au Lait designed its nursing covers with a patented rigid neckline that promotes bonding between mom and baby by allowing an unobstructed view of the baby during nursing. The covers are perfectly sized to give you the ultimate privacy, and they are available in a wide variety of beautiful prints in high-quality fabrics. Each cover also features internal terry cloth pockets that double as small item storage.

You can buy Bebe au Lait nursing covers and Bebe au Lait's Hooter Hiders for around $35. They're available at **BEBEAULAIT.COM** and through retailers and chains such as Babies R Us and Nordstrom.

enough to handle the resulting downpour, and besides, they were expensive. I had much better luck using thick, sanitary pads designed for overnight use. They were bulkier than the nursing pads, but they were less expensive, and they kept me from soaking my shirts several times a day.

Breastfeeding was wonderful, but challenging at times. I developed mastitis, and this was difficult for many reasons. I quickly received treatment, and I continued to breastfeed, which I loved.

—Leigh Andrea DeLair, MD, a mom of a two-year-old son and a family physician, in Danville, KY

I had really set out to breastfeed my son. But from the very beginning, breastfeeding was very challenging. It was extremely emotional for me; on some level it was even devastating.

My husband and I did everything in our power to make it work. Nine lactation consultants came to our home. I tried fingerfeeding, prepumping, hot towels—everything I could think of.

Then when my son was a few weeks old, I got such severe mastitis that I was hospitalized. My husband brought our son to visit me during the day, but I spent an entire week of nights without him. It was a life-changing experience. I understood what women go through to nurse and the lengths we go to fulfill our expectations. We can do everything in our power, but sometimes it just doesn't work out.

After I went home, I continued to pump for several months. It was pure misery for me. When I finally stopped and switched to bottlefeeding, that was the moment both my son and I started to thrive.

—*Wendy Sue Swanson, MD, FAAP*

When my baby was young and I was breastfeeding, I developed mastitis. It was horrible. I had read about it in all of the pregnancy books, so I was aware of the symptoms.

When my baby was 12 days old, I had just nursed her, but I started feeling really tender on the outer side of my left breast. I laid down for a nap, thinking it would pass. But I woke with a 104°F fever and aches and pains that felt like the worst case of the flu you could ever have.

My husband, who's also a doctor, started me on antibiotics. By the second or third day, I began to feel better. You can't mess around with mastitis; it can get very serious, very fast and can even be life-threatening.

—*Sadaf T. Bhutta, MD*

Breastfeeding was very hard. Lansinoh [a soothing nipple cream] was critical for me. My nipples were so denuded of skin that they were sticking to the breast pads. I bought Telfa dressing, which is the type of nonstick pads that we use for burn patients. After a while, I lost sensation in my breasts, and I didn't feel anything. I thought I wouldn't have sensation again, but I did after the skin grew back. It's amazing what we do for our kids.

—*Sonia Ng, MD, a mom of seven- and two-year-old sons, a pediatrician, and a sedation attending physician at the Children's*

Hospital of Philadelphia Pediatric Care and the University Medical Center at Princeton in Princeton, NJ, and the Pediatric Imaging Center in King of Prussia, PA

⁓

At 34, I was fairly old for a first-time mother. I was already well established as a baby doctor, and I had learned a thing or two about life. For the most part, maturity gave me a sense of self-reliance—even as a new mother.

I had not really given a thought to feeding my infant until he appeared. When he was about 30 minutes old, it seemed to me that it was time to nurse him, without my knowing much of anything about nursing. I did think that the baby and the breast seemed like an arrangement that probably would work itself out without interference, given a little bit of luck. I let the baby and the breast figure it out, which happened right away. My son was one of those wide-awake thinky babies, and it turned out he was really hungry.

There were on hand a variety of people—my husband and the hospital staff—ready to jump in and help if I needed a backup plan in case of a snag, so that was reassuring.

Nursing your own babies is, in my view, just about the best deal there is. If there is one experience on earth that summarizes that you have been there and played a role in the tide of life and known the depth of happiness, it is the experience of nursing your own babies. My aunt related to me that her four-year-old son, my cousin, ran home from a visit to their next-door neighbors, exclaiming in awe, "Mommy! Mommy! Mrs. Golden is feeding her new baby—with her *heart!*"

—*Elizabeth Berger, MD*

⁓

I really wanted to breastfeed, but I had breast reduction surgery, so I knew breastfeeding might not be possible. I tried *everything* to breastfeed my son, but in the end I didn't produce enough milk. I could pump about two ounces in 24 hours. I was just tiring myself out, and so I stopped and switched to formula.

—*Alanna Kramer, MD*

Rallie's Tip

I nursed all of my babies, and at least one of them had thrush.

Thrush is caused by the growth of a fungus, called Candida albicans, *on the tongue and elsewhere in the mouth. It's rather common in nursing babies, usually in the first few months of life. The fungus normally appears in creamy white patches in the mouth, but there can be variations of color. The patches can be painful, and if you scrape them lightly with a clean washcloth, they might bleed. Usually the patches appear on a baby's tongue or inner cheeks, and they can spread to the roof of the mouth, gums, and back of the throat. Because thrush can be painful, babies with thrush sometimes don't eat well, and they often cry more than usual.*

A very effective homeopathic treatment for thrush (when caught early while the infection is still very mild) is to open a capsule of probiotics, such as Bifidophilus, and sprinkle a tiny amount of the powder in the baby's mouth. Probiotics are beneficial bacteria that normally inhabit the skin, mouth, and digestive tract, and they help keep other, less desirable organisms (such as yeast) under control. Yeast organisms are also normal inhabitants of the skin, mouth, and digestive tract, and these organisms can proliferate when the population of beneficial probiotic bacteria is compromised in some way and diminished. Introducing additional probiotics, via the powder from a capsule, to the mouth increases the number of probiotic organisms in these areas, allowing them to bring the yeast organisms back under control.

Bottlefeeding

Bottlefeeding has many benefits, including for Dad. He gets to feed the baby too. The cost of formula can range from $54 to $200 per month, depending on the brand.

෴

I tried to breastfeed for around three weeks, consulting five lactation nurses over that time before I resorted to pumping. In the end, I don't think I was making enough milk for my son, and I couldn't stand it when my baby was hungry and crying. I simply switched over to the type of formula that my son's pediatrician recommended.

—Sharon Giese, MD, a mom of a two-year-old son and a cosmetic plastic surgeon in private practice, in New York City

After I returned to work, I pumped milk and froze it. I used the Playtex Drop-Ins system for bottles so that my nanny could easily transition from defrosting the freezer bags to the bottle.

—Stacey Weiland, MD

I breastfed my son, but to give myself more flexibility time-wise, I pumped often. I also supplemented my son's diet with formula when he was 4½ months old. He thrived.

—Leigh Andrea DeLair, MD

I had planned to breastfeed for the first six months, but unfortunately I was only able to breastfeed for approximately four months. Pumping

Mommy MD Guides-Recommended Product

AVENT Express II Microwave Sterilizer and AVENT Express Bottle Warmer

"I breastfed my babies, but I also gave them a bottle on occasion," says Lezli Braswell, MD, a mom of a six-year-old daughter and four- and one-year-old sons and a family physician, in Columbus, GA. "Two products that made this job much easier were the AVENT Express II Microwave Sterilizer and AVENT Express Bottle Warmer.

"The sterilizer made it simple to sterilize bottles without having to boil water," Dr. Braswell says. "It was easy to stack the bottles, nipples, and pump accessories into the steam sterilizer, add a little water, and microwave! Violà! Also, because you aren't supposed to microwave breast milk, the bottle warmer was a quick and convenient way to warm up a bottle of refrigerated expressed breast milk."

You can buy an AVENT Express II Microwave Sterilizer online and in stores for around $32 and an AVENT Express Bottle Warmer for around $46.

at work was challenging, and eventually my daughter preferred bottles to breastfeeding. Part of the learning process was that what I planned or expected wasn't always the way it worked out, and this was okay.

—*Kathleen Moline, DO*

Although I nursed both of my daughters for their first six or seven months of life, I found it helpful not to be rigid with only breast milk. Enfamil was heavier, and my daughters seemed to sleep better when they were "topped off" with a small bottle before bedtime.

—*Darlene Gaynor-Krupnick, DO*

During my sons' first years, I both breastfed and gave them bottles of either expressed milk or formula. This combination worked for us. I used a type of Playtex bottle with a silicone nipple that was very similar to the breast.

—*Jill Wireman, MD, a mom of 14- and 11-year-old sons and a pediatrician in private practice at Johnson City Pediatrics, in Tennessee*

For bottles and nipples, I swear by Dr. Brown's. When my older daughter was a baby, and I was going back to work, I had the hardest time getting her to take a bottle. I bought every type of bottle and nipple I could find. All that got me was a cabinet full of bottles and nipples!

The only nipple that my daughter would take was the one we brought home from the hospital nursery. Finally I took that nipple to Walmart and compared it to the ones on the shelf. The closest one I could find was Dr. Brown's. And that's what I've used ever since.

—*Sadaf T. Bhutta, MD*

I started out wanting to breastfeed. I was planning to pump between patients and between surgeries at work. My daughter was a champ, and even though she was growing, she always seemed hungry. She wanted to nurse constantly. I was exhausted and miserable, which decreased my milk supply. I couldn't imagine how I was going to keep this up and continue to work.

Finally, I allowed myself to switch my baby gradually to formula.

I felt guilty for a while, as if I had to explain my choice, until I realized that we were the only people who had to be comfortable with it. It was the best decision for us, and we have no regrets. She has been growing beautifully, and thankfully she has been healthy.

—*Rachel S. Rohde, MD*

The most difficult part during my baby's first year was breastfeeding. I tried to breastfeed my oldest daughter for months and months, but she wasn't getting enough milk. I had to start supplementing with infant formula, and a nurse recommended a clever device. It was a bottle that I hung around my neck with a tube I taped to my nipple. With this device, the baby was still suckling, but she was getting formula.

I wasn't able to nurse my twins because they ate every three hours! But I wanted desperately to nurse my youngest baby. After he was born, my milk didn't come in, so I started supplementing with formula. When I took my son for his one-week checkup, the pediatrician was horrified that I wasn't breastfeeding. When I went home, I was terribly depressed. A friend came to visit, and she told me, "You know you did a perfectly good job raising your other children; you should do what's right for you." That made me feel a lot better.

—*Penny Noyce, MD, a mom of 23- and 21-year-old daughters, two 21-year-old sons, and a 13-year-old son, the author of the preteen novel* Lost in Lexicon, *and an internal medicine specialist, in Weston, MA*

My husband was in charge of washing all of our babies' bottles and the breast pump attachments and breast cups. He would boil them and then set them on the counter on paper towels to dry. He was a big help!

—*Charlene Brock, MD*

My husband and I had vowed to ourselves that our daughter wouldn't be a finicky eater. We wanted her to be able to go anywhere with us and not to have to warm up her bottle every time.

She showed us! Once when we were at a restaurant, she wouldn't drink her bottle because the formula was at room temperature. Before this time she would drink her bottle anytime, anywhere, any temperature. We discovered that between me, my husband, and our babysitter, one of us had warmed up a bottle, and she decided she was going to demand a warm bottle from then on! We even had to warm up the cow's milk for a while when we switched her from formula to regular milk. We finally did break this habit, but it was rough!

—*Melody Derrick, MD, a mom of a 17-month-old daughter and a family physician in private practice with Central DuPage Physician Group, in Winfield, IL*

❧

I had major problems with breastfeeding. On some level, years later it still feels like the biggest disappointment and failure of my life.

I had difficulties from the start. In the hospital, I had eight different people giving me eight different theories on what the problem was. My nipples were sore and bleeding from the first day my baby was born.

Two days after my baby and I went home from the hospital (she was five days old), I had a lactation consultant come to our home. She was able to see the bigger picture and explain why my baby wasn't latching on. She saw that my daughter was really hungry, and she encouraged me to supplement with formula. Instantly, my daughter went from screaming all of the time to being content and sleeping, and her rather severe jaundice improved. She was a big baby who ate much more than most newborns. I was pumping six hours a day, and I was exhausted. I pumped about two-thirds of what she ate, and I supplemented the rest.

I had a healthy, big, growing baby, and breastfeeding and pumping were all-consuming and sapped the joy out of my time with my daughter. I *so* believed that *breast is best*, but I learned that if breastfeeding interferes with your ability to bond with your baby, or if your baby isn't growing or is constantly upset because she isn't getting enough nourishment, or if you feel yourself spiraling down into depression, then it's clearly time to consider other options. Breast is best—up to a point.

It's very difficult to choose a formula because there are so many options. I asked my friends who are pediatricians and moms, and they recommended Enfamil Lipil. That worked well for us.

—*Katja Rowell, MD*

⤳

When I went back to work after spending three wonderful months at home, I had to work fast to teach my first baby how to drink from a bottle. I was warned to introduce some of the feedings by bottle earlier, but I just didn't want to go to the trouble of doing that. It was so much easier to just flop down in a chair and nurse. Pumping breast milk and then putting it in a bottle and heating it just didn't seem efficient at the time.

I had to pay the price for procrastinating, though, when my baby completely rejected the bottle. I was to go back to work the next week, and when I realized the predicament I had gotten myself into, I became frantic. I called our pediatrician's office, and the nurse suggested that I offer the bottle for five minutes at a time. I was to let my daughter cry and fuss for 20 minutes, and then try again. I was to do this as many times as necessary.

"When she's hungry enough, she'll take it," the nurse assured me. On the fourth attempt, my baby grabbed the nipple of the bottle and drained the contents in record time. I didn't make that same mistake with my other two children.

—*Lesley Burton-Iwinski, MD*

Coping with Special Circumstances

There are many routes to motherhood, and there are as many circumstances as there are babies.

Each year approximately 120,000 children are adopted. Interestingly, that number seems to remain fairly consistent over time, remaining proportionate to the U.S. population.

According to *Twins* magazine, just over 3 percent of all births are twins. The U.S. birth rate for multiples rose 28 percent between 1990 and 1998. The number of triplet and higher birth multiples more than doubled in 1999, but it slightly declined in more recent years.

Another special circumstance is premature birth. Babies born before 37 completed weeks of pregnancy are premature. According to the March of Dimes, more than a half million babies each year (about 13 percent) are born prematurely. The premature birth rate has increased by more than a third since the early 1980s.

✎

My husband and I adopted our babies. We were fortunate to be there during our twins' births. Because the twins were full-term, we brought them home when they were only three days old. The only thing I missed was the pregnancy. That was fine with me because I'm not into all of that painful stuff.

—*Brooke Jackson, MD, a mom of 3½-year-old twin girls and a 14-month-old son and a dermatologist and medical director of the Skin Wellness Center of Chicago, in Illinois*

✎

Especially with twins, that first year is all about surviving. As a mom, I felt so much guilt. There's so much pressure to do this, don't do that: Buy organic, don't watch TV, and on and on. It was really a struggle for me. I felt so guilty and so worried that I would do the wrong thing. But in reality, especially in a baby's first eight months, you just have to do the best you can.

Now that my twins are 18 months old, I feel like I'm over the hump. Finally I feel like I can enjoy my kids! They're talking and interacting with me (or me and my husband), and at this age they're starting to give back. It's very satisfying. Now I love being a mom!

—*Jennifer Gilbert, DO, a mom of 18-month-old twins and an ob-gyn at Paoli Hospital, in Pennsylvania*

✎

We have twins, and that first year was like going from zero to 50 with no training. I had done my internship in pediatrics, so I wasn't scared of crying babies. What was difficult, though, was learning to do everything twice. A lot of people asked me how I did it. My answer is always, "I didn't know any better. You just do it!"

—*Brooke Jackson, MD*

⌒⌒

One of the most challenging parts of having twins was feeding them every three hours. My mother insisted on hiring a night nurse to give my babies their nighttime feedings for the first few weeks.

Not long after that, my mother-in-law came to stay for the summer. She rented a house nearby. She slept during the day and came over to feed the babies each night. It went very well!

—*Penny Noyce, MD*

⌒⌒

When my triplets were born, I felt so overwhelmed. I have a picture of myself in the recovery room after the C-section with all three of my babies. They say a picture is worth a thousand words, and the look on my face says it all, *Oh gosh, what am I going to do now?*

—*Sadaf T. Bhutta, MD*

⌒⌒

When my second son was born, he was critically ill. He was in the neonatal intensive care unit for six weeks. My husband and I spent every possible moment at his side. The nurses told me that it was a miracle that our son survived. They also said that my son was the feistiest infant they had ever seen. He's had that kind of energy his entire life. We were blessed that our son did fine.

—*Ann Kulze, MD, a mom of 22- and 15-year-old daughters and 20- and 19-year-old sons; a nationally recognized nutrition expert, motivational speaker, and family physician; and the author of the best-selling book* Eat Right for Life, *in Charleston, SC*

⌒⌒

My younger daughter was born nine weeks early. It was really hard; we barely got through it.

My husband and I tried to take the time to visit her as much as possible, while not feeling guilty about the time we couldn't be there. There's a lot of pressure to be at your baby's bedside every minute.

That's doable if you live locally and don't have any other kids! But otherwise, you can't be there all of the time.

We tried to reassure ourselves that our baby was in good hands and being well cared for. Not being there every single minute doesn't mean that you're a failure. I tried to remember that even if my baby had been at home with us, we still wouldn't be spending every single minute of every single day with her.

—*Kristie McNealy, MD, a mom of eight- and five-year-old daughters and three- and one-year-old sons and a blogger at KristieMcNealy.com, in Denver, CO*

My son was born at 29 weeks, 3 days. I had been on bed rest for a long time, and then my son was in the NICU for 56 days. It was very hard that the only two things I could really do for my son at that time were to pump breast milk and do kangaroo care, which is holding a baby skin-to-skin. Those were the only ways that I could be useful to him for his first few months of life.

Between the bed rest, C-section, and my son's prematurity, I had major problems with my milk supply. My son wasn't able to breastfeed while he was in the NICU, so I pumped 8 to 10 times a day to get enough milk to feed him through a tube and then eventually by a bottle. After my son came home, I was still trying to breastfeed him, and I also had to pump eight to ten times a day. It was exhausting. I didn't know how I could keep up that pace when I went back to work, so I called the lactation consultant from our hospital's NICU. As soon as she sat down with us, my son latched on like a pro. I still had to pump six to eight times a day to maintain my supply, but breastfeeding made the nights much easier.

On the other hand, the kangaroo care was wonderful. When you are skin-to-skin with your baby, it helps his growth. I was supposed to start a new job, but my employer encouraged me to spend time with my son instead of starting work. I'm so grateful to have had that time with my baby. I was in the NICU with him for 10 to 12 hours each day, and I spent as much of that time as I could holding my son and learning to care for him.

I remember sitting there thinking, *This is the one time in my son's life that I will have to really focus on holding him.* I really cherished that time. He's such a snuggly kid now, and I think it was because he was so used to being held the first few months of his life. He did grow pretty fast, and the nurses were convinced that kangaroo care helped.

Having a premature baby can be very isolating for a new mom. Most people think that bed rest is restful, but it was really one of the most stressful times in my life. I had a few friends who were amazing, but some of my closest friends seemed to disappear while I was on bed rest and after my son arrived. On the other hand, some people I barely knew provided tremendous support. Having a preemie in the middle of winter in Michigan is especially isolating. You aren't really supposed to take premature babies out in public, and it's too cold to go outside for fresh air. I'd hoped to take my baby on walks, but the reality of my experience didn't match my expectations at all. I felt so lucky to have a healthy baby, but I felt completely alone.

That first year was very hard. I didn't have postpartum depression, but I felt almost as if I was suffering from post-traumatic stress disorder. I've talked with other moms of premature babies who felt the same way. Having your baby in the NICU is so hard, and not knowing what is going to happen is so scary. This experience leaves a lasting mark on you.

—*Lennox McNeary, MD, a mom of a two-year-old son, a specialist in physical medicine and rehabilitation at Carilion Clinic, and a cofounder of the Mommy Doctors Bakery (makers of Milkin' Cookies), in Roanoke, VA*

Introducing Your Baby to Family and Friends

You've waited for this moment for a long time! What a wonderful opportunity to introduce your baby to your family and friends.

One of the most interesting introductions I've ever seen was my twins meeting each other. When my twins were born, my son had to stay in the NICU for a night, but my daughter got to stay with me in my hospital room. The next day, the nurse brought my son to my room. I put him in the bassinet with my daughter, and they stared at each other nose to nose, eyes wide open, for three hours. It was like they were wondering, *Where have you been? I've been with you for almost nine months, and suddenly you were gone! Good to have you back!*

It was fascinating that even as newborns, my twins were comforted by each other's presence.

As my twins became older, they started to become even more aware of each other. That was really fun! They would sit next to each other in their bouncy seats and just laugh hysterically together.

—*Ann Contrucci, MD*

When our twins were born, our oldest daughter was 21 months old. Before my husband brought our daughter to meet the babies, I tucked one stuffed bird under each baby's incubator. We explained to our daughter that the twins had each bought her a present. Our daughter was delighted. She never stopped to wonder how two babies who were confined to incubators had managed to go shopping.

—*Penny Noyce, MD*

When I was pregnant with our younger daughter, my husband and I lived 2,000 miles away from our families. We had two friends on call to watch our two-year-old daughter when I went into labor. But when I went into labor in the middle of the night, we couldn't reach either of these friends! So we packed up our daughter and took her with us to the hospital.

Thankfully, it was a quiet night in the labor and delivery department, and the nurses got crayons and colored with our daughter and then settled her into an empty bed to sleep. She missed the "scary" parts of her sister's birth. When our younger daughter was born and cried, our older daughter woke up and asked, "Is that my baby?" We asked our older daughter if she'd like to tell her sister her name, and she said, "It's Olivia Kate." It was very sweet.

—*Cheri Wiggins, MD*

My plan was to have my husband bring our son to the hospital to meet his baby sister. But some friends of ours were watching him, and he was having so much fun that we figured there was no sense hauling him in to the hospital for just a few minutes. Plus, I didn't want him crawling around on the hospital floor!

When my baby and I came home from the hospital, I was excited to introduce my children to each other. It was wonderful timing because it was my son's birthday, and we had lots of family and friends at our house. Most of the focus was on my son; the baby was also given love and attention, but we did what we could to make my son feel very special and important. We also bought a small gift for my son from his new sister, which went over very well with him!

—*Michelle Hephner, DO, a mom of a two-year-old son and eight-month-old daughter and a family physician in private practice with Central DuPage Physician Group, in Winfield, IL*

When my baby was born and came home from the hospital, my family and friends came to meet her. I was a little nervous about germs, and so when everyone got to our house, I made them wash their hands. After that, I relaxed about it, so I didn't make them wash their hands *again* before they held my baby. Unless they touched the dogs. Then they washed again!

—*Jeannette Gonzalez Simon, MD, a mom of a two-year-old daughter who's expecting another baby and a pediatric gastroenterologist in private practice, in Staten Island, NY*

When people come to visit and meet your baby, you don't have to entertain them. Stay in your robe! Then it's clear to them that you won't be entertaining them and that it's your job to be close to your baby. This is particularly important if you're breastfeeding, because newborns will be nursing quite frequently. Better yet, while your friends and family visit, if they want to clean and shop for you, let them!

—*Charlene Brock, MD*

We had a family party at Thanksgiving with my son when he was almost two months old. I'm Chinese, and Chinese people usually celebrate a baby's birth when the baby turns one month old, but I was too concerned that my son would catch a virus.

—*Sonia Ng, MD*

∽⌒⌒

I didn't have a baby shower before my son was born. It didn't feel right to receive gifts for a baby who wasn't born yet!

Instead, we had a baby party when my son was six weeks old. We invited 120 family members and friends, and everyone got to meet our son at once.

—*Sharon Giese, MD*

∽⌒⌒

My husband and I come from different religious backgrounds. Rather than having a christening, we had a baby-naming ceremony. Our baby wore something fancy that looked a bit like a christening gown. We invited all of our family and friends, and we spoke a bit about what it meant to us to have this wonderful new person in our lives and why we chose her name.

We held the ceremony at a restaurant, so we didn't have any housework either preparing for the event or cleaning up afterward. The baby-naming ceremony was a wonderful way to introduce our baby to the people we care for.

—*Ann V. Arthur, MD, a mom of a nine-year-old daughter and a seven-year-old son, a pediatric ophthalmologist in private practice at Park Slope Eye Care Associates, and a blogger at WaterWineTravel.com, in New York City*

∽⌒⌒

I had a very long first labor, more than 24 hours. So by the time the baby was born, I was really sick of being in the hospital. My husband and I got out of Dodge in a hurry and took our baby home with us on his very first day. Unbeknownst to us, all of our buddies were on the road, coming to the hospital to see us at the same time. By the time our friends arrived at the hospital, we had just burst in the door at our apartment with our newborn! The hospital redirected the whole crowd to our house, and everyone showed up 20 minutes later. It was great!

Like all mothers, I enjoyed explaining to the world how miraculous my child is, how *unlike* every other child. Other people do not always find this activity as much fun as the mother does. Mothers deserve the fun of explaining the miracle of their own children to an eager listener.

Motherhood is exhausting and uplifting; this is why mothers need lots of support as well as a listening ear. Someone needs to provide money and safety and backup. This is why there are families. Someone also has to share the exaltation of motherhood properly and reflect it empathically. This is *also* why there are families.

—*Elizabeth Berger, MD*

Coping with Crying

Babies cry at about 130 decibels. That's louder than a vacuum cleaner. And a lawn mower. And a chain saw.

In a given day, most babies cry for two to three hours. (They don't have hobbies, after all.) Babies cry for many reasons: They're hungry, tired, or hot. They need to burp, be changed, be swaddled. It's too loud. It's too quiet. It's a day of the week ending in Y.

When your baby cries, it shoots straight to your heart. Some moms describe it as feeling like their brains are spinning around in their skulls, or like a fire alarm going off in their heads. That's nature's way of making you want to soothe and calm your baby. Now.

? When to Call Your Doctor

It can be difficult to tell the difference between a baby's normal fussiness and more serious problems. If your baby is persistently irritable or has inconsolable crying jags, call your doctor. It's also important to call your pediatrician if your baby has fewer than six wet diapers in 24 hours. That could be a sign of dehydration and warrants medical attention.

When my older daughter was a baby, she cried a lot. I used skin-to-skin contact as often as I could. I took off her clothing, leaving her diaper on, and placed her on my chest. It helped to calm her down.

—*Eva Ritvo, MD, a mom of 20- and 15-year-old daughters, a psychiatrist, and a coauthor of* The Beauty Prescription, *in Miami Beach, FL*

When my babies cried, I made sure that they weren't hungry and I changed their diapers. If your baby cries, don't assume it's your fault! Remember that you *are* a good mommy and that you *are* doing things right.

—*Lillian Schapiro, MD, a mom of 14-year-old twin girls and an eight-year-old daughter and an ob-gyn with Peachtree Women's Specialists, in Atlanta, GA*

When my son was a baby, he cried a lot. He cried for hours and hours on end, and I couldn't figure out why.

Looking back now, I'm sure that part of it was that as a baby, my son didn't have any other way to express himself other than crying. But back then, it made me an emotional wreck. I felt helpless.

I'd put my son in his carriage and walk him around the hallways of our apartment building. If the weather was nice, I walked outside with him. Basically, I tried to cope with his crying as best I could. I sought advice from everyone I knew. Everyone had an opinion, but nothing helped. Finally, when my son was a few months old, he stopped crying.

—*Judith Hellman, MD, a mom of a 13-year-old son, an associate clinical professor of dermatology at Mt. Sinai Hospital, and a dermatologist in private practice, in New York City*

Some days my twins cried a lot. Sometimes one would cry, and just when I got that one calmed down, the other one would start. My husband and I joked that they had a conspiracy going.

Especially in my twins' first months, they just wanted to be held. And so I held them as much as possible. It's surprising how often my patients ask me if they're holding their babies too much and spoiling them. I say that in the first several months, you can't hold a baby too much.

The only way that a baby has to communicate his needs is by crying. So if your baby is hungry, tired, or lonely, the only way he can tell you is to cry.

—*Ann Contrucci, MD*

✑

It's a common misconception that if you hold your newborn too much, he'll become spoiled. That is untrue. Keep in mind, this is a tiny, brand-new human who has been living inside his mommy, listening to her heartbeat and voice for nine months. Then he pops out into this strange, huge world. Where do you think that baby wants to be? Where will he feel safe and comfortable?

In your baby's first few months of life, you should hold him, rock him, sing to him, and make him feel as loved and as comfortable as possible. If a baby younger than three months old cries, he's crying for a reason. Newborns need to be swaddled and held tenderly but firmly, to mimic the in utero environment. When your baby is 10 months old, it's a different story . . .

—*Hana R. Solomon, MD, a mom of four, ages 35 to 19, a board-*
certified pediatrician, and the author of Clearing the Air One Nose
at a Time: Caring for Your Personal Filter, *in Columbia, MO*

✑

I completed a fellowship in child abuse, and until I had my own child, I never understood why people might shake their babies. There was a moment when my first newborn was clean, fed, and dry, yet he was screaming for no discernible reason. Like all new moms, I was terribly sleep deprived, and all of a sudden, I got it. If I had no resources, no backup help, and I didn't understand the permanent damage it could cause, I could totally understand the urge.

Just realizing how the impulse could arise calmed me down a little, and of course having a husband to tag and say, "You're 'it'" meant my son was never in danger. But it gave me a lot of empathy for new moms who find themselves in less-than-ideal situations. Even in ideal circumstances, you don't appreciate how stressful that little bundle can be until you've lived it. I think this might cause a lot of guilt; first-time moms have been glorifying and idealizing the dewy gushing sweetness of holding their own precious babies. When the inevitable moment of irritation with your baby first arises, and despite your best efforts you can't make that sweet bundle quit crying, it's a big psychological disconnect. You might think, *Oh, no, I'm going to be a bad Mommy!*

One critical thing I learned is that when I was feeling overwhelmed, it was okay to put my baby in his crib and let him cry for a little while. A crib is a very safe place for a newborn. If you don't have anyone to hand the baby off to, it's even okay to put your baby on his back in his crib and walk around your house for 10 minutes. This gives you some time and space to calm down. And sometimes in those 10 minutes, babies fall asleep!

Humor also helps. I repeated to myself the line Holly Hunter says in the movie *Raising Arizona*, "Of course they cry! Babies cry!"

—*Amy Baxter, MD*

Trying a Pacifier

Check out the baby section of a store, and you'll see a dizzying array of pacifiers. They come in many shapes, sizes, and colors. Despite a bit of a bias in our society against pacifiers, the American Academy of Pediatrics (AAP) actually gives them the A-OK. Here are some benefits to pacifiers.

- Studies suggest that pacifier use during sleep might help to reduce the risk of sudden infant death syndrome.
- Pacifiers soothe fussy babies because babies suck to calm themselves down, even before they are born.
- If you need a distraction for your hungry baby, a pacifier can fit the bill, buying you a few minutes to find a place to nurse or warm a bottle.
- Pacifiers can help babies to fall asleep.
- When it's time to give up the pacifier, you can take it away. Not so with a baby's thumb!

But of course there's also a flip side. Early pacifier use might interfere with breastfeeding. Prolonged use might lead to dental problems, such as the teeth slanting outward or not coming in properly. Plus, babies who lose their pacifiers in the night cry out for help to get them back!

If you wish to breastfeed, the AAP recommends waiting to introduce a pacifier to your baby until breastfeeding is well established, when your baby is around one month old.

My son cried a lot in the first few weeks of his life before we found out that he had food allergies. During that time, the only thing that would soothe him was his pacifier. I know many moms hate them, but when you have a baby who will not stop crying, you have to do what you have to do. My son's pacifier was his special friend—as well as mine!

—*Saundra Dalton-Smith, MD, a mom of six- and four-year-old sons, an internal medicine specialist, and the author of* Set Free to Live Free: Breaking Through the 7 Lies Women Tell Themselves, *in Anniston, AL*

My kids all used "binkies" until they found their thumbs at around three months old. At that point, they sucked on their thumbs to self-soothe. I was fortunate to not have to go through the extract-the-binkie process.

—*Katherine Dee, MD, a mom of six-year-old twin daughters and a four-year-old son and a radiologist at the Seattle Breast Center, in Washington*

My daughter and I had a lot of difficulty breastfeeding early on, so I tried not to use a pacifier right away. I ended up bottlefeeding breast milk and formula, so eventually I did offer her a pacifier. It really helped her self-soothe and helped her go to sleep. She used a pacifier well into her second year, but only while she was going to sleep, and then I took it away without too much trouble. Her teeth did have that pacifier gap, but within six months of giving it up, her teeth were fine.

—*Katja Rowell, MD*

When my babies were small, they liked to use pacifiers. But I didn't like the idea of those pacifiers falling onto the ground. A simple solution is a pacifier clip. You can buy them in stores and online for a few dollars; they come in lots of neat colors and patterns. Clip one end to the paci and the other to your baby.

Be sure to choose one with a very short string, and never lengthen the string, to avoid strangulation, and don't put one on your baby if he will be unattended, such as when he's sleeping.

—*Lezli Braswell, MD*

∽

I tried to get my sons to take a pacifier, but they never would. I was quite tempted to use one myself at times though!

—*Rebecca Reamy, MD*

∽

My middle child wasn't interested in pacifiers at all. But it wasn't for lack of trying on my part! I went to Walgreens at 2 a.m. one night and bought one of each kind of pacifier they sold, hoping to find one that my son would like. It didn't work.

My oldest and youngest babies really wanted their pacifiers, though. In retrospect, I should have been more insistent about having my children stop using the pacifier at one year of age. I didn't do that with my older son, and he was still attached to his pacifier at age three. At that time, my husband and I made a big deal about saying, "What happens when you turn three? No more pacis!" It became a game. We'd sing the song, and my son would triumphantly whip the pacifier out of his mouth.

Just as we had trained my son, on his third birthday, we sang the song, he whipped it out, and we confiscated the paci and replaced it with a toy. That night he whimpered for it, but we said, "Oh, silly! Remember, you're a big three-year-old now! No more pacis!" So our son gave up his pacifier on his third birthday. I've found that pretty much anything works in parenting, as long as your will is stronger than theirs is!

—*Amy Baxter, MD*

Treating Jaundice

Jaundice is a very common condition in newborns. You might have been told by your mom that you were "a little bit jaundiced" as a baby. It's a condition in which a baby's skin and the whites of his eyes take on a yellowish tinge due to excess bilirubin in his blood. When your baby's body breaks down red blood cells, it produces bilirubin. Normally the bilirubin passes through the liver and is whisked out of the body through the intestines. But in newborns, bilirubin can build up faster than the liver can break it down. This happens because a baby's body is turning over red blood cells faster than an adult's body does, and the baby's liver might not yet have perfected its removal process. And so the baby's skin and eyes can start to look yellow.

Fortunately, the American Academy of Pediatrics is on the case. This organization recommends that all infants be screened for jaundice within a few days of being born. Your baby's doctor will take a teeny sample of your baby's blood, likely from his heel, and he will probably scream like his toenails are being pulled off. The doctor then will check the bilirubin level in your baby's blood.

?   ## When to Call Your Doctor
No doubt you spend lots of time looking at your beautiful new baby! If you notice your baby's skin color changing, call the doctor. Jaundice generally appears during a baby's second or third day of life. Interestingly, it begins at the baby's head and spreads down. So you'll spot the yellowing first on a baby's face and eyes.

Jaundice can get very serious, very quickly. High levels of bilirubin (above 25 mg/dL) can cause deafness, cerebral palsy, or other types of brain damage in some babies. Call your doctor right away if your baby's color begins to yellow, if your baby has a fever (any fever in a baby younger than three months), or if your baby starts to look or act sick.

Mild jaundice usually resolves on its own. But if a baby has high levels of bilirubin, he'll be treated with a special light to help his body get rid of the excess bilirubin. Mothers of infants with jaundice might also be urged to breastfeed more frequently, because this will help the baby pass more bilirubin in his stool.

My first baby was jaundiced, and that was the reason I went to medical school! After my son was born, we went home, and three days later I noticed that his skin was very yellow. I took him to our country doctor, who sent us to the hospital. When we arrived at the hospital, the nurses stripped my baby naked and took him away from me, with hardly any explanation at all. They put my son into a "light box," which was the treatment for jaundice at the time, and when I asked where I could pump breast milk, they showed me to a broom closet with a pull-chain light. That was my introduction to "real" medicine. At that moment, I realized that I could care for people better than that. And that's when I decided to become a doctor.

Now I know that full-term breastfed babies are at very low risk of developing any complications from high bilirubin levels. Hydration and exposure to sunlight is what I recommend for my patients, along with close monitoring. Taking the baby away from Mom and placing him in a light box for three days is not therapeutic for anyone.

—*Hana R. Solomon, MD*

My third baby came home from the hospital with a borderline-high bilirubin level. But when the pediatrician rechecked it the next day, the level was so high that we had to put him under lights at home for the next five days. Plus, we had to go back to the doctor every day to have his bilirubin level rechecked. It was very stressful.

I was very thankful that we could use the at-home treatment. A local home health company delivered a portable light set designed for treating babies with jaundice. There are two types of light sets. One type is designed to use when the baby is lying in his crib. I tried this type, and it was terrible because all my son wanted to do was breastfeed. He just lay there screaming whenever it was time for his light treatment. Fortunately, the home health company swapped out that contraption for a specially designed blanket that I could wrap my son in and hold him. That went a lot better!

—*Kristie McNealy, MD*

When my older son was born, my husband had moved ahead of us to another state where he was going to school. My mentor and her husband, who are both pediatricians, invited me to stay with them for the last few weeks of my pregnancy and the first few days of my son's life.

When my son was born, he looked a little orange. We three pediatricians assured ourselves that it was just his complexion. Breastfeeding wasn't going well, which is another symptom of jaundice, but we kept telling ourselves it would get better. We tried everything to get my baby to wake up and eat.

When my son was two days old, it dawned on us that he might be jaundiced. We took him to the clinic and took bets on how high his bilirubin levels would be. None of us were even close. His levels were really, really high. Pediatricians always tell new moms to watch their babies' skin for a change in color, because it could be a sign of jaundice. My baby's skin color never changed; he was orange when he was born! His bilirubin levels were probably very high from the beginning.

My son ended up back in the hospital at two days old, which is every parent's worst nightmare. He had to stay in the hospital under the bilirubin lights for around three days. We called those lights the "French fry warmer." My son was nice and toasty warm in the incubator with his eye protectors on, and he didn't seem to mind it a bit. I couldn't stand to stay in the same room, though, because the lights gave me a headache even with sunglasses on. My son's bilirubin levels came down enough in a few days that we could take him back home.

Fortunately, this experience would be very unlikely to happen today because all babies get a bilirubin check before leaving the hospital. But seven years ago, that wasn't the standard of care. Today my son is just fine.

—*Carrie Brown, MD*

I had to deal with jaundice in *all three* of my children. While it *completely* freaked me out with my first child, it definitely seemed much more manageable in my third child.

I distinctly remember that when my daughter was born, my mother commented on her perfect "peaches and cream" complexion and that she was so beautiful. (But she didn't look *at all* like me!) Within the first one to two days, however, my baby's complexion seemed to be less rosy and more pale. I have to say that I really did not notice that her skin or eyes were yellow, and that I was majorly *floored* when I was told that her total bilirubin was extremely high. (And here I was a new gastroenterology/hepatology fellow, specializing in diseases of the liver!)

Treatment of neonatal jaundice, when indicated, includes maintaining adequate hydration with frequent nursing and/or formula, and light therapy, also known as phototherapy. Several forms of phototherapy are available.

When my daughter was born, about 12 years ago, we had phototherapy lights installed over her crib. We had to put little felt "sunglasses" over her eyes to prevent any ocular damage, and we turned her from her front to her back at 10- to 15-minute intervals. She looked like she was catching rays in a tanning booth!

My boys were prescribed more portable phototherapy "vests" that were worn directly on their torsos and applied light to their fronts and backs simultaneously.

All of my kids required frequent rechecks of their bilirubin levels, which peaked and then dropped in less than a week.

For my daughter, I also had a visiting nurse come to our house. She gave me a card so that I could log the amount of time my daughter spent under the "bililights," how many minutes I nursed her, and how much formula I gave her each day. I was so freaked out about the whole situation that I stayed up the whole first night with her, and I was very diligent about recording everything. In the morning, the nurse's eyes nearly popped out of her head when she saw how much I had recorded! My baby's next bilirubin level had dropped like a rock! After being on call every third or fourth night for the previous four years, taking care of only one "patient" was a snap!

I think that my kids inherited the tendency to develop jaundice from my husband, although my mother-in-law vehemently denies it. However, she did relate a story that when my husband was born, he was so "nice and brown" because she ate so many carrots when she was pregnant, and that the pediatrician told her to keep him in front of a sunny window. I don't know, what do you think?

—*Stacey Weiland, MD*

Taking Your Baby Home

In all likelihood, after a few days—or weeks—in the hospital, you are anxious to go home. Now!

The hospital where my daughter was born had no set visiting hours, so we were bombarded with visits from family and friends. On the last day we were there, I asked everyone to please stay away so I could be alone with my husband and my daughter. It was wintertime and very cold, and we bundled our baby up. I had planned her going-home-from-the-hospital outfit way ahead of time. My husband pulled the car around to the front door, picked us up, and drove us safely home.

—*Jeannette Gonzalez Simon, MD*

I marvel at the fact that I had to go through four years of undergraduate college, four years of medical school, and four years of residency before I could see patients. Yet, they sent me home with a fragile newborn with no instruction at all after a few short hours. It didn't make any sense to me.

I quickly learned that my skill set at the time was zero. Being a doctor is easy compared with being a mother! Motherhood is so challenging because your emotions are involved. Plus, every time you figure one stage out, your child grows into a new one.

—*Eva Ritvo, MD*

My twins were born six weeks early, so they had to stay in the hospital for a few weeks. My husband and I spent as much time there as we could. We even took our older daughter with us, who was two years old at the time.

It was very difficult to be separated from my twins. Just about the time that I started to think, *I can't do this; it hurts me physically,* my twins were released to go home.

—*Penny Noyce, MD*

When my older son was born, it was freezing cold outside. At the time, my husband had moved ahead of me and the baby to another state for his PhD program. I had moved in with one of my mentors for a few months so I wouldn't be alone at the end of my pregnancy or after my baby's birth.

When my son was born, we bundled the little darling up, and we had a huge debate over how many hats you need to have on a baby's head in the middle of winter. My husband had installed the car seat weeks before, but my mentor went out ahead of me and the baby to make sure he had done it right. It was very funny to see this tiny, slender woman pushing down on the car seat with all of her might to make sure the seat was in good and tight. It was, and everything was fine.

—*Carrie Brown, MD*

∽◦

My daughter was born two days before Christmas, and we got to take her home on Christmas day. My in-laws came to visit shortly after. Our home was very neat and tidy, despite having a new baby in the house. I need it that way to function. My in-laws walked in and put their stuff all over the place! I ran to my room and shut the door. My husband came up to check on me, and he found me crying in the closet.

My husband asked me, "What's wrong?"

"They put stuff on the table!" I sobbed.

There was no logic, but for a woman who just had a baby, this was a very normal reaction!

—*Alanna Kramer, MD*

∽◦

My parents are from Italy, and our family tradition is to avoid buying anything for the baby before he's born. Back in the village, after a baby is born, the aunts, uncles, and grandparents make meals for the new parents, build a crib, knit stockings, go shopping, and totally outfit the nursery.

My husband and I kept that tradition. We didn't buy a stitch of baby clothing or a single item for the baby. When I was pregnant, my mom would ask me, "You didn't go looking at baby things, did you?"

But once our baby was born, we realized, *There's no village here to help us! Where are all of those little old ladies now?*

At the time, my husband was a fellow in a maternal-fetal medicine program, so he was quite busy. But in the days after our daughter was born, he raced all over town, buying diapers, clothing, sheets, furniture, decorations—everything our new baby needed.

My husband did a phenomenal job. He's a very gifted decorator, and the nursery turned out beautifully. It also was a blessing that he was so involved in the process of getting ready for our baby. He was very invested.

But that certainly wasn't the *easy* way to prepare for a new baby. Sometimes the ideas that command us and the traditions we're bound to are illogical. It's important to question those things instead of sticking to a tradition that no longer makes sense.

—*Lisa Dado, MD*

Recovering from the Birth

In the movies, after a woman gives birth, she's slim, cheerful, and pain free. This is not the reality for most new moms!

After delivery, you're a new person, and you probably feel like one too. Your emotions might be running amok due to dramatic changes in hormone levels.

Even if you're not breastfeeding, your breasts might feel full and sore, engorged from milk. If you are breastfeeding, your nipples might feel tender.

For a few days after your baby is born, you might experience painful contractions of your uterus. These are called afterbirth pains. They are often more intense with second and subsequent deliveries. Acetaminophen (Tylenol) might help.

If you've had a vaginal delivery, you might feel sore from tearing or from having an episiotomy. Holding an ice pack on the sore spot for 10 minutes at a time can help. While you're in the hospital, you might ask the nurses for some acetaminophen (Tylenol).

If you had a C-section, you'll likely be in the hospital for a few extra days. But the nurses won't let you lie around; they'll have you up on your feet within around six hours of your surgery. You'll be given pain medication as needed. Most women experience the greatest soreness 48 hours after delivery. Take care to keep your incision clean, and don't be alarmed if it itches after the first week. That's a good sign of healing.

Many months without a menstrual period will catch up with you now. Whether you've had a vaginal delivery or a C-section, you'll probably have vaginal discharge, which will begin bright red and heavy, then fade to white or yellow, and finally stop when your baby is around two months old.

You might feel constipated—and be dreading your first bowel movement after delivery. The first one might be painful, but it should get better after that. Hemorrhoids might be causing you discomfort as well. Try to drink water and eat foods with lots of fiber, such as fruits and vegetables.

Your legs and feet might be swollen. It helps to elevate them as often as possible. (Go ahead, put your feet up!)

It's not uncommon to feel hot and cold flashes as your body adjusts to new hormone levels and blood volume. Your body's thermostat could be out of whack for a few days. There's not much you can do about this besides layering up and down as necessary.

Your body has just accomplished a miracle. Be kind to yourself!

&

My deliveries were all vaginal, and my recoveries were quick. As an ob-gyn, there weren't any surprises there for me. I healed quickly, and the recovery was straightforward. Now breastfeeding on the other hand . . .
—*Siobhan Dolan, MD*

&

My recoveries from both of my sons' births went pretty well, even though the delivery of my second son was horrible. I laid on the couch a lot and used a lot of Tucks Pads and ice.
—*Carrie Brown, MD*

&

What unbelievable changes our bodies go through when we have babies! Somehow, it seems that I was better prepared for the changes that occurred during the pregnancy than the changes I was in for postpartum. After my baby was born, my hair started to fall out, my skin became extremely dry (especially my palms and soles), and I think that my vagina thought we were going into menopause. It was so dry and irritated down there that I thought I had a yeast infection.

I just rode these changes out. I am lucky that I have a lot of hair, so my hair loss wasn't really noticeable. I used a lot of Lubriderm moisturizer on my skin, and when I finally agreed to have sex with my husband, we used some K-Y Jelly. After a few months, all of these problems went away.

—*Stacey Weiland, MD*

One of the many positive things about having a fully natural birth is I didn't have to recover from any medications or heal from any stitches.

I was surprised by the intensity of afterbirth pains, especially with my second son. I tried taking Tylenol, but that didn't even touch the pain! I took homeopathic remedies called caulophyllum and cimicifuga, and those took away the discomfort.

After I got home, I had a short time of recovery and convalescence. For the first month, I stuck close to our home to give myself time to get my strength back and bond with my baby. I felt that by taking that month to relax, away from the normal activities of life, I was able to regain my strength sooner.

—*Lauren Feder, MD, a mom of 17- and 13-year-old sons, a nationally recognized physician who specializes in homeopathic medicine, and the author of* Natural Baby and Childcare *and* The Parents' Concise Guide to Childhood Vaccinations, *in Los Angeles, CA*

I had a C-section, and the recovery was very difficult. I had never had surgery before, and I didn't realize how important all of those abdominal muscles are until the doctor cut through them to get my baby out.

The recovery was painful, and even easy things like positioning my baby to nurse were hard. But I'd go through all of that pain all over again, even knowing how bad it was, because having my daughter is so worth it.

—*Christy Valentine, MD, a mom of a five-year-old daughter, a specialist in pediatrics and internal medicine, and the founder of the Valentine Medical Center, in Gretna, LA*

I didn't plan to have a C-section, but I ended up needing to have one. The recovery was more difficult than I had expected. For the first few weeks after my daughter was born, I felt very wounded.

In the hospital, the beds and chairs are hard and adjustable, and that's actually better than soft furniture after a C-section. I thought that it would be great to get home to my comfortable house, but I found that it was better to sit on a high, hard chair and put my feet up on a nursing stool. That was much easier to get out of than a soft couch or bed.

Another thing that helped me to get comfortable nursing my daughter was my Boppy nursing pillow. It helped me to get my daughter into a good position to nurse. It took a few weeks after my C-section before I started feeling better.

—*Dina Strachan, MD*

? When to Call Your Doctor

During the postpartum period, call your doctor or midwife right away if you develop a fever of 100.4°F or higher, bleed enough to soak more than one sanitary pad per hour or pass large clots, have a new pain or swelling in your legs, experience painful urination or the sudden urge to urinate, develop a foul-smelling vaginal discharge, have a C-section or episiotomy incision that becomes red or swollen, or have hot, red, sore breasts or cracking and bleeding nipples.

Both of my boys were born by C-section. After my older son was born, my husband brought him over to me to hold. But I had such terrible chills, which is common after having a C-section, and I was shaking so badly that I didn't want to hold my son for fear I'd drop him.

Later, I was in a painkiller haze, so I had to be careful holding him. It didn't take me long to get over this, and I had a lot of family around to help me hold him if I needed it. The shakes passed fairly quickly, mostly in the recovery room. The medications I was prescribed made me tired and sleepy, so I had to make sure I timed the medications for when I had help with the baby.

The recovery was tough. I always needed to support myself when I got up or down. I'd lean on my husband or the arm of the chair. After my second son was born, my three-year-old son would help pull me up. That was a lot better than doing it all by myself, and it made my three-year-old feel like he was needed. It also gave me a chance to bond with him and hold his little hand too.

—*Leena Shrivastava Dev, MD*

RALLIE'S TIP

I wasn't one of those beautiful, glowing pregnant ladies. I was swollen and puffy and enormous! I gained nearly 60 pounds with my first pregnancy, mostly because I wasn't able to exercise very much in the last trimester. I was just too huge. In retrospect, I probably ate just a tad too much too!

I couldn't wait to start working out again. I had an episiotomy with my first baby, and my doctor warned me not to start exercising until I'd had a chance to heal. Of course I didn't listen to him. I started exercising the first week after delivery, and I ended up pulling loose the sutures. It was really painful, and it took me forever to heal. If I had just listened to my doctor in the first place and waited another week, I would have been able to return to my regular exercise routine a lot sooner. As it turned out, I had to wait an extra month while my body healed. With my second baby, I didn't even think about working out until a month after I had delivered.

Discovering Your Baby's Personality

Does your baby seem like a blank slate? We didn't think so either!

It's fascinating how babies have their own personalities. You really notice this with twins. Even as a newborn, my son was more alert and interactive, while my daughter would stare off into space for long periods of time. I actually worried about that, but it turns out she's just fine. From the very beginning, there was such a contrast between my kids.

—*Penny Noyce, MD*

It was clear early on that my twins were high-maintenance babies! They needed to be held a lot. But it's interesting how they had distinct personalities even in their first few months of life. My son, for example, was a little more demanding regarding getting fed and being picked up. It needed to happen *now*!

—*Ann Contrucci, MD*

I am always amazed at how different two people can be when they come from the same parents. Our sons have completely different personalities. What works to soothe one may not work at all on the other. You always have to be ready to change your strategy.

—*Saundra Dalton-Smith, MD*

I know it sounds corny, but I was totally in love with my baby, and I was absolutely ecstatic to discover her personality and watch her develop new skills. Believe it or not, she developed a sense of humor at three months. Watching her laugh uncontrollably, especially at dogs and the antics of a five-year-old whom she adored more than anyone in the world, was truly one of the most amazing experiences of my life.

—*Stuart Jeanne Bramhall, MD*

One of the biggest lessons I've learned is that kids have their own way of being. Even though you *think* you're bringing them up, they're really bringing themselves up with your help. You can't change them into someone they are not.

For example, my son is very laid-back and slow-paced, and I'm the kind of person who does everything quickly. I'm always telling my son, "Come on, move faster!" but he can't. It's not him. He doesn't function that way. Let your kids be who they are.

—*Judith Hellman, MD*

It is amazing how babies' personalities are so apparent, and so different, starting at such early ages. My older daughter was always very happy-go-lucky and easy to please. She wanted to help and to get along with everyone. My second daughter, on the other hand, came home on the Fourth of July. Either the date, or her DNA, or both seemed to have an effect on her personality. She was a firecracker from the beginning. She had abundant energy that just needed to be channeled in the right direction. My son's temperament was easy-going and flexible. He was happiest when everyone was getting along.

All children have wonderful qualities, and they also have plenty of opportunities to grow. The same is true for us parents as well! Our job is to help our children recognize and develop their gifts even while we continue to discover and claim our own. We need to support and encourage our children with positive discipline, using mistakes as opportunities to learn and successes as a means to build a sense of competence and capability. Treating both ourselves and our children with compassion is vital.

—*Lesley Burton-Iwinski, MD*

◌◌◌

I really feel that you can tell from the moment your kids come into the world who they are. I don't think that they are blank slates. They're born with their own temperaments.

When my son was a baby, I could tell he was a very different kid from my daughters. For example, I knew that he needed me to have a longer maternity leave than my daughters did; he needed more time with me. I remember going to my boss and asking for another month of leave. It was a pretty brave move, but it was very important to me. It was a hard decision for me to make because my son is my second child, and I thought, *I'm a well-greased mom. I should be able to make this transition.* But my son was a big baby who drank a lot of milk, and even then he was slower to make transitions.

The key is that what worked for one child might not work for the others. Each child is unique, and you must be flexible with that.

—*Nancy Rappaport, MD*

Changing Diapers

For some reason, disposable diapers feel like a relatively new invention. But actually, they were invented in 1949 by a mom who made them herself and sold them at Saks Fifth Avenue in New York City. She got $1 million for the patent rights. Today, the diaper industry is a $17 million *a year* industry.

Now might be a great time to buy stock in Procter & Gamble. In babies' first years, they go through around 2,788 diapers. But interestingly, the cost difference between disposable and cloth isn't as great as one might think. Estimates show that disposable diapers cost approximately $50 to $80 per month, using a diaper service also costs approximately $50 to $80 per month, and washing your own cloth diapers costs only slightly less at around $25 to $60 per month.

Costs aside, there's a huge debate about the environmental impact of disposable versus cloth. It's estimated that 5 million tons of untreated waste and 2 billion tons of urine, feces, plastic, and paper are added to U.S. landfills each year as a result of disposable diapers. It takes around 80,000 pounds of plastic and 200,000 trees each year to make the diapers for American babies. On the other hand, washing cloth diapers can add about two extra loads of laundry to the average household a week. That's a lot of extra time, energy, and water.

It's a tough choice, but the great thing is, nothing says you can't change your mind or be flexible if one option isn't working.

One thing that's not disputable is that you will be changing a lot of diapers. Newborn babies typically need 10 to 12 diaper changes each day. That number goes down as a baby grows. From the age of one month to around five months, babies need to be changed around 8 to 10 times a day, and then more like 8 times a day after that. Until they potty train, that is, which might feel like a million years from now but will be here before you know it!

RALLIE'S TIP

A baby's first few diaper changes can be tricky. That's because meconium, a thick, dark green, tar-like substance that lines your baby's intestines before birth, can be a real challenge to remove from your newborn baby's tender bottom. Normally, meconium is expelled with the stool in the first two to three days of life.

I found that olive oil works beautifully. It helps remove the messy meconium without scrubbing and tugging. Olive oil is very gentle, so it cleans without irritating your baby's sensitive skin.

My Diaper Genie was great. I kept it in my baby's nursery, right next to the changing table. When you put the diapers in it, it wraps them up into sausage-link-like packages. My older son thought it was the funniest thing to drag the diaper-sausages through the house and outside to the trash. It's perfectly clean, so that was just fine with me—one less thing for me to do!

—*Jill Wireman, MD*

I never thought I would need a Diaper Genie, but it has been key. We empty our trash frequently, so I thought we could get away with a small trash can and bags; how much volume could a few diapers create? We were shocked at how many diapers one little baby could use, how bad they could smell, and how much they could weigh!

We keep the Diaper Genie right next to our baby's changing table in the nursery. It helps tremendously with the smell. (Although when you dispose of subsequent diapers, you might get a whiff of the last change!) We sometimes bag the poopy diapers in extra bags within the Diaper Genie. It can accommodate a few days' worth of diapers. Using the Diaper Genie is definitely more expensive than just taking diapers out to the trash immediately, but it's a time- and nose-saver.

—*Rachel S. Rohde, MD*

I completely understand why people use cloth diapers. New babies go through so many diapers in a day, and disposable diapers are so expensive! But I use disposable diapers. I used to counsel my patients on the importance of changing diapers frequently to prevent diaper rash, but I can see how some parents might try to change their babies' diapers less frequently because disposable diapers are so expensive. It's super important to change diapers often to prevent rash. Luckily, we've been rash free so far!

My husband and I have also found that it's important to use the right size of diaper for our baby. When we were transitioning from newborn size to size 1, we went through so many onesie changes every

Mommy MD Guides–Recommended Product
Pampers Swaddlers

"I buy Pampers," says Sadaf T. Bhutta, MD, a mom of a five-year-old daughter and three-year-old triplets and an assistant professor and the fellowship director of pediatric radiology at the University of Arkansas for Medical Sciences and Arkansas Children's Hospital, both in Little Rock. "I believed those other diaper companies' ads that say their diapers are cheaper but work just as well. I tried them, and it's not true. Stuff leaks. Plus a lot of those cheaper diapers are hard and stiff. That's not good to put on a baby's bottom! Pampers are soft, and they don't leak. I initially used Swaddlers, and then I moved on to the Cruisers."

You can buy Pampers Swaddlers in stores and online, for $25 to $35 a box.

day because the diapers were still too big for our baby and didn't fit her right. Urine and poop would leak out of the sides all the time!

—*Jennifer Bacani McKenney, MD*

I found that disposable diapers were easier than cloth, especially when we were away from home. I did have some cloth diapers, but I used them as catch-all cloths, not as actual diapers.

I also found that using disposable diapers made the transition from diapers to pull-ups much easier. We mainly used Pampers diapers, but we also used a biodegradable brand called gDiapers. They are better for the environment, which made me feel better about choosing to use disposable diapers.

—*Christy Valentine, MD*

A lot of people have an aversion to using cloth diapers, but my husband and I found that using cloth diapers saved a lot of money. It was relatively easy and saved our children from chemical irritation related to paper diapers. We used paper diapers only at night and while traveling. Plus, we saved our landfills from all the extra garbage. Washing diapers is really no different from running a load of laundry like any other clothes that need washing.

—Michelle Storms, MD, a mom of 24- and 20-year-old sons and a 21-year-old daughter, the assistant director of the Marquette Family Medicine Residency Program, in Marquette, MI, and a member of the health professionals board for Intact America

I'm a little old-fashioned, and I used cloth diapers with all six of my babies. When we went out, I put plastic pants on top of the diapers to keep them from leaking. Many people are scared to use cloth diapers, but it's really easy. Plus, I'm sure I saved thousands of dollars on diapers.

When I changed a diaper, I rinsed it off if it was dirty, and then I put it into a bucket with a bleach solution in it. The bucket had a step-on lid so it wasn't open to air—nor accessible to the baby. We kept the bucket under a cabinet or in a corner so that it was out of the way. Once the bucket was full of diapers, I dumped the diapers and the bleach solution into the washing machine.

It was a lot of washing! But I think using cloth diapers really helped to prevent diaper rash. My kids had only about one case of diaper rash each.

Back then, it was actually hard to find cloth diapers, but now there are lots of places to buy them.

—Susan Besser, MD, a mom of six grown children, ages 26, 24, 22, 21, 19, and 17, a grandmom of one, a family physician, and the medical director of Doctors Express-Memphis, in Tennessee

When my third child was about a year old, my second child was taking quite a long time to potty train, and my husband and I were talking about having a fourth baby, I decided we were spending way too much money on diapers.

A good friend of mine had used cloth diapers with her first baby. I remember saying to her, "You're crazy!" But a few years later,

I reached out to her for advice on how to use cloth diapers myself. I started researching cloth diapers, and I discovered that there are many options out there. Some of the cloth diapers today look and work much like disposable diapers.

I don't use them, though. Instead I use the flat, square diapers with covers like your grandmother would have used. Because I have several kids in several sizes, that works best for me.

Rather than using pins, I use a fantastic invention called Snappi (SnappiBaby.com). It holds the diaper on without pins. I do have a few diaper pins in case of emergency. You can't run to Walmart and buy Snappis if you need them.

I keep a few disposable diapers on hand in case I have a babysitter who doesn't have experience using cloth diapers. But I far prefer using cloth diapers—and the fact that we don't have to buy diapers all of the time.

—*Kristie McNealy, MD*

I think a lot of moms-to-be feel so frenzied about being prepared that they buy things they don't really need. One thing I found not so helpful in my baby's first year involved diaper changing—the wipe warmer.

I bought a butt wipe warmer, but I didn't know when I bought it that you have to keep it filled with water. With so much else to do, that felt totally overwhelming to me. Plus, it didn't seem to make any difference to my daughter whether the wipes were warm or not.

—*Katja Rowell, MD*

Caring for Your Baby's Umbilical Cord Stump

It's one of so many things moms don't think about before having kids: A baby's belly button starts out as an umbilical cord stump about an inch long. It might look terrible, but the umbilical cord doesn't have any nerve fibers, so it doesn't hurt your baby at all.

Usually a baby's cord stump falls off in 10 to 14 days—but not before it changes from yellowish green to brown to black.

Don't be alarmed if you see some crust or dried blood near the stump. That's a normal part of the healing process.

In the hospital, your baby's doctor and nurses will tell you how to care for your baby's cord stump. In all likelihood, they'll recommend leaving it alone for the most part. Just wash it with water, and maybe a bit of baby soap if it somehow gets dirty. It's best to give your baby a sponge bath until the stump falls off.

Keep your baby's cord stump as dry as possible. Change wet diapers quickly so they don't irritate your baby's skin. It helps to fold the diaper down a bit so that it doesn't rub up against the cord stump.

Don't tug or pull on the stump. Be patient; it will fall off all on its own in time.

∽

It's interesting that the recommended care for the umbilical cord stump changed as the years went by. For my first baby, the pediatrician told me to clean it with rubbing alcohol swabs a few times a day. By the time my fourth baby was born, the advice had changed to "do nothing." I don't know if it was a coincidence, but my fourth baby got an infection in that area, and he needed to be on antibiotics when he was three days old.

Until my babies' umbilical cord stumps healed, I was careful to keep the top of their diapers folded down so the diapers wouldn't rub it or irritate it. With my fourth baby, I used cloth diapers, and I bought the type of cloth diaper with the lowest rise so it didn't come up over my baby's belly button.

—*Kristie McNealy, MD*

RALLIE'S TIP

When my oldest son was born, his umbilical cord stump seemed to take forever to fall off. If a new mom tells me that her baby has a similar problem, I recommend putting some olive oil on the baby's umbilical cord stump. It's one of the traditional practices for babies in some cultures. Studies have shown that the use of olive oil on babies' umbilical stumps is safe and effective, and helps it fall off earlier. In one study, researchers in Turkey found that at 10 days after birth, umbilical cord separation had occurred in almost three-quarters of the infants receiving treatment with olive oil, compared to only half of the infants who were not treated with olive oil.

The umbilical cord stump area can become infected, so you want to inspect it carefully. I'd look at the area at each diaper change and watch for redness or drainage.

When my middle son's cord stump fell off, I noticed a little red blood that looked fresh—not just the dark black dried blood that is typical. Our pediatrician explained that granulation tissue had formed there. Granulation tissue forms when our bodies heal wounds, and this new tissue sometimes bleeds. Our pediatrician treated the area with a little silver nitrate in the office. Silver nitrate chemically cauterizes the wound, and it's applied with a stick that looks like a long matchstick.

My son tolerated it just fine. It was just a little hiccup in his first few weeks of life.

—*Amy Thompson, MD*

Caring for Your Son's Circumcised —Or Uncircumcised—Penis

If you have a new baby boy, by this point, you've already decided if he will be circumcised or not. A circumcision surgically removes the foreskin, exposing the glans, or top, of the penis. Around 55 to 65 percent of newborn boys in the United States are circumcised. The rates are highest in the north central region, and lowest in the western states.

Whether your son was circumcised or not, it's important to keep his penis clean with water. Avoid soaps and bubble baths because they can be irritating.

If your son was circumcised, don't use diaper wipes on his penis until his incision heals. Wiping with diaper wipes could slow the healing process. For the first five days or so, until the incision heals, put Vaseline or A+D Ointment on the incision each time you change your baby's diaper. This keeps the skin around the incision from sticking to the diaper. It usually takes about 7 to 10 days for the incision to heal completely. The skin around the incision might appear a little red and swollen initially, and a scant yellow discharge or crust after a few days is normal.

〜

I was raised Jewish, and it was incredibly important to me that my boys be circumcised in our home. Of course, it's a personal choice, and you have to weigh the benefits and risks of doing it and not doing it.

As the circumcision healed, I applied Vaseline or Triple Paste to the end of his penis so that the skin wouldn't adhere.
—*Hana R. Solomon, MD*

〜

My younger son wasn't circumcised because neither his dad nor his brother was. I didn't want him to think he was different. I made the decision not to circumcise because we don't have any first-degree family members with a history of urinary tract infections or urinary reflux. Everyone should make their own decisions, but you should know that if you change your mind and decide to have your son circumcised later in life, he might require general anesthesia during the surgery.

To care for my son's un-circumcised penis, I just rinsed it without trying to pull back the foreskin, which can cause tearing and scar tissue formation. I just wiggled it in soapy bathwater, and then rinsed him off.
—*Sonia Ng, MD*

My sons were not circumcised. Our pediatrician advised us to simply make sure to clean the penis at each diaper change, but not to retract the foreskin. Once our boys started potty training, I watched them closely to make sure the urine stream was coming out appropriately, and not ballooning up the foreskin because this can be a sign of a condition called phimosis. When my sons are around age three, we start to teach them how to gently retract the foreskin so that they get used to doing that and cleaning themselves properly.

—*Amy Thompson, MD*

⟜

My husband and I chose not to circumcise our sons because we felt that circumcision is harmful and unnecessary. Circumcision removes the foreskin of the penis, which is meant to protect the glans from urine and feces. It also

? When to Call Your Doctor

If your son was circumcised, his penis will likely be wrapped in gauze after the surgery. Call your doctor right away if you notice persistent bleeding or more than a quarter-size spot of blood in your baby's diaper. Also call if you see signs of infection, such as a fever (any fever in a baby younger than three months old or a fever of 101°F or higher in a baby three months old or older), increasing redness, worsening swelling, pus, or blisters. With quick intervention, almost all circumcision-related problems are easily treated.

protects the glans from chemical irritants in disposable diapers. The intact penis requires no special care and does not need to be retracted by parents or physicians, contrary to what many are taught. A baby's penis should just be wiped off on the outside similar to the way a girl's labia are cleaned.

We simply gave our boys regular baths. When our sons were around three years old, they learned that their foreskins could retract, which allowed them to clean themselves while bathing. The foreskin should never be forcibly retracted since this can lead to major problems. Our sons have never had an issue keeping themselves clean, and their foreskins have never been a problem. They have often asked us why anyone would remove "the best part" of a penis.

—*Michelle Storms, MD*

Going to the Doctor

It's a good bet that the pediatrician or family physician you've so carefully chosen for your baby will have stopped by to give your baby a checkup while you're in the hospital. This is a great time to ask the doctor any questions you have.

Newborns have very frequent well baby visits. Your first visit will probably be when your baby is only a week or two old. The nurses at your pediatrician's office will weigh and measure your baby and check his head circumference. You might want to bring along a baby book or small notebook because it's fun to jot down these numbers to keep track of them as your baby grows.

At your baby's first visit, the doctor will also check his vision, hearing, and reflexes and give him a head-to-toe examination.

༄

I had interviewed a couple of doctors before I chose my son's pediatrician. Some things I like about my pediatrician's group are that it has a very good cross-coverage schedule and early morning drop-in hours at their office. Also, they don't let newborns wait in the waiting room. Instead, newborns are taken straight into the exam rooms. I also like that the exam rooms each have different themes, and they're all very visually stimulating to babies.

I'm not a pediatrician, and I learned early on that even doctors have to lean on their pediatricians. I had to take a leap of faith and trust what my pediatrician was telling me. It doesn't mean that you can't do your own research about your baby's symptoms. But you can't become a pediatrician online!

—*Sharon Giese, MD*

༄

Being a doctor did not prepare me for being a mother. Like my friends who are also doctors, I had thought that we'd have an advantage over moms who aren't doctors, but we really don't. Medical school doesn't prepare you for having a crying baby. If anything, it made me more paranoid.

I am careful not to be my baby's doctor. If someone needs to look in her ear, it's not going to be me. I'm taking her to her doctor. I keep those two parts of my life completely separate. I'm her mother, not her doctor.

—*Jeannette Gonzalez Simon, MD*

When to Call Your Doctor

Don't hesitate to call your baby's doctor if you have concerns. The type of people who become pediatricians and family physicians in general don't mind middle-of-the-night calls. If they did, they would have become accountants instead. No one calls H&R Block for tax advice at 2 a.m.

The following are concerning and warrant a call to your baby's doctor.

- Fever (any fever in a baby younger than three months old or a fever of 101°F or higher in a baby three months old or older)
- Excessive drowsiness, which can be a sign of infection
- Problems with the eye, such as white discharge, which can be a sign of pinkeye
- Extreme floppiness
- Unusual jitteriness
- Runny nose, which can be a sign of a cold that can be dangerous for a newborn
- Very loose or watery stool, which can be a sign of illness
- Dry mouth, lack of tears, or reduction in urine (fewer than six wet diapers in 24 hours), which can be signs of dehydration

I don't want to be my own baby's doctor. I always feel it's better to have an objective opinion, so my husband and I took our daughter to her doctor when we had concerns.

I remember the first time (and only time so far) that my husband and I decided to call the pediatrician on-call about a concern. I was so glad I called her; I was very relieved.

That experience also reminded me that as a doctor, sometimes the most valuable thing a doctor can provide is reassurance and a little peace of mind.

—*Kathleen Moline, DO*

∞

I had a wonderful pediatrician, and I never tried to be my children's doctor. I firmly believed that I chose the best pediatrician to take care of my kids, and I let that pediatrician take care of them based on what he thought was best.

I've always believed that the stupidest question is the one that's not asked. And so I asked my kids' pediatrician everything I had a question about. If it was after hours, I didn't hesitate to call the answering service.

—*Sandra Carson, MD, a mom of two grown sons and the director of the Center for Reproduction and Infertility of Women and Infants Hospital, in Providence, RI*

∞

It's such a judgment call whether or not to take your baby to the pediatrician. This is even the case for parents who are also doctors.

One day, after taking my baby for a walk in the park, I noticed that she had a red dot on her cheek. Because I had done my medical training in an area of the country where Lyme disease is common, I was sure that the red bull's-eye on her cheek was a sign of Lyme disease.

I called the hospital's help line, and they said that they had never had a case of Lyme disease, but I had better bring my baby in. At that point, I took a breath and decided it was probably just a zit. That was exactly what it turned out to be.

—*Lillian Schapiro, MD*

I was the primary doctor for my kids. We had a very meager income at that time, and we really couldn't afford to go to a pediatrician for well baby visits. Fortunately, my babies were very healthy.

—*Lauren Feder, MD*

Just as some doctors are better than others, it's important to know that some *hospitals* are better than others. I was very aware which hospital was the best one in our city. One night when my daughter, who has asthma, was in distress, I drove to the children's hospital, passing another hospital along the way, with my daughter vomiting in the backseat. I knew that even though the drive was longer, my daughter would be better off at the better hospital.

—*Nancy Rappaport, MD*

Getting Shots

Most children receive many vaccinations. This can be hard on the baby, and also on the mom. Generally, babies get shots at birth and when they are two, four, and six months old. It's a great idea to maintain a record of your baby's vaccinations. Some doctors' offices will give you a small card, and the nurses are usually happy to write the vaccines on it, just as they do on your baby's medical chart.

Sadly, a recent study in the *Journal of the American Medical Association* reported that more than a third of U.S. babies were behind on their vaccinations by more than six months during their first two years. This means these children were unprotected from serious diseases.

It's not easy to watch your baby get shots. I'd just try to hold my baby down, soothe her as best I could, and hope we got a nurse who was really quick!

After it was over, I'd scoop my baby up and give her a big hug, and I always had her bottle ready. My daughter was never a pacifier baby, but once she had her milk, she'd calm down really quickly.

—*Jeannette Gonzalez Simon, MD*

Mommy MD Guides-Recommended Product
Buzzy for Shots

The number of recommended vaccinations has risen exponentially over the past decade: Children now get more than 20 vaccines by the time they're two years old. Yet only 6 percent of pediatricians use any kind of pain management before or after giving children vaccinations. Is it any wonder that 30 percent of kids are severely needle phobic?

Amy Baxter, MD, a mom of 13- and 10-year-old sons and an eight-year-old daughter, the CEO of MMJ Labs, and the director of emergency research of Children's Healthcare of Atlanta at Scottish Rite, in Atlanta, GA, invented a terrific product called Buzzy, which is a reusable pain-relief device that eases the pain of shots, splinters, and scrapes.

"I knew that the body could stop pain naturally using something called gate theory," Dr. Baxter says. "If you bang your knee and then rub it, the pain stops; if you smash your finger and then shake it, it helps the pain; or if you burn your finger and then stick it under cold running water, it quits hurting."

Buzzy combines cold temperature and vibration to block the transmission of sharp pain in the body, just as putting a burned hand under water makes it feel better. To use it, parents freeze the included ice pack and take it with them to the doctor's office in a Cold-to-Go bag or sandwiched between two freezer packs. When the nurse is ready to give the shots, the freezer pack is slipped into an elastic band behind Buzzy, the vibrator is switched on, and the ice and vibration are applied together above the site of the shot. Buzzy stays on during the needle stick to keep disrupting the pain signal in the nerves. You should leave Buzzy on the skin for at least 15 seconds after the shot, or up to a minute or so for extra numbing.

You can buy Buzzy online for $34.95 at BUZZY4SHOTS.COM.

Babies get a lot of shots their first year. It's important to go to a pediatrician who's willing to work with you and teach you about the best way to prepare your baby for shots, such as giving the baby a dose of acetaminophen (Tylenol) beforehand. It's best if the medication is given about 30 minutes before the vaccination, or perhaps when you're walking into the doctors' office. (Talk with your doctor before giving your baby this or any medication.)

Cuddling or breastfeeding while your infant gets shots also reduces distress. I found it helpful to bring a toy along to the doctor's office to distract my baby—red, black, and white toys for the two-month shots and brightly colored toys for the four- and six-month shots. A plastic toy, as opposed to a stuffed toy, is great because you can wipe the germs off afterward.

—*Amy Baxter, MD*

When my boys were babies and got their shots, I would let the nurse put a Band-Aid on the needle mark so it wouldn't bleed. But at my son's 12-month finger stick, the nurse put a Band-Aid on his finger. As soon as we got into the car, he pulled it off and put it into his mouth! Besides being a choking hazard, a Band-Aid is not a good thing for a baby to chew on!

We use Buzzy. (See "Mommy MD Guides–Recommended Product: Buzzy for Shots.") My husband took our younger son for his flu shot (without taking Buzzy) while I was at work. When our older son realized what was going to happen, he cried, "What about Buzzy?!"

—*Rebecca Reamy, MD*

I had my babies get all of the recommended vaccinations, and I have no regrets. I'm a huge believer in immunization. I believe that immunization ranks up there along with clean water in terms of being one of the biggest public health achievements of the 20th century. Yes, there are risks, but there are risks to everything. That argument doesn't sit well with me. There's a reason we don't see polio or certain other diseases anymore, and that's because we give immunizations.

Parents need to be very careful where they get their information regarding immunizations, as there are a lot of inaccurate and unfounded "facts" out there. The MMR/autism controversy is the perfect example: I believe the study it was based on is questionable. Unfortunately, it has probably led to some of the increase in measles we've seen, due to children not getting that vaccine. I don't regret immunizing my kids at all.

—*Ann Contrucci, MD*

❧

For a baby's first year, vaccinations are a really big issue. When my kids were babies, I did a great deal of research about each and every one, and I made choices to have them get some shots, but not get others. My decision depended upon the child and also upon the vaccine. I don't think it's wise to say universally that every kid should get every shot.

I think that we Americans are making a mistake to assume we all should receive the same vaccinations. We aren't a herd of cows! Before my kids were given any shots, I'd ask the doctor the following questions.

• Is this vaccine safe? How do you know that?
• For a particular vaccine, how many people were involved in the scientific study that led to the conclusion that the vaccine was "safe"?
• What are the risks to my baby if he doesn't get the vaccination?
• What are the risks to my baby if he *does* get the vaccination?

If our pediatrician had told me that he didn't have the time to explain all of this to me, I would have found a new doctor.

—*Hana R. Solomon, MD*

❧

My husband and I chose not to vaccinate our babies. It was never an issue with schools because we are permitted exemptions in California.

—*Lauren Feder, MD*

Stocking Your Diaper Bag

The phrase "don't leave home without it" brings on new—and multiple—meanings when you have a baby.

During our babies' first years, my husband and I were always upgrading our diaper bags. Our favorite was a backpack that had a fold-out changing pad. It made it so easy to change our babies' diapers anywhere.

—*Penny Noyce, MD*

❧

Make sure that you *never* leave home without diapers, which I did many times by the time I had my third child.

—*Lillian Schapiro, MD*

❧

While my husband and I were at work, our daughters stayed with either my parents or my in-laws. We sent the girls with a fully stocked diaper bag each day, with diapers, wipes, formula, and a change of clothes. But we also kept a supply of diapers, wipes, formula, and clothes at each house. It was handy that my parents and in-laws never minded throwing a load of baby clothes in the wash if need be.

—*Siobhan Dolan, MD*

❧

The advice I would offer for moms going on an outing of any kind is to be prepared! Always bring diapers, wipes, juice, snacks, quiet toys, and bottled water for yourself. I also always kept a change of clothing for any clothing catastrophe that might happen while we were away.

My diaper bag was fairly large, and it had a couple of pockets on the outside, which were handy. I found it very helpful to choose a diaper bag that fit underneath my stroller because those bags get to be so heavy to carry.

—*Lesley Burton-Iwinski, MD*

❧

Rather than worrying about keeping my diaper bag stocked, I kept a bag in my car. In fact, to this day, I keep a change of clothes for all of us in a bag in the car. I also keep baby wipes and hand sanitizer in the car. When my kids were potty training, I kept changes of underwear.

It's funny how diaper bags often get *smaller* with second kids. With my second child, rather than carrying a diaper bag, I'd just throw a diaper and some wipes into my purse.

—*Michelle Paley, MD, PA, a mom of two and a psychiatrist and psychotherapist in private practice, in Miami Beach, FL*

Keeping Your Baby Happy and Safe in the Car

There's good reason the hospital won't let you take your baby home without a car seat. Motor vehicle crashes are the number one killer of children from ages 1 to 14. About half of the deaths in children younger than five years involved children who were unrestrained. Where children were restrained, improper use of car seats was reported in 80 to 95 percent of cases. Injuries requiring hospitalization are even more common, and many involve the head, neck, and spine. Some of these injuries inflict permanent damage.

It is never safe to hold your baby in a moving vehicle. The forces in a crash can be hundreds of pounds or more, far too great for you to hold on to your baby.

The good news is that car seats are very effective for reducing deaths and injuries. Experts agree that the safest car seat is the one that you will use correctly each and every time you put your baby in the car. His life depends on it.

❧

In the car, my son had a stuffed elephant and lion that dangled from the car seat handle. When he was older, we got him rattles that he could chew and a musical mobile. He usually fell asleep very easily in the car.

—*Sonia Ng, MD*

It's maddening to be in the car and have a baby—or two babies—screaming. The one thing that saves us is we have a DVD player in the car. That has made a world of difference on long car trips. It keeps us sane.

—*Jennifer Gilbert, DO*

I didn't have a DVD player in my car until my kids were about nine years old. It got to the point that I couldn't keep them from fighting on long trips unless I let them watch TV. Before that, we listened to books on tape. They didn't understand all the words, but I was entertained.

—*Melanie Bone, MD, a mom of four, ages 16, 15, 14, and 13, a grandmom of one grandson, a gynecologist, the founder of the Cancer Sensibility Foundation, and the author of the syndicated column Surviving Life and the book* Cancer, What's Next?, *in West Palm Beach, FL*

I found that when my son was old enough to eat finger foods, giving him a snack kept him very entertained at home and in the car. It took him so long to pick up a piece of food and get it into his mouth that it kept him occupied for a long time.

Once when my son was about 14 months old, we drove to visit family, and I gave my son a closed container of Gerber Puffs snacks. He was getting fussy, and we had another 15 minutes of driving left. I thought he would shake the container and use it to make noise. Little did I know that he was able to remove the lid. When we arrived, it looked like a Puffs explosion! He had eaten some of the Gerber Puffs as well. Had I realized that he would be able to take the lid off, I would have found something else to use for entertainment.

Often we will give him a few snacks—maybe three to five pieces—but I wouldn't want to have an entire container at his fingertips again due to the choking risk. Now we bring books and toys to occupy him.

—*Michelle Hephner, DO*

My sons were both good car passengers. I think it helped that we trained them at an early age. It was routine for them. They'd sometimes fight getting into the car seat, but once they were in, they did just fine.

For that first year when they have to ride facing backward, I had a mirror mounted on the back window so that when I looked in the rearview mirror, I could see my son's face.

—*Jill Wireman, MD*

I had one of those mirrors that stick to the back window of the car so I could look into my rearview mirror and see my baby's face. It didn't turn out to be such a great safety feature for me. One day, I almost rear-ended the car in front of me because I was so busy admiring my baby in the mirror! How ironic: I almost crashed into someone because of a safety device. I took the mirror out of the car that day.

One travel product that I had bought for my daughter that didn't even make it out of the box was the car seat cover that you're supposed to put over the seat to keep it from getting too hot. Life at the time was too overwhelming for me to give it a try.

—*Katja Rowell, MD*

Two days after my older son was born, my husband left to go back to school in another state. My mom had come to help me with my baby, and two days later, we packed up and drove to meet my husband in our new home.

Most new babies are good car riders. They sleep most of the time. The only challenge for us was that we had to stop along the side of the road in the middle of winter so I could breastfeed. Other than that, the long drive was uneventful.

—*Carrie Brown, MD*

Even as an infant, my son wouldn't nap. I used to load him up in the car and take him for long drives, hoping that would lull him to sleep. He would poke himself in the face and tug on his ears, anything to stay awake.

But I tried anyway. Even though my son wasn't sleeping, that time driving in the car was very peaceful for me.

—*Alanna Kramer, MD*

Before our triplets were born, my husband and I would make fun of our friends who drove minivans. "Soccer moms," we'd call them.

When we found out we were having triplets, we already had an older daughter. My husband searched in vain for a vehicle other than a minivan that could accommodate four car seats. Guess what we ended up buying? A minivan.

Truth be told, I love our minivan. The doors open wider than those on other vehicles, and you can easily move the car seats in and out without killing your back or hitting your head. It's very convenient for all four kids, and we even have room for a set of grandparents if they want to come along somewhere.

—*Sadaf T. Bhutta, MD*

❧

My husband and I are both physicians, and he is actually trained as a biomedical engineer as well, but believe it or not, for the first three months of our oldest daughter's life, we actually had the car seat installed wrong!

I think that probably the best advice is to have a certified Child Passenger Safety (CPS) technician look over your car seat to ensure that it is properly installed. You can find lists of certified CPS technicians and Child Seat Fitting Stations on NHTSA.gov and SeatCheck.org or by calling 888-327-4236 or 866-SEATCHECK (866-732-8243).

—*Stacey Weiland, MD*

❧

When our daughters were small, I drove north to work, but my husband drove the girls a half hour south to my parents' or his parents' houses, so the girls could stay with their grandparents while we were at work. To keep the babies happy in the car, my husband had every kind of string-thing invented to keep the bottles, pacifiers, sippy cups, and snacks within the girls' reach.

In the car, they'd listen to kids' music like Raffi. My husband really loves Steely Dan, and so they'd listen to that also. Now that our daughters are older, they have fond memories of their commutes with their dad. It was good bonding time for them.

—*Siobhan Dolan, MD*

RALLIE'S TIP

My babies were usually pretty happy riding in the car when they were newborns. In fact, they were probably much happier than I was. I didn't like not being able to see them while they were in their rear-facing car seats and I was driving. I got one of those mirrors that you put on the headrest of your backseat, but that was to keep me happy, rather than my babies. They couldn't care less if I could see them, because they couldn't see me when they were in their rear-facing car seats, and that seemed to worry them a bit.

I found that my boys were happiest in the car when they could hear my voice. I didn't have a cell phone when my kids were babies, so there was no chance of having a real conversation with another adult. So I had one-way conversations with my babies. I told them about my day, or I ran through my to-do list with them. When I ran out of things to talk about, I would sing—badly. But they loved it! As long as they could hear me, they were happy little passengers!

Dressing Your Baby Comfortably

Soft cozy onesies, itty bitty booties, who can resist baby clothes?

I grew up playing with Barbie dolls, and I was looking forward to dressing my babies. I loved dressing them up and taking them out. But because I had boys, there were definitely limitations to what I could do.
—*Sandra Carson, MD*

I prefer to dress my sons in cotton clothing. Cotton fabric breathes easily and thus minimizes the drying of underlying skin.
—*Amy J. Derick, MD*

Most of the time, when my twins were small, I dressed them in those one-piece sleepers. I just changed them as necessary throughout the day. The one-piece sleepers were especially good when we went out, because they kept the baby's legs and feet covered and warm. If you put on pants and socks, you get a gap of bare skin!
—*Jennifer Gilbert, DO*

I really don't like pink. Plus it seemed like such a waste not to put the onesies my son had worn on my daughter in the beginning. So my daughter wore quite a few of my sons' baby clothes. I got yelled at by the grandmother though!

Now as luck would have it, my daughter's favorite color is pink—and sparkly.

—*Alanna Kramer, MD*

∽

It's such a hassle to change a baby's clothes. My daughter wore a coordinated outfit to come home from the hospital and for holiday photos, but that was about it!

Instead I tried to make dressing my baby simple for me and comfortable for her. My daughter lived in Carter's snap-front outfits almost the entire first year of her life. I had about 15 of them. Those snap-front outfits were easier for both of us. I like to wear comfortable clothing, and I wanted my baby to be comfortable too.

—*Katja Rowell, MD*

∽

There are so many cute baby girl outfits. It's hard to stop buying them! My daughter has lots of clothes. I'm a big Carter's fan. There's a Carter's store near me, and I think the clothes are very good quality.

People tend to give a lot of zero- to three-month baby clothes as presents, and babies outgrow them so quickly. Plus clothing doesn't always turn out to be appropriate seasonally. I kept the tags on everything, and I exchanged quite a few small outfits for larger sizes if I had the wrong size for the wrong season. My husband used to tease me that I was at Carter's returning things all of the time.

—*Jeannette Gonzalez Simon, MD*

∽

When my kids were babies, my favorite clothing brand was Osh Kosh. Everything mixed and matched, so I didn't have to think about it.

Dressing my boys was so simple: Grab a pair of pants and a shirt, no big deal. Little girls were more complicated. Their frilly dresses were so cute, but once they started to crawl, they'd get tripped up by their skirts. Also they skinned their bare knees, so I often put leggings on under their skirts.

—*Susan Besser, MD*

Washing Baby's Clothes and Bedding

Americans wash 35 *billion* loads of laundry each year. No doubt, moms do far more than their fair share of that!

One important tip: Don't use fabric softener on your baby's pajamas. It can damage the flame-retardant chemicals.

I used Ivory Snow to wash our baby's clothes.
  —*Cathie Lippman, MD*

With my first baby especially, I tried to do *everything* by the book, including using those so-called baby detergents. All I can say is that they just didn't clean my children's clothes well. So after I used up the first few containers, I returned to Tide. My kids never had any problems with contact dermatitis.
  —*Stacey Weiland, MD*

When washing and drying clothing, I avoid using fabric softener and dryer sheets. I want to minimize or eliminate any chemical residue that might irritate my sons' sensitive skin.
  —*Amy J. Derick, MD*

Even when my daughter was a newborn, I washed all of our family's clothes together. But rather than washing my baby's clothes with our regular detergent, I switched to hypoallergenic soap. I also double-rinsed every load to make sure to get rid of the soap residue. My husband has sensitive skin, so this worked really well for our family.
  —*Katja Rowell, MD*

I work full-time, and my husband helps out a lot around the house. After my daughter was born, I was off work for about 10 weeks on maternity leave. I quickly learned not to let the laundry pile up. I'd try to wash at least one load a day.
  —*Michelle Hephner, DO*

Thank goodness, we had our own washing machine when my baby was born because I was washing clothes all of the time. I don't have any tricks to make it faster or easier. Just accept the fact that the washer runs at least one load every day. It's easier to keep up with laundry that way.

—*Susan Besser, MD*

I buy enough clothes so that I don't have to do laundry every day. Plus, I delegate the laundry to my babysitter. For a few hours each day, she only has two of our four children to watch, and that's when she washes the laundry.

—*Sadaf T. Bhutta, MD*

I use cloth diapers on my babies, and I do my diaper laundry pretty much every day. I do have enough diapers to last longer than one day if I have a "washing machine emergency," though.

I like to air-dry the diapers outside on a line when the weather's nice. We just had a blizzard here, but I can line-dry diapers a good eight months of the year.

—*Kristie McNealy, MD*

To protect our baby's mattress, a pee mat was ultra important. We have four mats, just in case. They weren't that expensive, and they save sheets.

There is also a product that our friends used called a crib saver. Our friends' baby threw up very often, after every feeding. The crib saver is a lightweight cover that can easily be removed and washed after the baby vomits.

—*Sonia Ng, MD*

Asking for Help

It's all too fitting that "mother" and "martyr" both begin with *m*. Call it pride, call it stubbornness, but a lot of moms are reluctant to ask for help—or even to accept help when it's offered. But why? If someone asked you for help, wouldn't you be happy to give it?

When people offer to help, let them!

—*Michelle Hephner, DO*

During my daughter's first year of life, I had an incredible amount of support from female friends and a male nanny who lived with us when my daughter was 3 to 12 months old. It also helped for me to go back to work part-time—both to get out of the house and to experience adult interactions.

—*Stuart Jeanne Bramhall, MD*

I'm a very organized person, and my husband is even more so. Plus, he *likes* to organize things. I think that the key when asking for help is to identify what a person likes to do, and then ask him to do that. My husband likes organizing our daughter's clothing, so I say, "By all means, go for it!"

—*Jennifer Bacani McKenney, MD*

With twins especially, I just couldn't do everything by myself. Thank goodness, my husband was quick to help. In the middle of the night, for instance, I'd nurse one twin, and then he'd change her diaper and put her back to bed while I nursed her brother. My husband was very helpful. He jumped right in, and he was just as sleep deprived as I was!

It can be hard to ask for help, but if anyone offers to make a meal, do some laundry, cut the grass, or take your baby on a walk, say, "Yes!" You will still be a superparent!

—*Ann Contrucci, MD*

Communicating what you need is critical, and communicating that with your partner is a bit of an art. It's hard to ask for help, but you have to learn to do that as a mom. I've learned to keep a positive attitude, and when I ask my husband for help, I try to do it gently, but directly. We girls say a lot of things, but sometimes with men, it's better to be direct and to the point.

It also helps to be supportive of my husband. I like to say, "You're great at this, can you help me?" I think sometimes husbands get scared, and that's when they escape to watch TV. You have to involve them and make them feel good about helping.

—*Gabriella Cardone, MD*

RALLIE'S TIP

When my youngest sons were babies, I finally learned how to ask my husband for help. He was really happy to pitch in, but he had trouble figuring out exactly what needed to be done. Instead of asking him simply to "help me out," I finally realized that I should tell him exactly what I wanted him to do. So instead of asking something like, "Can you help me clean up around the house?" I'd have better luck saying, "Honey, would you mind emptying the dishwasher and putting the stroller back in the closet?" I was hesitant to be so specific at first, because I thought he would feel that I was bossing him around. As it turned out, he was really relieved not to have to read my mind, and he enjoyed knowing that the work he did around the house was important and appreciated.

❦

I'm used to taking care of a lot of things myself, and it was not easy for me to ask for help. However, several friends and family members insisted that *now* is the time to accept any help that's offered. I feel like that saved me. Family and friends brought food and other necessities to the house and sat with my daughter for a while so that my husband and I could get some rest. Accepting others' generosity was crucial.

—*Rachel S. Rohde, MD*

❦

Because I was so dreadfully sleep deprived, I learned early in my son's life to say "yes" to help. I think that the biggest mistake new moms make is not asking for help. You can't be good to yourself—or to your baby—if you're in a constant state of exhaustion.

If a friend asks if she can come over and hold your baby so you can lie down, or if your mom wants to bring over dinner, say, "Yes!" It's okay!

—*Heather Orman-Lubell, MD, a mom of 10- and six-year-old sons and a pediatrician in private practice at Yardley Pediatrics of St. Christopher's Hospital for Children, in Pennsylvania*

When my younger son was born, I was living far away from my family, and my husband was working in a PhD program in another state. My aunt wasn't working, and she told me to call her when I went into labor and she would come to help me with my new baby. That was wonderful! It was great to have her help me with the baby so that my older son didn't feel abandoned to some stranger in the woods. My aunt changed my baby's diapers and rocked him. She pretty much did everything for him for a few weeks, except breastfeeding!

This gave me more time and energy, so that when my two-year-old son was awake, I could engage him, and he didn't feel like his whole world was turned upside down by the baby. I think when a mom has to do everything for a new baby, her older child can feel resentful. My experience with my second baby was totally different from my first, but because I had such wonderful help, it was okay.

—*Carrie Brown, MD*

When my first son was born, my mother, aunt, and mother-in-law all came to help. They were wonderful, but having three very strong female personalities in my house was very interesting. I was very grateful for their help and advice, but for the first few weeks, I felt sad. How could they know what to do for my baby better than I did? I felt they were much better at soothing him than I was, and I was wondering why I couldn't get it right. I felt such a disconnect between what I thought my knowledge base would be and what it actually was. Medical books don't tell you how to calm a crying baby in the middle of the night! I can see why so many women get frustrated and feel overwhelmed.

When they all went home, my husband and our baby settled into our groove. Around six months later, my family came back to visit for Christmas. By then, my husband and I knew all of the nuances of caring for our baby, and I didn't have those feelings of inadequacy anymore.

—*Amy Thompson, MD*

I think new moms are often reluctant to ask for help. In almost every culture from the beginning of time until now, new moms would be surrounded with experienced helpers. The first time around, you don't know everything you need to know, and you can't do it all by yourself. When things aren't going smoothly, it's easy to get frustrated and feel like a failure.

I think it's helpful to make a list of the people who offer to help you. Then don't be afraid to call those people on the list! This will keep you from feeling overwhelmed. When people offer to help, they're generally sincere. It's important to get over your pride and ask for it.

When my babies were small, I took friends up on their offers to bring meals and to come and hold the baby for half an hour. When your baby is colicky and cries for hours on end, having someone else hold him for a spell is a huge relief.

—*Amy Baxter, MD*

We were totally unprepared when we got home with our daughter. I had a complicated C-section, and I was in so much pain that I needed my husband to help me pick her up and position her for feedings. We also had major breastfeeding problems that kept us working on nursing every 15 minutes around the clock. We were prepared in terms of diapers and stuff for the baby, but we forgot about us! I remember crying and eating granola bars and drinking water because we ran out of food!

My husband and I had this idea that we would bond with our baby and establish breastfeeding during the first week of her life, so we hadn't arranged to have any help until a week after she was born. We ended up calling our friends to bring us milk, take-out food, and even sanitary pads! So, stock up your freezer and fridge, and ask friends if they can bring meals over. Line up any help you might need in advance, such as a grocery delivery service. It didn't take long for me to go from feeling very competent to learning how to ask for help. It was humbling! Don't be too shy to ask for help!

—*Katja Rowell, MD*

As women, especially women physicians, we're trained to believe we know it all. But the reality is that it's impossible to know it all, and that is perfectly fine. I recommend seeking out people who are experts.

For example, when I started to breastfeed, I found a lactation consultant to teach me how to nurse my baby. We've been friends ever since, and she's a wealth of knowledge about all aspects of parenting.

As soon as I was able to, I had a babysitter come to my house to help me with my baby. I chose an older woman who had been babysitting for children for decades. She taught me so much.

A little later, I took my son to Mommy-and-me classes, where I met a psychologist who's become a lifelong friend and great resource. There are so many sources of help around us. The trick is to get out there and meet them.

—*Cathie Lippman, MD*

My biggest challenge during my baby's first year of life was that there was no one I felt I could ask for help. When our older son was a newborn, my husband had graduated from his MBA program, and I graduated from medical school, and we moved far away from our families to start our new jobs.

It's so ironic: When our family was nearby, we didn't want their help; we wanted our own space. After we moved far away, we felt so alone. We wondered, *Why did we ever refuse their help?* Our moms had helped us a lot, and they would have gladly helped us even more. It was very stressful and challenging to have a baby, new jobs, and a new house with no family or friends nearby to ask for help.

I often called my mom to ask her for advice. Luckily, I was also a pediatric resident, and I had access to attending physicians. These physicians were educating me, and I truly trusted them, so I had the health part down. But it was wonderful to ask my mom for advice on practical things like doing laundry and cooking meals with a baby, and how long it would take for the hard part to pass!

—*Leena Shrivastava Dev, MD*

Giving a Sponge Bath

Doctors recommend giving babies sponge baths until their umbilical cord stumps fall off. Some moms bathe their babies in their kitchen sinks. Be sure to keep a hand and a close eye on that slippery baby. It really is worth the cost of a baby bathtub. Some are even hinged so they fold up, which is great for storage.

Before you get your baby anywhere near that water, gather all of your supplies: washrag, soap, towel, pajamas. It's simple to store all of your baby supplies right in the baby bathtub.

∽⌒∽

My son was a very tiny baby. I remember that I was so scared that I would drop him or break him. I was literally afraid I was going to do something wrong, and something horrible would happen. For his first bath, I asked my mother to come over, and she showed me how to bathe him.

—*Judith Hellman, MD*

Mommy MD Guides-Recommended Product
Aubrey Organics Shampoo

Despite the fact that babies aren't playing in mud puddles, there's a huge industry of baby soaps and shampoos. Although many brands are commonly sold in grocery stores, a brand that's a little less common but worth considering is Aubrey Organics. Their Baby & Kids Shampoo and Baby & Kids Bath Soap cleanse gently, while chamomile and balm-mint soothe and hydrate baby's hair and scalp.

Be careful to keep the shampoo out of your baby's eyes because it's not a "no tears" formula, and it will sting. Also, it doesn't lather up. However, the ingredients that make a shampoo or soap "no tears" or super sudsy are chemicals you might not want anywhere near your baby!

You can purchase Aubrey Organics online and in health food stores. An eight-ounce bottle of the shampoo or the soap costs around $8.50.

My sister was a nurse in the hospital's NICU, and she came over and helped me give my first child a first sponge bath, showing me how to do it. It can be so helpful to have someone experienced around for these scary first-time things.

—*Michelle Paley, MD, PA*

∽

I give my sons two short baths each day. Avoid long baths that can dry out the skin.

—*Amy J. Derick, MD*

∽

When my second son was born, my mom was convinced that I didn't bathe him often enough. My first son got a bath every two days, but with my second I was so swamped that he probably only got a bath once every 10 days. But his skin looked fantastic!

—*Wendy Sue Swanson, MD, FAAP*

∽

When my babies were little, I didn't stress out about giving them baths every day. If I was too tired, or they had runny noses or I didn't have anyone to help, bath time simply would not happen that day. Infants aren't running around sweating or getting muddy. They can live without a bath every once in a while. You just have to let go of little things sometimes, to keep your sanity.

—*Sadaf T. Bhutta, MD*

∽

When I gave my baby a bath, I used Johnson and Johnson's baby wash. It's gentle and safe, and you can buy it practically everywhere.

—*Leigh Andrea DeLair, MD*

∽

My favorite parenting tips: Make sure you have enough baby soap before you start the bath. Have your towel ready before you get the baby wet.

—*Lillian Schapiro, MD*

Sending Out Birth Announcements

Some things in life make you want to climb to the top of a 32-story building and shout from the rooftop. Having a baby is one of them.

A huge baby announcement industry has sprung up to accommodate this sense of unabashed joy. You can choose simple cards or make-it-yourself elaborate keepsakes, and everything in between. If you go the elaborate route, be sure to check with your post office to see if your announcements require extra postage to mail.

ᘒᓌ

When my son was born, I sent an e-mail announcement to the family. It was simple and quick.

　　—*Sonia Ng, MD*

ᘒᓌ

Because my daughter was born near Christmas, I sent out combination birth announcement/Christmas cards. You could do this if your baby is born near any major holiday, such as Halloween or Easter. It saves a little time and money.

　　—*Jeannette Gonzalez Simon, MD*

ᘒᓌ

A photographer came to our residence and took photos of our new baby. We included some of the photos with birth announcements. Don't delay having photos taken. After a few weeks, babies can show neonatal (or baby) acne.

　　—*Amy J. Derick, MD*

ᘒᓌ

I knew we'd be busy after our baby's arrival, so I took our wedding invitation address list, added some friends and colleagues, and made a file of mailing labels ahead of time. A few weeks after our baby was born, I ordered birth announcements online from Shutterfly. I had very little energy for anything but taking care of our newborn, so it was great to have the labels ready to go.

　　—*Rachel S. Rohde, MD*

ᘒᓌ

Before my kids were born, I bought plenty of stamps and printed out mailing labels on my computer for our friends and family. This made it much easier to get the birth announcements out soon after my babies were born.

　　With my first child, I was really quick to get out thank-you cards too. But I cut myself a lot more slack on this after my second child was born.

—*Michelle Paley, MD, PA*

⌀

For my first baby, I created handmade, beautiful, elaborate birth announcements, printed on fine cardstock and decorated with stamps, ribbons, and a photo. My second baby was born premature and had to stay in the NICU for several weeks, so I was too overwhelmed to send out announcements. After my third baby was born, I just printed out announcements on an online service.

A few weeks ago, my dad called me and said, "I don't think we ever got a birth announcement for your youngest."

"That's because I never sent one," I replied. Life just gets so hectic; you just do the best you can!

—*Kristie McNealy, MD*

Adjusting Your Insurance Policies

Having a new baby sure does generate a big to-do list. One more thing to add to your list is to make sure to adjust your insurance policies, both health and life. If your job situation has changed, you might want to adjust your automobile insurance too.

It's very important to find out when and how you should add your baby to your health insurance policy. Read the fine print because some policies have only a small window of time in which a baby can be added to a policy after his birth. After that, no coverage will be provided.

For your life insurance, it's a good idea to re-evaluate your needs and to appoint a guardian for your baby if something happens to both you and your husband.

⌀

When my daughter was born, it was very easy for us to change our health insurance policy to add coverage for her. I think working with the insurance company was more of a challenge when I was pregnant than it has been since my daughter was born.

—*Christy Valentine, MD*

I'm self-employed, and so it was important that my husband add our daughter to his health insurance plan. At one of our OB appointments, the office staff gave us a heads-up that we needed to call the insurance company before our baby was born, which we did.

We still have to update our life insurance, though! I have to bring that up to my husband. There's so much to think of when you have a baby!

—*Jennifer Bacani McKenney, MD*

It's important to get your new baby on your health insurance plan right away. If you forget, don't worry. Your pediatrician's office will remind you at your baby's first visit!

Most babies don't need life insurance. Parents, however, need to adjust their life insurance to provide for the baby if something happens. I did it very soon after my first baby was born. My husband and I chose the person who would be our baby's guardian in the event we both died. We wrote a codicil to our will on a piece of paper and put it into our safe-deposit box with our will.

—*Melanie Bone, MD*

Deciding Where Your Baby Will Sleep

Some parenting decisions are a great divide. Deciding where your baby will sleep is one of them. According to the American Academy of Pediatrics (AAP), studies of co-sleeping show that it can be hazardous under certain conditions. Some of the studies have shown a correlation between bed sharing and sudden infant death syndrome (SIDS) among women who smoke. Another study showed that the health risks associated with bed sharing were greatest for infants younger than 11 weeks old. The more time a baby spends sleeping with a parent or parents each night, the greater the danger. It's especially dangerous for infants to sleep with an adult on a couch.

The AAP has concluded that the safest place for an infant to sleep for the first six months of life is in a crib in the parents' bedroom.

Our older daughter slept with us for a while. She wasn't a good sleeper, and it was so hard going back and forth between the nursery and my bedroom, so I gave in and let her sleep with us. When my daughter was 2½, we moved into a new home. To make the transition easier, we gave her our bed, and we got ourselves a new bed! (We needed a new bed anyway.) That finally got her out of our bed!

—*Cheri Wiggins, MD*

My son slept with me from birth. I still sleep with him, but it's not what I tell parents to do as a pediatrician. I tell people not to co-sleep because of the risk of SIDS. Do as I say, not as I do—and please don't tell our pediatrician.

The big joke with my family was that my son weighed 22 pounds at nine months, and they were afraid he would roll over onto *me*.

—*Sonia Ng, MD*

When I was around seven months pregnant, I was thinking about buying a crib. But my yoga teacher had talked with me about the family bed. I remember thinking, *Isn't that just for people in other cultures?*

But then I read the book *The Family Bed* and learned that even in this country, families all slept together until the Industrial Revolution.

So I never did buy a crib. My sons slept in our bed until they were around five years old. By five, they were ready to move into their own beds.

—*Lauren Feder, MD*

For the first year of my twins' lives, they woke every two to three hours, every single night. Before they were born, my husband and I had vowed they'd never sleep in our bed. In fact, I advised parents in my pediatric practice not to allow their babies to sleep in their beds. But my husband and I did what we had to do to get some sleep, and so our twins ended up in bed with us. Usually, they both would fall asleep on my chest after nursing. I don't recommend sharing your bed with your baby. It's certainly not my first choice!

After sleeping in one bassinet together for their first two months of life, my twins then slept in their car seats next to each other beside our bed. (The twins actually cried more if they weren't next to each other.) Then we moved their car seats a few feet away from our bed into a nearby sitting area. Then we moved the car seats into their nursery, but we still kept them on the floor. Then we put their car seats into their cribs. Finally, when they were around four months old, they began sleeping in their cribs in the nursery. They were so bonded that it was actually hard for me to put them into separate cribs. It was quite a unique introduction to sleeping in cribs.

—*Ann Contrucci, MD*

For both of my sons, the biggest issue in their early years was sleep. Neither of them was good at staying in their beds and sleeping. I know all of the right things to do. I read all of the books, but my sons clearly *didn't* read them. My husband and I joke that our crib was barely used; we passed it off to another family practically new.

—*Jill Wireman, MD*

Before my daughter was born, I bought a co-sleeper , which I put right next to the bed. I loved it because it made breastfeeding my daughter at night so much easier. I worried that if I had to get up out of bed and walk to another room, I'd drop her because I was so tired. The co-sleeper was great for her first few months.

Transitioning my daughter out of the co-sleeper was not so great, though. When she was able to sit up, I moved her to her crib in her own room to sleep. She screamed for hours. It was very hard. I broke the rules by picking her up sometimes until she fell asleep. I did what I had to do so that I could also get some sleep. In a few weeks, she got used to sleeping in her crib.

—*Dina Strachan, MD*

Before our baby's due date, my husband and I had readied the house for her arrival. Although we had a crib in her nursery down the hall, I had so much pain after the delivery that it was difficult for me to rise from the bed, much less walk down the hall and back every hour or more often. A Pack 'n Play next to the bed was very helpful for those times when I was home without help.

—*Rachel S. Rohde, MD*

RALLIE'S TIP

When my husband and I were expecting our second child, we worked for weeks getting the nursery ready. Our oldest son was 13 years old, so we didn't have baby things left that we could use. We had to start from scratch. We painted and decorated the nursery, and we bought a beautiful new crib, and I couldn't wait to see my new baby sleeping there. As it turned out, he was born four weeks early, and he was so tiny! When I brought him home, I couldn't bear the thought of putting him in the nursery all by himself. My husband and I hadn't thought to buy a bassinet to put in our bedroom, so on that first night at home, my sweet little baby slept in a big laundry basket beside my bed. He slept in our room for about four or five weeks before I felt comfortable moving him to the nursery.

Sleep is always a challenge with babies. When your baby is first born, especially if you're nursing, it's easy to have him right beside you in a bedside crib.

But I think one of the best things my husband and I did was moving our son's crib into his own room. We did this when he was around five months and he no longer needed a nighttime feeding.

We also turned off his baby monitor and left the doors to both of our rooms open. That way we could hear our baby if he cried, but we couldn't hear every little sigh. Now instead of us waking our son every time we rolled over, and him waking us every time he made a noise, we were able to distance ourselves just enough that we wouldn't disturb each other.

That one small change really helped reduce our baby's middle-of-the-night wakings.

—*Nancy Thomas, MD, a mom of a 22-month-old son who practices general obstetrics and gynecology in Covington, Louisiana, with Ochsner Health System*

Our daughter is a better sleeper than our son was. When I was in the hospital with her, I let the nurses take her to the nursery at night so I could get some sleep. I feared what was coming when we got home!

My daughter's room is a little farther down the hall than my son's room. I was nervous about that at first, but I think it's turned out to be a good thing. I don't hear every single little move she makes and then rush in to her. The first night my daughter was home from the hospital, she woke to nurse, and then she went right back to sleep.

—*Michelle Hephner, DO*

When my triplets were first born, they all slept in one crib in our master bedroom on the first floor of our home. But after they outgrew that arrangement, I wasn't comfortable having them sleep on a different floor of our home than I was sleeping on. So I moved everyone to our second floor, even though we have a perfectly nice master bedroom suite on the first floor! Thank goodness we have three bedrooms upstairs, so my husband and I took one, our older daughter took the second, and the triplets shared the third.

—*Sadaf T. Bhutta, MD*

I believe you should put your baby in his crib his first night home from the hospital and always have him sleep in his own room.

My children are 21 months apart. We had a big decision: Do we move our son out of his crib, or do we buy a second crib? Practicality won out, and two months before our daughter was born, we moved our son into a big boy bed. We also got him new furniture to match, and our daughter got all of the nursery furniture.

We didn't move our son out of his room, however. I felt that as the older child, he might already feel like he was losing so much. I didn't want to take away his bedroom too. I felt that it offered him security and comfort. That was a big deal to me. I think that a baby's room is the most comfortable place for him; he should sleep in that room from the beginning. So we moved the crib and nursery furniture into my daughter's new room.

—*Alanna Kramer, MD*

My twins slept in the same cradle in the same room for a while. Then we moved them into the same crib. After that, they slept in different cribs, but still in the same room.

This worked out great. Surprisingly, they didn't keep each other awake. One twin didn't seem to care a bit if the other twin was crying. When they were older and they both woke up, they would stand in their cribs and throw their stuffed animals at each other until the animals all wound up in a pile in the middle of the room.

—*Penny Noyce, MD*

Before our twins were born, my husband and I decided to put both of their cribs in the same room. In hindsight, I'm not sure that was the best decision because I think they wake each other up. But my husband isn't very handy. He'd have to take a crib apart to move it to another room, and that's not going to happen!

—*Jennifer Gilbert, DO*

My husband and I tried different strategies to get each of our children to sleep. My first baby sometimes slept in his crib, and sometimes in my arms as I was trying to breastfeed.

My second baby had worse reflux than the others. And perhaps because of that, he fell asleep most easily in his car seat, which kept him more upright. During my son's first two months of life, we kept his crib in our room next to our bed, and we put our son inside his car seat, and his car seat inside the crib!

Our third baby didn't sleep well in her crib. So my husband and I scooted down in our bed to make a space above our heads, and our baby slept there. That minimized any danger of her rolling out of bed, me rolling onto her, or her getting trapped in the covers. We pretty much did whatever worked to get our kids to sleep.

—*Amy Baxter, MD*

As with all new parents, my husband and I had to adjust to our children's unpredictable sleep schedule.

We set up a separate nursery with a crib, changing table,

dresser, and rocking chair. I also set up a twin bed in the room. This worked out great for nights when I was up late feeding the baby, and we could lie down together and cuddle. I could even catch a few zzzz's while the baby slept in the crib, and I wouldn't be far away when she woke up.

I also set up a bassinet in our bedroom next to our bed and used it for the first six weeks or so. Bassinets come in a lot of different styles. My friend had one that actually had a little door on the side that could open up right next to your bed.

My husband and I actually kept the babies in our bed *a lot*. I almost felt like I was paralyzed when I had that little warm bundle next to me, and my husband was as well.

I nursed all three of my children, and I would sleep wearing a nursing nightgown with a nursing bra underneath. During the night, I would move the baby from one side to the other so that she would have access to both breasts.

—*Stacey Weiland, MD*

Getting Your Baby to Sleep

Whoever coined the phrase "sleeping like a baby" had a really good sense of humor. Maybe she didn't have kids!

A newborn might sleep up to 16 hours total each day, but that's probably only for a few hours at a stretch. Breastfed babies tend to get hungry more frequently than bottlefed babies, and it's not uncommon for them to nurse every two hours for their first few weeks of life.

Sleep safety is very important. The only thing that should be in your baby's crib or bassinet is the baby, the mattress, and a tight-fitting crib sheet. That means no toys, pillows, blankets, or bumpers. Be sure there's nothing nearby with a cord or string, such as window blinds.

The American Academy of Pediatrics (AAP) recommends that babies be placed on their backs to sleep, not on their stomachs or even their sides because from this position, they can roll over onto their stomachs. Experts believe that when babies

? When to Call Your Doctor

If you are concerned by how much—or how little—your baby is sleeping, give your baby's doctor a call. If your baby is hard to rouse from sleep and doesn't want to eat, call your doctor immediately.

sleep on their stomachs, they might rebreathe their own carbon dioxide or suffocate on soft bedding. Since the AAP announced this recommendation in 1992, the incidence of sudden infant death syndrome has decreased by more than half.

Sweet dreams!

⁓

Don't underestimate the power of swaddling. New moms need to know how to do this! Ask the nurses in the hospital to give you a crash course. Then get those babies snug as a bug in a rug. Babies sleep so much better when they're nice and warm and snug.

—*Jeannette Gonzalez Simon, MD*

⁓

One baby product that I found to be indispensable during my baby's first year was the baby swaddler blanket. It had Velcro on it, and it wrapped perfectly around her so she was swaddled when she went to sleep. It was invaluable!

—*Melody Derrick, MD*

⁓

When your baby is born, buy an industrial-size box of earplugs. When our first baby was born, my husband and I took turns wearing earplugs at night. That way, at least one of us would have a good stretch of sleep.

—*Ellen McDonald, MD, a mom of four sons and an internist in private practice, in Pasadena, CA*

⁓

When my twins were infants and they were eating every three hours, my partner and I did what we called a sleep feed, feeding them in their sleep right before we went to bed. This bought us a couple more hours of sleep.

—*Katherine Dee, MD*

For my older daughter, the book *The Happiest Baby on the Block* was indispensable. The five S's technique worked wonders: swaddling, sideposition, shushing, swinging, and sucking. It was magic.

One thing that surprised me about my baby and my lack of sleep was that I didn't mind losing sleep. When something else wakes me in the middle of the night, I get resentful. But when my baby woke me up, I didn't mind getting up for her.

—*Robyn Liu, MD, a mom of seven- and four-year-old daughters and a family physician with Greeley County Health Services, in Tribune, KS*

A major sleep challenge for me was that my daughter wanted to play after her 2 a.m. feeds. On a friend's advice, I took her into bed with me after 2 a.m. feeds, and she went right back to sleep.

One thing I found indispensable for my baby's first year was an extra thick pair of pajamas with feet. I always worried about the risks of sudden infant death syndrome with blankets.

—*Stuart Jeanne Bramhall, MD*

The first month is terribly difficult. Embrace the fact that you will not sleep through the night for a LOOOOOOONNNGG time.

When my son was first born, my husband wrote "It gets better" on Post-it Notes and placed them all around our house. They reminded me that there was a light at the end of the tunnel.

The first month was the hardest for me because it was such an adjustment. After that, I think it gets easier—or at least you get used to the exhaustion!

—*Silvana Ribaudo, MD, a mom of a five-year-old son and a two-year-old daughter and an assistant clinical professor at the Columbia University Medical Center, College of Physicians and Surgeons, and at ColumbiaDoctors Eastside, both in New York City*

I was pretty sleep deprived those first few years of my baby's life. I relied upon my residency experience; all of those sleepless nights were great training for motherhood. I remember once I was complaining to a nurse about how I'd been up most of the night, sleeping a few restless hours rocking my son in the rocking chair.

The nurse gently, and wisely, said, "Well you know, looking back, those are the times that I cherish most." After that, I had a better attitude about it. I realized that my son wasn't going to be this age for long.

—*Jill Wireman, MD*

My daughter was a big baby, and perhaps that helped her sleep better. She was sleeping through the night by the time she was 7½ weeks old.

Our bedtime routine also might have helped. Each night, we moved a space heater into our bathroom to warm it. Then my husband gave my daughter a bath, and I followed with a massage. (I took a class when she was six weeks old.) After that, my husband or I gave her a bottle, and then put her into her crib. The first time we did that routine, she slept through the night. We didn't want to mess with success, so we did the same thing every night, and it worked!

—*Katja Rowell, MD*

When my son was born, friends told me, "You've been in residency and on call so much that sleep deprivation with a baby will be nothing. You're used to it!" They were completely wrong.

For my son's first seven weeks of life, he had his nights and days mixed up. So he slept all day and was up all night. He wanted me to stand and hold him all night. My husband and I were going crazy. I'd make it until around 4 a.m., then I'd go crying to my husband and say, "It's your turn now. I can't take it anymore."

To make matters worse, we lived in a house with squeaky wood floors. I'd finally get my son to sleep, lay him in his crib, tiptoe out of the room, and then "Squeak!" My son would wake up and start crying again.

Finally when my son was around eight weeks old, he started to sleep better. We didn't really do anything different to make that happen. I think he was just ready.

—*Michelle Hephner, DO*

My baby wasn't sleeping for long stretches at night—only for around an hour and a half at a time. I was concerned that maybe I wasn't producing enough milk to keep her satisfied at night. So I started to pump some extra, and I gave her a bottle of breast milk in addition to nursing her before I put her to bed. The first night that I tried it, my baby slept for four hours straight! I felt like a new woman after sleeping that long!

After about a week of doing this, I found that I wasn't producing as much breast milk. I couldn't pump enough to feed her during the day while I was at work *and* give her an extra bottle of breast milk at night. This was really stressful for me.

My husband and I discussed adding formula at night, but in my head I thought that meant that I was failing as a breastfeeding mom. After discussing this with our baby's family physician, she told us to

Mommy MD Guides-Recommended Product
Miracle Blanket

A small study in *Pediatrics* shows that swaddling helps infants sleep longer and better. Wrapping babies up snug as a bug in a rug mimics the tight fit of the womb. Experts hope that swaddling also encourages parents to put their babies to sleep on their backs, which helps to prevent sudden infant death syndrome.

Even tiny babies can be Houdinis-in-the-making and wriggle their way out of blankets. And then those loose blankets in the crib can become a hazard. Mindi and Mike Gatten, parents of three sons, invented a very unique swaddler with a clever design that babies have a hard time escaping. The Miracle Blanket is simple to use, and it's very comfortable for babies to wear. The blankets are made of 100 percent cotton, come in several colors, and one size fits up to four months. They come with a 100 percent lifetime satisfaction guarantee. You can buy Miracle Blankets online for around $30.

go ahead and give the baby an ounce or two of formula at night. She said it was important that I didn't stress out about breastfeeding and that I needed to sleep as well. The doctor told us, "Even though you're giving her a little bit of formula at night, she's still a breastfed baby." That was really important for me to hear, and now both my baby and I are sleeping great.

—*Jennifer Bacani McKenney, MD*

The fatigue with a new baby is like nothing I had ever experienced. I went into parenting thinking, *I've been an intern. I can do this!* But it's different when you're not getting good sleep every single night.

After the first few sleepless weeks, my husband and I worked out a schedule. I'd breastfeed the baby each night around 8 p.m., and then go to sleep. My husband would stay up to give the baby a bottle at 11 p.m., and then he'd go to sleep. Then I'd wake up the next morning with the baby. That way, we'd each get a nice stretch of sleep.

—*Heather Orman-Lubell, MD*

A major challenge for me during my twins' first year of life was sleep deprivation. When you have two little babies and you still have to work and be "on your game," it's hard.

To cope, my husband and I took sleep shifts. Rather than us both being up all night and miserable, one of us went to bed at 9 p.m. and slept until 2 a.m. The other slept on a couch in the nursery and tended to the babies when they woke up. Then we switched. At least that way, we were each guaranteed to get four to five hours of good sleep. It worked out beautifully. We both felt we could function on four to five hours of uninterrupted sleep.

—*Brooke Jackson, MD*

My son was a very fussy baby. He wouldn't sleep on his back. For months, he slept in either his bouncy seat or his car seat, which we placed in his crib.

As soon as my son could roll over and sleep on his belly, he was much happier, and then he started to sleep in his crib. He slept through the night when he was 10 weeks old. The first time he slept through the night, I woke up in a panic thinking something had happened to him!

My daughter, on the other hand, was a good sleeper from the beginning. For her first four months, I slept in a bed in her room so that I could get up and feed her without waking my husband or our son. After four months, my husband asked, "Are you ever coming back to bed?"

"It's quiet here!" I said. "Nobody snores."

—*Alanna Kramer, MD*

⁓

My son was a horrible sleeper. It was so frustrating to me that my patients had babies who slept through the night when they were just eight weeks old! That's not the norm, but I would get so angry, wondering, *Why isn't my baby sleeping through the night?* I went back to work when my baby was 10 weeks old, and he still wasn't sleeping through the night. He didn't sleep through the night until he was four months old. My husband and I were exhausted.

The reality is "sleeping through the night" is defined as one six-hour stretch of sleep. You might not like that definition, but a six-hour stretch will feel like forever when you've been getting only two- or four-hour stretches of sleep.

If you have a baby who's doing better than the norm, don't tell anyone!

—*Ari Brown, MD, a mom of two, a pediatrician with Capital Pediatric Group, and the author of* Baby 411, *in Austin, TX*

⁓

My mom told me that I didn't sleep through the night until I was around 18 months old. So when my daughter didn't sleep, my mom jokingly told me that it was my own fault.

My husband and I tried everything to get our daughter to sleep. We used *The Happiest Baby on the Block* methods, and we tried a hammock bed. We even tried to let her cry it out, but she was stronger than we were. She finally started to sleep through the night when she was 22 months old.

—*Cheri Wiggins, MD*

I was never a rock-or-feed-your-baby-to-sleep person. I wanted my kids to learn how to soothe themselves and fall asleep on their own. I did let them cry to fall to sleep.

Swaddling helped a lot. My babies loved to be swaddled—rather tightly. My daughter wanted to be swaddled until she was over two years old. At that point, she didn't let me wrap her arms in, but she liked having the lower half of her body wrapped tightly in a blanket. I think it feels cozy to kids.

I liked the book *The Baby Whisperer*, and I followed her cycles of eating, activity, sleeping, and then "my time." I also liked the book *Healthy Sleep Habits, Happy Child*. At one point, the author suggested, contrary to common sense, that when kids start waking up too early in the morning, they might need to go to bed earlier, rather than later (as we might have imagined). He suggested that at times, a child might need to go to sleep at 6:30 p.m. *No way*, I thought. But I tried it out of desperation, and it worked. Sleep begets sleep. It didn't last long, and yes, it was disruptive for our lives to have to get them in bed so early in the evening, but each of my kids went through this phase, and the author's advice helped.

—*Michelle Paley, MD, PA*

Our biggest challenge during our twins' first year was getting them to sleep. You'd think getting a baby to sleep would be so natural, but it isn't! Our babies didn't sleep through the night until they were 11 months old. They woke up to nurse every two to three hours, every night. Initially, they were so tiny (they were a bit preemie) that they needed to eat every two to three hours. Later, waking up so often was just habit, and the only way they knew to get back to sleep was to eat for comfort. The biggest mistake we made was probably not allowing them to self-soothe, so that they could put themselves back to sleep on their own. The process of fixing this was very painful! Their first year is a blur to me, with lack of sleep being a big contributing factor!

Looking back, I think that how a baby sleeps has a lot to do with his temperament. High-maintenance kids just don't sleep a lot. And both of my babies were very high maintenance. Sometimes, there's not much you can do but just have a sense of humor, grin and bear it, and get through it. Because you will!

—*Ann Contrucci, MD*

⟡

Before I had my daughter, I'd visit friends who were moms, and their babies were always sleeping. I expected my baby to sleep a lot too, but she didn't. One thing I learned about my daughter early on is that she doesn't need a lot of sleep.

Turns out my daughter is a bit of a night owl like me. When we went to visit friends, their babies would be sleeping, but my daughter would be wide awake. This actually made it easier for me to take her places and spend more time with friends.

I talked to my baby's pediatrician about it, and he said that as long as she was getting a total of 10 hours of sleep during naps and at night, all was just fine.

—*Dina Strachan, MD*

⟡

One thing that I found very interesting is that babies prefer different conditions for sleep. Once you figure out what your babies like, it makes getting them to sleep much easier.

For example, my older daughter liked to be swaddled in a blanket. My younger daughter, on the other hand, slept in her undershirt and diaper with the ceiling fan blowing on her, legs and arms splayed out! If I tried to swaddle her, she'd kick and scream.

One of the best baby items we owned was our swing. It was a godsend. My older daughter would fall asleep in it, and then I'd transfer her to her crib.

With our first baby, my husband and I bought a swing that you had to crank. After that, we bought a battery-operated one. I made sure that I had spare batteries on hand at all times. I didn't want to run out of batteries in the middle of the night!

—*Lisa Dado, MD*

⟡

I have four children, and I can tell you that every single kid is different as far as sleep goes. I think if there was a single sleep solution that worked for every baby, someone would have written the book on it and she would be a trillionaire.

If what you are doing to get your baby to sleep isn't working, it doesn't mean you're doing it wrong. It just means it doesn't work for your kid. Simply try something else.

—*Kristie McNealy, MD*

Resuming Birth Control

Sleepless nights and all that crying are probably enough to keep you from wanting to have another baby right about now. And that's *your* sleepless nights and *your* crying, not the baby's! But not wanting to have another baby right now doesn't mean Mother Nature doesn't have other plans. So resuming birth control is probably a very good idea.

If you're breastfeeding, you shouldn't take birth control pills containing estrogen, so you'll want to have a different plan for contraception, such as using condoms, an IUD, or a diaphragm.

Speaking of diaphragms, they need to be refitted to your body after your pregnancy or anytime that you lose or gain 20 percent of your body weight.

If you're not breastfeeding and you want to use oral contraceptives but the cost is a concern, talk with your ob-gyn. She might have samples she can give you. Or consider going generic. When you first begin using a birth control pill, be sure to use a backup form of birth control until you're sure the pill is working properly and you're not having any breakthrough bleeding. Your insurance company might allow you to buy enough birth control pills for three to six months for one co-pay when you use a mail-order prescription program.

❧

My husband and I decided to use condoms after our baby was born. Breastfeeding isn't a reliable form of birth control! My husband had read in his daddy books that new moms can have trouble with vaginal dryness, so he bought lubricated condoms. He was right. Even though I had a C-section, I still had that problem.

—*Jennifer Bacani McKenney, MD*

I had a hard time getting pregnant with my first son, and so I had expected that getting pregnant would be hard the second time too. It was quite a surprise when I got pregnant with my second son without trying. I had only one period in the year and a half between the delivery of my first son and my second pregnancy.

Looking back, I don't know why I was so surprised. When my mother got pregnant with me, she was using three forms of birth control at the same time. And I still happened.

—*Carrie Brown, MD*

I was so stressed out when I was a resident and a gastroenterology fellow, and even the first several years in private practice, that I actually developed an infertility condition called hypothalamic amenorrhea. I took the drug Clomid to get pregnant with my first two children. Because of my infertility issues, my husband and I stopped using birth control. Besides that, I had read that nursing was at least a "partial" form of birth control, so I figured that I was covered.

As it turned out, my birth control strategy apparently didn't work very well, because I became pregnant with my third baby a month after I stopped nursing my second baby. My second baby's major colic issues were quite a stimulus for my husband. He got a vasectomy when our third baby was three months old!

—*Stacey Weiland, MD*

RALLIE'S TIP

If you aren't ready for another baby, make sure you're using an effective method of birth control! I found out that I was pregnant again when my middle son was just six months old. I was nursing and I hadn't had a period since my delivery, so I felt certain that I was "safe." Wrong! Of course it all worked out just fine, and I wouldn't change a thing now, but having two babies in two years is one of the hardest things I've ever done, physically and emotionally. To this day, when I see pictures of myself looking a bit dazed and frazzled and holding those two little boys, I think, How in the world did I do it?

Chapter 2
2nd Month

Your Baby This Month

YOUR BABY'S DEVELOPMENT

Your baby is developing at her own rate, in her own time. These days, she still sees the world a little fuzzy. Her optic nerve, which transmits information from her eyes to her brain, isn't functioning like an adult's. Also, the cones of your baby's eyes, which perceive color, aren't yet completely operational. Right now your baby probably sees similar colors, such as red and orange, as the same color. That's why black-and-white patterns catch her eye more quickly.

Your baby is still quite nearsighted. Right now, she sees objects best that are around 8 to 15 inches away. This is one reason why she gazes so lovingly at your face when you cradle her in your arms.

As this month goes along, your baby will become more and more interested in what's going on in the rest of the room. She'll study your face, and then she'll shift her focus to look past you to something in the background. Then she'll more than likely shift back to gaze at you again.

Around two months, your baby's tightly clenched fists are starting to loosen—as if she's preparing to explore her world. If you place a small toy, such as a rattle, in your baby's hand, she might be able to hold onto it, and she won't want to give it up. If the toy makes a sound, your baby might not yet realize that she's the one making the noise though!

Your baby's feeding schedule at two months is probably still very erratic. Despite that, she's probably gaining about half a pound a week.

Babies at this age start to spend more time awake and alert, but they still sleep around 16 hours each day. Because they can't distinguish day from night, the sleep is still divided between night and day. The time is tipping more in your favor, though, because at around four weeks old, a baby usually sleeps only 6¾ hours during the day and 8¾ hours at night.

Around this time, your baby can probably lift her head about 45 degrees when she's on her stomach. Your baby's head control is improving, and she might be able to keep her head steady when you hold her in a sitting position. Some babies at this age can roll over, one way only.

Babies at this age start to explore more and more with their hands, reaching, batting, and swatting. Although your baby tries to reach for things, she misses most of the time.

Your baby's main method of communication is still crying. At two months, most babies cry more than two hours each day. For most babies, crying spells peak at about six weeks, and then gradually decline.

By two months, about half of babies can recognize their parents. They react differently to their parents than to other people by smiling more quickly. Around this time, your baby can start to respond to a smile with one of her own. She might have added a new way to communicate: sweet little baby coos. These soft, wonderful sounds are a baby's first attempts to communicate her joy. Toward the end of this month, some babies' grunty sounds become more vowel-like and musical. Your baby also might be able to blow bubbles. She might start mimicking your facial expressions now.

You might be able to see signs of your baby's temperament around now. Is your little one feisty, calm, active, relaxed?

Taking Care of You

Sleep as often and as much as you can. A well-rested mom is a healthier mom. Sleep improves mood, memory, immunity, cardiovascular health, and more. Sleep: It does a body good.

Justification for a Celebration

You made it through the first month!

Playing with Your Baby

Besides being just plain fun, playing with your baby is critical to her development. Through play, babies explore their surroundings, understand their place in the world, develop motor skills, and learn social skills.

❧

Gymboree was great fun for the first year for my daughter—and for my husband and me.

> —*Darlene Gaynor-Krupnick, DO, a mom of five- and two-year-old daughters, a female urologist fellow trained in pelvic reconstruction and neurology, and the inventor of Valera, a USDA-certified organic vaginal lubricant, in northern Virginia*

❧

I loved introducing new things to my son. The excitement on a baby's face when he sees himself in the mirror, that first smile, first tooth, first words, first steps—all of the new adventures of the first year were a great experience.

> —*Saundra Dalton-Smith, MD, a mom of six- and four-year-old sons, an internal medicine specialist, and the author of* Set Free to Live Free: Breaking Through the 7 Lies Women Tell Themselves, *in Anniston, AL*

❧

I loved getting to know my babies in impromptu moments, such as while they were on the changing table and while I was reading stories to them. I also loved going for walks and talking to the children about what we saw. They became very observant, and they loved the routine of getting up, having breakfast, going for a walk, watching Barney, playing, eating lunch, napping, and then going for an outing.

> —*Lesley Burton-Iwinski, MD, a mom of 20- and 18-year-old daughters and a 14-year-old son, a retired family physician, and a parent and teacher educator with Growing Peaceful Families, in Lexington, KY*

❧

When I played with my babies on the floor, I always placed them on a cotton receiving blanket, rather than directly on the carpeting.

Direct contact with carpeting can flare eczema.

—*Amy J. Derick, MD, a mom of two-year-old and nine-month-old sons and a dermatologist in private practice at Derick Dermatology, in Barrington, IL*

❧

My younger son loved Baby Einstein videos and puzzles. He also loved watching his brother have playdates. He was very interested in other children. At two months, he liked to try to swat the baby gym toys and would often fall asleep on the mat. I guess it was very exhausting.

—*Sonia Ng, MD, a mom of seven- and two-year-old sons, a pediatrician, and a sedation attending physician at the Children's Hospital of Philadelphia Pediatric Care and the University Medical Center at Princeton in Princeton, NJ, and the Pediatric Imaging Center in King of Prussia, PA*

❧

My husband and I are fans of books and building blocks. That first year, babies don't need elaborate toys. They love simple things they can shake and bang.

—*Heather Orman-Lubell, MD, a mom of 10- and six-year-old sons and a pediatrician in private practice at Yardley Pediatrics of St. Christopher's Hospital for Children, in Pennsylvania*

RALLIE'S TIP

When my babies were little, I always felt as if I had a hundred things to do, and at least half of them needed to be done immediately. There were clothes to wash and fold, floors to sweep, meals to make, and phone calls to return. It was a challenge for me to put all these pressing tasks completely out of my mind for 15 or 20 minutes so I could focus my entire attention on playing with my babies, but I did it.

I always tried to avoid multitasking when we were playing. I think it's really important for parents to spend time with their babies, one-on-one, talking to them and making eye contact with them without distraction. I believe that when children have their parents' undivided attention for short periods of time on a regular basis, they're less likely to be clingy when their parents need to focus their attention elsewhere, such as when they're making a phone call or writing an e-mail.

~

My youngest son is nine months old, and he's really into large motor activities, such as walking. His favorite things to do are setting up toys and knocking them down and playing with toys that have buttons to press, keys to turn, or lights that light up. Anything that shows cause and effect really fascinates him right now.

One thing that *all* of my boys love to do is dance. I turn on some music or my boys get out their kid instruments and play "music." We have guitars and drums, and they're happy as long as noise is being made. I see a garage band in our future.

—Amy Thompson, MD, a mom of four- and two-year-old and nine-month-old sons and an ob-gyn at the University of Cincinnati College of Medicine, in Ohio

~

My husband works in New York City, and he has a long commute after a long work day, which means he's away from home for most of the day.

My daughter was born in the middle of winter when my son was 21 months old. One day it was too cold for us to go outside and play, and I was going stir-crazy in the house. To make matters worse, my son didn't want to play with any of his toys!

In desperation, I took out a box of tampons, and my son played with those tampons for hours! He took the wrappers off, pulled the tampons apart, and stacked them up. He was entertained, my baby was entertained watching him, and I was happy!

—Alanna Kramer, MD, a mom of an eight-year-old son and a six-year-old daughter and a pediatrician with St. Christopher's Hospital for Children, in Philadelphia, PA

~

During that first year, it's so much fun to share the world with your baby and to share your baby with the world. Everything is fascinating to an infant—discovering pots and pans or leaves on plants is fun! An old sock is fun! A slice of orange is fun!

I remember going with my baby to an outdoor nighttime party at a neighbor's house. There were big candles on the garden wall. I remember my son sitting quietly on my lap, staring at and considering those flames with a serious look on his face for what seemed like an eternity of meditation. It was one of the most vivid experiences I had as a new mother, seeing my offspring—who wasn't old enough to stand or to say a word—having complex thoughts about the dancing fire and experiencing a whole drama inside his little head. I felt for the first time the pang of separation, knowing that he would grow to think a world of thoughts unknowable to me.

The world becomes known to the child through the mother's sharing of it—tasting the same cookie, patting the same stuffed bear. The child's world becomes animated when a mother shares her experiences.

—Elizabeth Berger, MD, a mom of a 28-year-old son and a 26-year-old daughter, a child psychiatrist, and the author of Raising Kids with Character, *in New York City*

During my daughter's first year, we went to some early childhood classes that were offered locally by the state. We got a lot of great play ideas there, simple things like rhymes and songs. Because my husband and I were new in town, the other moms were my best source for finding out where the family-friendly activities were.

To find these kinds of classes and activities, ask other moms at the playground and ask your child's doctor. You can find programs for dads, too, such as dads-only playgroups. These can be invaluable for stay-at-home dads.

One of my favorite activities for older babies is to give them a bag of big pompoms from the craft store. You have to supervise your baby while she's playing with the pompoms, of course, but she'll love putting them inside toilet paper rolls, filling boxes with them, and sorting them. A bag of pompoms would keep my daughter entertained for hours.

—Katja Rowell, MD, a mom of a five-year-old daughter, a family physician, and a childhood feeding specialist with FamilyFeedingDynamics.com, in St. Paul, MN

Wearing Your Baby

On one hand, the word *babywearing* seems a little bit silly, like your baby is an accessory or a handbag. But on the other hand, *babywearing* is a lovely word. You're wearing your baby close to your body, close to your heart.

Mothers' instincts run deep, and when a baby cries, our instincts tell us to pick that baby up, *now!* We're often rewarded when our babies stop crying and snuggle contentedly into our arms.

Moms don't need a study to prove that carried babies are happy babies, but scientists in Montreal were determined to find out anyway. A team of pediatricians studied 99 mother-infant pairs. The first group was told to carry their babies in baby carriers for at least three hours a day, and they were encouraged to carry their babies as often as they could. The other group was given no specific guidance about carrying their babies. After six weeks, the babies in the more-often-carried group cried 43 percent less than the babies in the less-often-carried group.

Some experts believe that babies who are "worn" in slings and other carriers learn more. These babies spend less time crying, and in their "free" time, they spend more time learning.

A generation ago, moms simply carried their babies on their hips. Today, you have an aisle full of carriers as near as the closest baby supply store. You'll find a dizzying array of slings, front carriers, and back carriers. There's even a Hip Hammock for larger babies. (See "Mommy MD Guides–Recommended Product: Playtex Hip Hammock" on page 449.)

If you plan to carry your baby a lot, take your time choosing a carrier. Look for one with soft shoulder padding and lower back support. Follow the weight limits closely. Heed the safety instructions carefully: Make sure to use the proper settings so that your baby doesn't fall out. Always be sure that your baby is positioned in the carrier so that she can breathe.

⁓

The most valuable baby item I had in the first three to four months of my baby's life was my baby sling. When my girls were little, the sling was amazing. I could take them out with me but keep them completely covered and protected from the public. The baby sling allowed me to keep my hands free, and it covered the post-delivery belly!

—*Marra S. Francis, MD, a mom of seven-, six-, and four-year-old daughters and an ob-gyn, in The Woodlands, TX*

During my baby's first few months, I loved my baby sling. It was so nice to just bundle my baby up in the sling and be hands-free.

—*Melody Derrick, MD, a mom of a 17-month-old daughter and a family physician in private practice with Central DuPage Physician Group, in Winfield, IL*

Wearing my babies was a very positive experience. I remember when my one son was about six weeks old, and we were at a small dinner party. He was lying in his baby sling, which was wrapped around my body. One of the guests at the dinner party didn't even know my son was there until his tiny hand emerged from the sling!

I highly recommend baby slings, but not upright baby carriers, which can strain your back.

—*Lauren Feder, MD, a mom of 17- and 13-year-old sons, a nationally recognized physician who specializes in homeopathic medicine, and the author of* Natural Baby and Childcare *and* The Parents' Concise Guide to Childhood Vaccinations, *in Los Angeles, CA*

I had a BabyBjörn and a baby sling. When I put my daughter in the sling, I found that she felt too heavy and I felt off balance. Plus people often mistook her for a pocketbook!

The BabyBjörn kept my daughter closer to my core. That was most comfortable for me.

—*Dina Strachan, MD, a mom of a five-year-old daughter, a dermatologist and director of Aglow Dermatology, and an assistant clinical professor in the department of dermatology at Columbia University College of Physicians and Surgeons, in New York City*

My younger daughter was the easiest baby, except that she never wanted to be put down. I first used a homemade sling, and later I got an Ergo baby carrier. That allowed me to wear her around, and she was just fine with that. You can buy Ergo carriers at ErgoBabyCarrier.com for $115 to $145.

—*Robyn Liu, MD, a mom of seven- and four-year-old daughters and a family physician with Greeley County Health Services, in Tribune, KS*

We were penniless when we had our kids, so lots of their stuff were hand-me-downs. A friend gave us one of her old cloth carrying gizmos. It tied around the grown-up's waist and also around the neck, with the baby sitting, feet dangling through leg-holes, slung against the grown-up's chest. This was quite a while ago, but at that time these were simple carriers with no metal or plastic parts. You could throw it in the washing machine. I passed it on to another parent when our kids outgrew it. Our kids never used strollers. We always carried them.

—*Elizabeth Berger, MD*

I really liked my BabyBjörn. My daughter was a chubby baby, so I could only carry her in the BabyBjörn for about three months before the weight started to hurt my back. When my husband and I went out, he would have to carry her in the BabyBjörn, or we would put her in the stroller instead.

—*Jeannette Gonzalez Simon, MD, a mom of a two-year-old daughter who's expecting another baby and a pediatric gastroenterologist in private practice, in Staten Island, NY*

To carry both of my twins around at once, I strapped two of those front carriers to myself! I don't recall double ones being available at the time; that would have been much easier.

I loved those carriers because they kept my babies all snuggled up, nestled right next to me. Sometimes that was the only thing that soothed them.

—*Ann Contrucci, MD, a mom of 12-year-old boy-girl twins who works as a pediatric emergency physician, in Atlanta, GA*

We had a soft carrier by Becco that we used nonstop for about two years. I couldn't have functioned without it!

My husband preferred the BabyBjörn, but I didn't like that as well. It was actually nice that we each had our own carriers, because then we didn't have to keep readjusting the straps to fit.

—*Cheri Wiggins, MD, a mom of four- and two-year-old daughters, a specialist in physical medicine and rehabilitation at St. Luke's Magic Valley, and a cofounder of the Mommy Doctors Bakery (makers of Milkin' Cookies), in Twin Falls, ID*

Rather than putting my babies into slings or carriers, I really liked just carrying them in my arms. For the first time in my life, I was glad to have big wide hips. Babies fit nicely on hips.

—*Lillian Schapiro, MD, a mom of 14-year-old twin girls and an eight-year-old daughter and an ob-gyn with Peachtree Women's Specialists, in Atlanta, GA*

Pumping and Storing Breast Milk

Breast milk is an amazing substance. It actually has antibacterial properties that help it to stay fresh. Some people call breast milk "white blood." It takes a lot of time and effort to pump and store milk, so you'll want to do it as efficiently and carefully as possible to maximize all of that. The good news is the production of breast milk works by the principle of supply and demand: The more you pump, the more you produce.

Pump whenever it is convenient for you. You could pump after your baby eats, between feedings, or when you're away from your baby.

There are many options to pump milk, from simply expressing it by hand to buying or renting a hospital-grade pump. Simply put, the trade-off for lower cost is lower efficiency. By spending more, you'll gain efficiency.

Recently, the Internal Revenue Service said that it is reclassifying breast pumps as medical care purchases. That means they can now be deducted from income on IRS tax forms as medical expenses.

Once you pump the milk, it can remain at room temperature safely for only four to six hours. You'll want to get it in a refrigerator as soon as possible, where it can safely stay for 72 hours, and possibly even as long as eight days. Any longer, you'll need to freeze it, although frozen milk has less effective antibacterial properties than refrigerated milk. Breast milk can stay safely frozen for six months, and possibly even as long as a year.

Before you store your milk, take a cue from the dairy industry and date it.

According to the La Leche League, the best containers for storing milk are glass or hard-sided plastic containers with well-fitting tops. Be sure the plastic containers don't contain bisphenol A (BPA).

Like water, breast milk expands as it freezes. When you put the milk into the container, leave about an inch of space at the top to allow for expansion. Plastic bags can leak or break. Consider

Mommy MD Guides-Recommended Product
Medela Pump in Style

"The one product I found most indispensable during my babies' first years was my Medela breast pump," says Bola Oyeyipo, MD, a mom of three-year-old and six-month-old sons, a family physician in private practice, and the owner of SlimyBookWorm.com, in Highland, CA. "I used the Medela Pump in Style. It was a little expensive, but worth every dime. The suction and motor of the breast pump have endured two babies, 2½ years apart."

You can buy Medela Pump in Style breast pumps in stores and online for around $280.

how much your baby drinks at a time, and freeze that amount in each container.

It's easy to thaw frozen milk. If you can plan ahead, put it in the fridge overnight. If you forget, thaw it under water. Begin with cool water and slowly increase the temperature until it's at feeding temperature. Don't refreeze thawed milk because it might lose even more beneficial properties. Thawed milk will keep in the fridge for 24 hours.

Don't microwave milk. It can reduce some of the beneficial properties. Plus, microwaving can create hot spots in the milk that can burn your baby.

If you pump milk at work and need to store it until you get home, the law is on your side. According to the U.S. Centers for Disease Control and the U.S. Occupational Safety and Health Administration, breast milk can be stored in a common refrigerator at a workplace or day care center. It does not require special handling or storage in a separate place.

〜

I had a double Medela breast pump, and I pumped twice during every shift I worked at the hospital. It's amazing what we do for our kids.
—*Sonia Ng, MD*

My Medela breast pump was my saving grace. When I went back to work, I could go home and nurse my baby at lunchtime, and I pumped at other times during the day. My pump was fast and efficient. Within 10 minutes, I'd be done and have milk stored to use later. It was an expensive pump, but it was well worth it.

—*Jill Wireman, MD, a mom of 14- and 11-year-old sons and a pediatrician in private practice at Johnson City Pediatrics, in Tennessee*

❧

I returned to work three months after my baby was born, and I was still breastfeeding. I know that I would not have been successful at breastfeeding if it were not for my breast pump. I purchased a Medela Advanced Backpack Pump. It was small enough to carry back and forth to work but still efficient enough to pump plenty of milk in less than 10 minutes.

—*Saundra Dalton-Smith, MD*

❧

One of my biggest challenges in my baby's first year was combining nursing with work, since I was away from home for up to 13 hours each day. I would get up early in the morning to use the Medela pump, and I was happy to do it.

It was motivating for me to know that I was giving my child the benefits of breast milk. I would pump again at lunchtime and before bedtime. I gave my daughters breast milk for the first six to seven months of their lives.

—*Darlene Gaynor-Krupnick, DO*

❧

The breast pump was the greatest first-year investment ever! I tried a few, and the one I liked best by far was the Double Up Breast Pump made by the Natural Choice Company. I have loaned it out to at least three other mothers over the years, and it is still in the back of one of my kitchen cupboards. That reminds me that it's probably time to give it away—or retire it to a museum. I'm sure the newest models are more attractive!

—*Lesley Burton-Iwinski, MD*

One of the best purchases I ever made was a high-quality breast pump. I bought a Medela Pump in Style. It was battery powered, and I even bought a car charger for it. I've joked that my husband bought the charger at Radio Shack, but you can buy them on Medela's website (Medela.com).

—*Carrie Brown, MD, a mom of seven- and five-year-old sons and a general pediatrician who treats medically complex children and specializes in palliative care at Arkansas Children's Hospital, in Little Rock*

During my daughter's first year, I was working very long hours. I woke up early each morning and nursed her before I went to work, and it was nice bonding time. I also pumped at work. My pump was built into a shoulder bag, and it was my constant companion that year. Pumping took a lot of effort, but it was well worth it. Because I was away at work so much, it was very meaningful for me to pump milk for my baby. It was my way of being there for her.

—*Siobhan Dolan, MD, a mom of 15- and 12-year-old daughters and a 10-year-old son, a consultant to the March of Dimes, and an associate professor of obstetrics and gynecology and women's health at Albert Einstein College of Medicine/Montefiore Medical Center, in Bronx, NY*

One of the most difficult things for many working moms is pumping at work. I was fortunate that the pediatric hospital I worked at had lactation rooms. The lactation room has a hospital-quality pump and a sink. While I was working at the hospital, I could go to the lactation room, pump, and even clean up afterward. That arrangement made pumping very easy.

The trick was finding the time to pump. It's not easy for some moms to let down their milk for the pump. I found that it helped to take my phone with me and look at the photos and videos of my son stored on my phone. It also helped if I stuck to a schedule. I tried to follow a routine, and your body learns to prepare for that.

—*Rebecca Reamy, MD, a mom of six- and one-year-old sons and a pediatrician in emergency medicine at Children's Healthcare of Atlanta, in Georgia*

I breastfed all of my babies for at least a year. I pumped and collected breast milk so that during the first six months of my babies' lives, if they did get a bottle, it was pumped breast milk.

When I was breastfeeding my baby on one side, I often leaked on the other side. I used milk cups, which are also sometimes called breast shells, to collect that leaking milk. Between that and pumping, I was able to collect a freezer full of milk in a few months.

To make the whole collecting, storing, and feeding process easier, I put the milk in plastic, disposable Playtex nurser liners and fastened them with twist-ties. I doubled-bagged the milk and put it in the freezer. Then when it was time to use the milk, I'd thaw it in warm water.

—*Charlene Brock, MD, a mom of 28-, 25-, and 23-year-old sons and an 18-year-old daughter and a pediatrician with St. Chris Care at Falls Center, in Philadelphia, PA*

I had my daughter when I was completing my fellowship in gastroenterology, and I remember asking my attending physician if I could go to the bathroom to pump. He thought I was going to lift weights! Sometimes I would be so busy that I couldn't even find the time to pump. I always had to wear heavy sweaters to absorb milk leaks. One time I was scoping a patient with a bleeding ulcer, and the milk ran all the way down into my socks!

Learning how to pump was interesting. I chose the Medela Pump in Style breast pump. The carrying case is pretty discreet looking. It's easy to clean, and it has roomy pockets for storing ice packs, pumped milk, and bottles. With the Medela, I could either plug it in or use the battery pack, and I could pump both breasts at once. All of the equipment is washable. Dealing with the bags was a little difficult for me, and I did have some spills. Sometimes I would just store the milk in the freezer in the small bottles instead of using the bags.

—*Stacey Weiland, MD, a mom of a 12-year-old daughter and 7- and 5-year-old sons and an internist/gastroenterologist, in Denver, CO*

Even though I breastfed my daughter, I also pumped milk. That way, if I couldn't get home from work to breastfeed my daughter, at least she could have a bottle of breast milk.

I used bottles with collapsible baby bottle liners. I thought they were the best invention ever! They're sterile, and they kept my daughter from taking in a lot of air when she nursed. My daughter was a hungry baby and a very fast eater, and those collapsible bottles really helped. Plus, even back then, they didn't have any bisphenol A (BPA).

—*Debra Jaliman, MD, a mom of a 19-year-old daughter, a dermatologist in private practice, and an assistant professor of dermatology at Mt. Sinai School of Medicine, in New York City*

Because my son was born prematurely, I pumped breast milk exclusively for the first few months of his life. Cleaning that breast pump was a huge task!

I recommend that all moms who pump breast milk buy multiple sets of the pieces that need to be cleaned. I had three sets of horns so that I didn't have to wash them immediately. Extra horns aren't expensive, and for the time I saved it was well worth the cost.

I used cloth diapers with my son, so I had purchased "wet bags" for his soiled diapers. I quickly learned that these wet bags were perfect for transporting both clean and used pump parts to and from work. I also had an AVENT bottle sterilizer. I used that to clean my breast pump parts.

—*Lennox McNeary, MD, a mom of a two-year-old son, a specialist in physical medicine and rehabilitation at Carilion Clinic, and a cofounder of the Mommy Doctors Bakery (makers of Milkin' Cookies), in Roanoke, VA*

Transitioning to the Tub

Rub-a-dub-dub, look who's now in the tub!

Doctors recommend that babies transition to the tub after their umbilical cord stumps fall off.

Tub safety is critical. Babies can drown in any amount of water. Never leave a baby or child unattended in a tub for even a second. That means that when your baby's in the tub, you'll have to leave the doorbell unanswered, and let the phone ring. Bath time gives you an excellent opportunity to sit and connect with your baby. You're right there, at eye level, so it's the perfect time to talk. Even though your baby can't answer you yet, she loves looking at you and hearing the sound of your voice.

Interestingly, in a recent poll, almost one-third of dads surveyed said that they never, ever give their babies a bath. Another third of dads said they bathe their babies only "when my wife asks me to." The last third of dads said they bathe their babies either every day or once a week.

⁓

Once my babies' umbilical cord stumps fell off, I started bathing them in the infant tub. I have tried several versions of this tub. My favorite one has a padded hammock that attaches to the plastic tub. I used the hammock attachment for the first three to four months, and then transitioned to the incline tub. At six months, I used the sitting side tub. I placed this inside of the empty bathtub until my baby had very good control of his core body muscles at approximately 9 to 10 months. Being inside the bigger tub helps with splashes and cleanup after the bath. It also gets the baby used to sitting in the tub area and looking out at us.
—*Amy Thompson, MD*

⁓

My daughter screamed at each and every bath time. On a friend's advice, I took her into the bathtub with me when I had my bath.
—*Stuart Jeanne Bramhall, MD, a mom of a 30-year-old daughter and a child and adolescent psychiatrist, in New Plymouth, New Zealand*

⁓

When my twins were infants, I loved bathing them in our kitchen double sink. I have lots of great photos of the two of them grinning from ear to ear, up to their waists in water. It was the most fun, convenient, and efficient way to give them their baths.

—*Penny Noyce, MD, a mom of 23- and 21-year-old daughters, two 21-year-old sons, and a 13-year-old son, the author of the preteen novel* Lost in Lexicon, *and an internal medicine specialist, in Weston, MA*

Both of my kids have sensitive skin, so for their baths, I used Cetaphil cleanser, rather than soap. Afterward, I'd give them a massage with safflower oil, which kept their skin moist. It was a nice, peaceful activity for both of us.

—*Michelle Paley, MD, PA, a mom of two and a psychiatrist and psychotherapist in private practice, in Miami Beach, FL*

When bathing my sons, I use a shampoo/body wash combination that has no fragrance. I use no bubble bath.

My philosophy is to avoid having unnecessary chemicals come in contact with my sons' sensitive skin. I keep baths short because long baths can dry the skin. After my sons bathe, I apply a thin coat of Aquaphor Baby ointment.

—*Amy J. Derick, MD*

When my older daughter was born, we were living in a tiny rental house that was drafty and let cold air inside. When my daughter got a bath, it was a massive production. I'd go into the bathroom, turn the space heater on, turn the hot water on, and gather all of the supplies. Once the room was warm, my husband would run our daughter in and quickly bathe her before she caught a chill. Bath time actually turned out to be a fun family event.

   — *Cheri Wiggins, MD*

I have four kids, so we have no time for prolonged play in the tub. We have a good routine: Get in, soap up, rinse off, and get out! I am usually done with bath time for all four of my children in about 30 minutes. My mom is also a physician, and she came to stay with me after my babies were born. She really helped me with their baths when they were little and slippery.

   — *Sadaf T. Bhutta, MD, a mom of a five-year-old daughter*
   and three-year-old triplets and an assistant professor and the
   fellowship director of pediatric radiology at the University
   of Arkansas for Medical Sciences and Arkansas Children's
   Hospital, both in Little Rock

For bath time, we have a floating tugboat thermometer, and I use it to make sure the water temperature isn't too hot before I put my son into the tub. I always keep my hand under his neck to help support his head. When my son was young, I kept all his bath stuff very close to the tub during bath time: towels, diaper, clean clothes, Aquaphor, Desitin, and a rattle to distract him. I also kept a space heater in the bathroom to warm up the room if I needed to. If you use a space heater, remember you should never leave it on unattended.

   I bathed my son once every two days until he was six or seven months old because he had eczema. After he started feeding himself, he got a little bit stickier, so we went to once-a-day baths, with extra wiping of the face and washing of hands.

   — *Sonia Ng, MD*

RALLIE'S TIP

I've always loved the smell of baby lotion, and I kept my first son slathered in the stuff. Thirteen years later, I still loved the smell of baby lotion, but by that time I had graduated from medical school, and I was more educated and concerned about chemical ingredients in lotions. When my second son was born, I found a 100 percent natural and organic brand of cocoa butter at my local health food store to put on my son after his bath. It didn't smell like baby lotion, but it was just as delightful. To this day, when I smell cocoa butter, I think of babies! Excessive exposure to water and soap at bath time can lead to dry skin. Applying cocoa butter after bath time safely and effectively soothes and moisturizes your baby's skin.

In my work as a physician, I have seen many drowning victims. In one case, a baby drowned in ½ inch of water in a tub.

When my kids were young, I was especially careful at bath time. I gathered up all of my bath supplies first—pajamas, diapers, washcloths, and soap—before I started filling the tub with water. I bathed all three kids at the same time so I knew where everyone

Mommy MD Guides-Recommended Product
Aquatopia Safety Bath Time Audible Thermometer

You probably turned your water heater temperature down to 120°F before your baby was born. If you're wondering what the temperature of your hot water is, simply run the water until it's as hot as it gets, fill a coffee mug, and insert an instant-read thermometer.

But even if your heater is set correctly, your baby can still be hurt in an overly hot tub. There are many bath thermometers on the market, but this one is especially handy. It has a digital display to show the temperature, and if the temp drops too low or goes too high, it beeps. It's shaped like a green turtle on a yellow life preserver.

You can buy Aquatopia Audible Thermometers online for around $12.

was, and I closed the bathroom door so no one could escape!

While my kids were in the tub, bathing them was the only thing I was doing. I didn't answer my pager or my phone. I focused 100 percent of my attention on that bath.

—*Lisa Dado, MD, a mom of three children, ages 21 to 16, a pediatric anesthesiologist with Valley Anesthesiology Consultants, and a cofounder and CEO of the Center for Human Living, which teaches life skills and martial arts training, in Phoenix, AZ*

Preventing and Treating Cradle Cap

Such an odd name for a very common problem. About half of all babies get cradle cap. When a baby gets cradle cap, you might see a yellow, greasy scalp with flaking skin. Even though it's called cradle cap, it can extend to a baby's face and neck, especially along a baby's eyebrows and behind her ears.

We used Dove soap, and we gently washed my son's hair for cradle cap. He didn't have much.

—*Sonia Ng, MD*

Our baby had a few bouts of cradle cap. I tried what had been recommended—using baby oil to get it off—but her hair looked really greasy even after shampooing! I decided to let the cradle cap resolve on its own, and it did.

—*Rachel S. Rohde, MD, a mom of a five-month-old daughter, an assistant professor of orthopaedic surgery at the Oakland University William Beaumont School of Medicine, and an orthopaedic upper-extremity surgeon with Michigan Orthopaedic Institute, P.C., in Southfield, MI*

All three of my sons got minor cases of cradle cap. I tried to prevent it by gently brushing their hair with soft baby brushes and washing their scalps with baby shampoo in the tub after their umbilical cord stumps had fallen off. I'd shampoo my babies' hair, really froth up the bubbles, and then gently scrub their scalps.

Cradle cap is a collection of old, dead skin cells and secretions. I was able to treat it and prevent it from building up and looking really bad!

—*Amy Thompson, MD*

Both of my sons had cradle cap, which is actually eczema on the scalp. Cradle cap usually resolves itself, but you can apply mineral oil to the scalp and thus lift skin flakes for subsequent washing away. During my sons' "cradle cap" phases, I washed their hair twice each day.

—*Amy J. Derick, MD*

My baby hasn't had cradle cap. Because it's so cold, she's had some very mild flaking on her scalp. We wash her hair only about once a week because the air is so dry.

—*Jennifer Bacani McKenney, MD, a mom of a two-month-old daughter and a family physician, in Fredonia, KS*

RALLIE'S TIP

My babies didn't have cradle cap, but it's a relatively common condition that many new parents find worrisome. In most cases, it doesn't seem to bother babies nearly as much as it bothers their parents. Cradle cap creates white or yellow patches of crusting or scales on a baby's scalp. Although it usually isn't serious, most parents don't like seeing it on their precious newborns.

Although the exact cause of cradle cap isn't known, one contributing factor might be hormones that pass from the mother to the baby before birth. These hormones cause an excessive production of oil (sebum) in the oil glands and hair follicles.

Using a dab of olive oil is a safe and effective way to gently loosen and wipe away the scales of cradle cap from your baby's scalp. Natural plant compounds called phenols in olive oil have anti-inflammatory properties, which can help reduce redness, inflammation, and irritation of the scalp.

Preventing and Treating Skin Conditions

With the skin being our largest organ, it's not surprising that it's susceptible to a variety of pesky conditions. To make things even more challenging for babies, their skin dries out much faster than an adult's. Two very common skin conditions in babies are baby acne and dry skin. Rashes are also very common. (See "Preventing and Treating Rashes" on page 219.)

Baby acne is very common, especially in baby boys. It's caused by hormonal changes, and it typically appears during a baby's first three or four weeks of life. Most babies develop baby acne on their foreheads, cheeks, and chins. It looks like small red bumps. Not surprisingly, it often looks redder and a little worse when a baby is fussy or after a warm bath. There's not much you can do to prevent it, and the best treatment is simply time.

When to Call Your Doctor

Talk with your baby's doctor at her next visit if you're concerned about her skin, if her baby acne is getting worse, or if she still has baby acne at three months old.

In most cases, millia will resolve without treatment, but call your baby's doctor if she still has it at three months.

Some babies also develop tiny white bumps on their faces. These are called millia, and they also will simply go away in time without treatment.

My daughter had neonatal acne, and it was really hard for me to just wait and not do anything. I kept looking for treatments that would take away the rash on her face, but alas, I had to wait almost a year until it went away on its own.
—*Melody Derrick, MD*

It is common for newborn babies after several weeks to show neonatal (or baby) acne. My sons had this experience. Mild neonatal acne will resolve itself, but severe neonatal acne can leave scars and should be examined by a dermatologist.
—*Amy J. Derick, MD*

My fourth child had bad skin. He was one of those babies whose hair fell out in chunks with big patches of scalp attached to it. For a while, he looked like an old man with a bad comb-over. His hair all grew back, and today he has beautiful hair.
—*Penny Noyce, MD*

I love Cetaphil—the wash, lotion, and cream. It's safe, and it's great for kids with normal skin and also for babies with eczema. I *still* use it on my kids, who are 10 and six years old.
—*Heather Orman-Lubell, MD*

My daughter had very dry skin. I discovered that even the gentle or all-natural baby soaps made her skin very pink and dry.

Instead of using baby soaps all the time, I put a few drops of almond oil into her bathwater, and I washed her with soap only once a week. I found a brand called Vanicream that I really liked. I used the Vanicream bar soap for bathing my daughter. After her bath, I used the lotion. It comes in a big pump dispenser, which is really handy. Two days after we started using the Vanicream, my daughter's skin cleared up, and she never had problems with dry skin again.

—*Katja Rowell, MD*

RALLIE'S TIP

I've always tried to avoid putting products that contain lots of chemicals on my children's skin, and mine too, for that matter! The skin is the body's largest organ, and many substances that are applied to a baby's body are easily absorbed by the skin and make their way into the bloodstream. So it makes good sense to avoid applying any substance to your baby's skin that you wouldn't want to end up in her body.

One safe substance to use on your baby's skin is olive oil. The oil is edible, and it's also wholesome and health-promoting. Because olive oil is edible, I've always felt really good about putting it on my children's skin as a moisturizer.

Many baby skin products, such as petroleum-based oils and lotions, contain ingredients that don't fit the "wholesome and edible" description. Unlike olive oil, you probably wouldn't be tempted to sprinkle these products on your salad! As it turns out, there might be ingredients in some baby lotions, wipes, shampoos, and other products that we wouldn't intentionally choose to put in or on our babies.

It's also a good idea to avoid products that contain ingredients that are likely to be allergenic, such as nuts or eggs. In a study conducted at Children's Memorial Hospital in Chicago, IL, researchers found that more than a quarter of 293 over-the-counter children's skin care products tested contained at least one common allergenic food ingredient, including cow's milk, egg, soy, wheat, peanuts, and tree nuts.

Treating a Fever

In adults and older children, fever can be your friend. It helps to elevate body temperature, killing off viruses and bacteria and speeding healing reactions.

But in a baby, it's another story. If your baby is younger than three months and develops any fever, call the doctor. It could be a sign of a serious illness.

❦

Fortunately, we haven't had to deal with a fever yet, but here's advice I usually give my patients: If your baby is younger than a month old and has a fever, you should always take her to the doctor because one-month-old babies should not have fevers. If her doctor decides that no other treatment is needed, acetaminophen (Tylenol) or ibuprofen (Motrin) might be recommended in the appropriate dosages. (Talk with your doctor before giving your baby this or any medication.)
—*Jennifer Bacani McKenney, MD*

❦

I always watched my daughter carefully for signs of fever, such as glassy eyes, red face, and decreased activity. One day when my daughter was a little less than a year old, she felt very warm, and I took her axillary temperature (under her arm). It was high, so I checked it again rectally. That of course was even higher, over 103°F.

We were out of town at the time, which added a whole other dimension of concern. I rushed my daughter to the emergency room. The folks in the ER drew blood, collected urine, and checked for viruses. Thank goodness, my daughter was fine.

I found generally that ibuprofen (Motrin) worked better for my daughter's fevers because I didn't have to give it as often as I did acetaminophen (Tylenol).
—*Christy Valentine, MD, a mom of a five-year-old daughter, a specialist in pediatrics and internal medicine, and the founder of the Valentine Medical Center, in Gretna, LA*

❦

It's important to know that if a baby two months old or younger has a temperature higher than 100.3°F, your doctor may feel compelled to order a lumbar puncture [which involves placing a needle into the space surrounding the spinal cord and removing a bit of spinal fluid] to rule out meningitis. I tried to prevent my son from getting sick—and having a fever—at all costs.

My brother-in-law traveled on the New Jersey Transit to visit us when the baby was five weeks old. He came in and reached for the baby. I screamed. I did not allow people to touch the baby if they had a cough, congestion, or a rash, even if they washed their hands.

I did take my son plenty of places after he turned a month old, but I didn't allow anyone to touch him except my husband. My older son was allowed to kiss the baby on the top of his head. I allowed my older son to hold the baby after he came home from school, but only after changing his clothes and washing his hands. If my older son had to cough, he would turn his head away from the baby. He was very good with his little brother.

—*Sonia Ng, MD*

? When to Call Your Doctor

If your baby is younger than three months old and has any fever, call your doctor right away.

If your baby is three months old or older and has an oral temperature lower than 100.4°F, offer rest, comfort, and fluids to keep her comfortable. If your baby's temperature is 100.4°F or higher, you might give an appropriate dose of acetaminophen (Tylenol). (Talk with your doctor before giving your baby this or any medication.) If the fever doesn't respond to the medication or lasts longer than one day, call your doctor. If your baby is older than three months and her temperature is 101°F or higher, call your doctor right away. In the presence of other concerning symptoms, such as poor feeding, a new rash, or decrease in activity, call your doctor right away, even if your baby's body temperature is only slightly above normal.

The cause of febrile seizures is a very rapid rise in a baby's body temperature, as opposed to a high fever that mounts over an extended period of time.

During my babies' first years, I was very judicious with the acetaminophen (Tylenol) and ibuprofen (Motrin). These medicines are not magic cure-alls, and I learned through my patients that all medications have side effects, even medications that seem harmless.

After my babies were older than three months, I'd give them medication if they had a fever higher than 100.4°F, depending on how they looked. If they had a 100.4° fever and looked awful, I'd give them Tylenol or Motrin. But if they had a 100.4° fever and were playing and eating, then I'd worry less about it and I wouldn't give them medication. I'd check it again in about 30 minutes or so to see if it was going higher or lower. (Talk with your doctor before giving your baby this or any medication.)

—*Leena Shrivastava Dev, MD, a mom of 14- and 10-year-old sons, an assistant professor of medicine at Drexel University College of Medicine, and a general pediatrician, in Philadelphia, PA*

During my sons' first years, they did get a few fevers. My philosophy is that in older babies, fever is our friend; it's not really a bad thing. A fever is your immune system's way of fighting off an infection. I understand that fever causes most parents to worry. Most of the phone calls I get from parents are about fevers.

As long as my over-three-month-old babies looked at me, made eye contact, and interacted with me, I didn't even treat fevers under 101°F. Those low-grade fevers help the body to fight off infection.

If a child over three months of age has a fever over 101°, though, I'd recommend taking off the baby's clothes, giving him an age- and weight-appropriate dose of acetaminophen (Tylenol), and getting plenty of fluids into him. (Talk with your doctor before giving your baby this or any medication.) If a child is less than three months old and has a fever, it is important to speak to your doctor right away to get your baby evaluated as soon as possible. Fever in a baby this age can be a sign of a serious infection and needs to be addressed immediately.

To check my kids' temperature, I used an axillary thermometer. That's probably the least trendy type, but it was best for me. I've never invested in fancy thermometers. We're very low-tech at our house.

Truth be told, it's not really all that important what the exact temperature reading is; what's more important is whether the baby has a fever. I take the baby's axillary temperature, by placing the thermometer under the baby's arm, and if it's greater than 99.4°F, the baby has a fever—because you need to add a degree to an axillary temp. If it's below that 99.4°F, there is no fever. If a newborn's axillary temperature is over 100°F, parents should take the temperature again with a rectal thermometer because it's more accurate. If the rectal temperature is 100.4°F or higher for an infant less than three months old, call your child's doctor right away.

—*Jill Wireman, MD*

⁓

I had to take my son to the emergency room when he was two months old because he had a very high fever.

I don't use ear thermometers because most kids don't like them, and I don't think they're very accurate. Instead I use the type of thermometer you swipe across the forehead. That's the best way to get a read on a kid. Putting a rectal thermometer in her butt sucks for the baby and for Mom too.

When in doubt, I've always taken my kids' temperature. I take it at the drop of a hat. I've learned from experience that a fever can be their only symptom of an illness, and it can make them feel very crummy. Once when we were hiking in the Olympic Mountains, my daughters were both behaving abominably. When we got back to the car, I took their temperatures, and they were both around 102°F. (Yes, we took the thermometer on vacation!) I felt bad because I didn't know they were sick, but at least then I had an explanation for their behavior!

—*Katherine Dee, MD, a mom of six-year-old twin daughters and a four-year-old son and a radiologist at the Seattle Breast Center, in Washington*

Dealing with a sick child can be extremely stressful, particularly for new parents. Fortunately, the medicines are all flavored these days, so it is generally not difficult to get babies to take them.

One thing that has changed since we were kids is that aspirin and all products that contain aspirin *should not* be given to children under the age of 20 years old, due to the risk of Reye's syndrome, a condition that can cause fatal liver failure.

With a physician's recommendation, children can be given acetaminophen (Tylenol), but it's essential to check the label for proper dosage based on weight and age. Pediatricians might also recommend giving ibuprofen (Motrin) to babies after the age of six months, using weight and age to determine the proper dose. For lingering persistent fevers, some pediatricians recommend alternating Tylenol and Motrin so that your baby doesn't get too much of either medication. (Talk with your doctor before giving your baby this or any medication.)

When a child has a fever, it's important to maintain adequate hydration. Research suggests that for every 1 degree increase in body temperature, there's a 10 to 15 percent increase in the baby's metabolic rate and a significant loss of body water. Depending on the baby's age, pediatricians might recommend offering babies fluids such as Pedialyte or chicken soup.

—*Stacey Weiland, MD*

Protecting Your Baby from the Sun

We have such a love-hate relationship with the sun, and this achieves new heights when you have a baby to care for. Babies' skin is so fragile and delicate that it's especially vulnerable to the sun.

The American Academy of Pediatrics (AAP) urges parents to keep babies under six months old out of the sun. In particular, limit sun exposure between 10 a.m. and 4 p.m., when the ultraviolet (UV) rays are strongest. Give babies plenty of shade, under a tree, umbrella, or canopy. Dress your baby in clothing that covers most of her body. Clothing made from fabric with a tight weave is best because it helps reduce the skin's exposure to UV light. Not sure if your fabric measures up? Hold it up to the light to see how much light shines through. The less light, the better. To protect your baby's face and eyes from the sun, put a hat on her.

If there's no shade in sight, the AAP gives the A-OK to put sunscreen on small areas of a baby's skin, such as her face and the back of her hands.

For babies older than six months, you should apply sunscreen to all exposed skin. As you have likely noticed, having a baby takes a lot of the spontaneity out of life. You have to plan ahead because you need to apply the sunscreen 30 minutes before going outside so that the skin will have time to absorb it. Sunscreen wears off after swimming, sweating, and even just from soaking into the skin. Be sure to reapply it every two hours.

It's critical to protect your baby's eyes from the sun too. Because an infant's pupils don't shrink at bright light, more than 75 percent of the ultraviolet radiation that she's exposed to enters her eyes, compared with only 10 percent for an adult.

～ℰ⁓

I live in Florida, and sunburn is a big concern here. A baby can get sunburned by spending just five minutes in the sun. I was careful not to take my babies outside in the sun between 10 a.m. and 2 p.m. We went out to play or exercise early in the morning or later in the evening.
—*Melanie Bone, MD, a mom of four, ages 16, 15, 14, and 13, a grandmom of one grandson, a gynecologist, the founder of the Cancer Sensibility Foundation, and the author of the syndicated column Surviving Life and the book* Cancer, What's Next?, *in West Palm Beach, FL*

～ℰ⁓

My husband and I took our babies to the beach early and often. By about six months, they were able to sit on the beach and play in the sand. To keep them safe in the sun, we set up a tent for them to play under, and we also used lots of sunscreen and hats. And it's not like we left them sitting in the sun for hours!
—*Alanna Kramer, MD*

My daughter had very sensitive skin. We took her to Grand Cayman with my in-laws when she was about six months old. I slathered her in some SPF 50 baby sunscreen, and she developed the most horrific rash! I don't know if it was an allergy to the lotion or a heat rash, but she had to be inside for most of the trip, which was unfortunate. After that experience, we tried several other brands of sunscreen, and she seemed to do the best with Coppertone Water Babies SPF 50.

—*Stacey Weiland, MD*

Mommy MD Guides-Recommended Product
K&J Sunprotective Clothing

Think your baby's delicate skin is safe under her onesie? Think again! No standard onesie or T-shirt provides adequate protection from the sun during daily play—and certainly not on a day at the beach. Regular cotton has an ultraviolet protection factor (UPF) of about 5. Most of the sun's harmful rays go straight through it.

To complicate matters, the American Academy of Pediatrics (AAP) recommends using only a minimal amount of sunscreen on babies younger than six months.

But the danger of sunburn is very real. Just one blistering sunburn in childhood doubles a person's lifetime risk of melanoma, which is a potentially fatal form of skin cancer.

The best way to protect a baby from the sun's rays is with sunprotective clothing, yet some sun-protective clothing contains chemicals. K&J Sunprotective clothing, invented by Mona Gohara, MD, a dermatologist and a mom of four- and two-year-old sons, is chemical free. These shirts have a UPF of 50, and because they're made of very tightly woven fabric, they block 99 percent of the sun's harmful rays.

K&J T-shirts are printed with fun graphics and cute sayings such as "I scream for ice cream." They're available in sizes zero to three months to 6T, and they cost $22 each. You can buy them at **KJSUNPROTECTIVECLOTHING.COM**.

In Miami, we're big on skin cancer protection. I keep sunscreen in my car at all times. I try to put it on my kids every day, even now that they're in school.

I used to buy the more popular sunscreen brands. But I've read about potential hazards of the chemicals in some sunscreens. I don't know how much of that is real, but now I choose more natural products, such as Blue Lizard. My daughter also likes Purple Prairie Organic.

—*Michelle Paley, MD, PA*

RALLIE'S TIP

My middle son was very sensitive to the ingredients in baby sunscreen when he was younger, and his skin would break out in a rash whenever I tried to slather him up before taking him outside. I finally gave up on the sunscreen lotions and protected him from the sun the old-fashioned way. I dressed him in a hat and lightweight clothing that covered his arms and legs, and I used the umbrella on the stroller to shade him from the sun.

By the time my son was about a year old, his skin wasn't quite as sensitive, and he was able to tolerate sunscreen without breaking out in a rash, as long as I washed it off his skin an hour or two after putting it on.

For each of my babies, I had a favorite lightweight pair of pants and lightweight, long-sleeved shirt that they could wear to protect them from the sun. I also had a blanket and a sling made out of sun-blocking fabric. A friend of mine made the sling, and she kept the "tail" of the sling long so that I could drape it over my baby's face. You can also buy UV-protective blankets and stroller covers online.

—*Kristie McNealy, MD, a mom of eight- and five-year-old daughters and three- and one-year-old sons and a blogger at KristieMcNealy.com, in Denver, CO*

Before my sons were six months old, I didn't put any sunscreen on them at all. Instead, I used sun avoidance, such as having them play under a tent at the beach. I also dress my sons in sun-protective clothing. (See "Mommy MD Guides–Recommended Product: K&J Sunprotective Clothing.")

When to Call Your Doctor

If your baby develops a rash after being in the sun, call your doctor. Your baby might be experiencing an allergic reaction to the sunscreen.

If your baby shows any sign of sunburn, such as redness or blistering, call your doctor right away or take her to an emergency room for evaluation. Because sunburn can lead to serious dehydration or infection, it can be life-threatening in infants and babies.

After my sons were older than six months, I used Neutrogena Baby sunscreen because it's a physical blocker, not a chemical sunscreen.

—*Amy J. Derick, MD*

As a dermatologist, I was always more freaked out about skin things than nonskin things. Even though I had to pass the dermatology board exams to practice medicine, I would all of a sudden forget everything I had learned when it came to my own kid.

Both of my babies were very sensitive to the sun, and they developed rashes whenever they were in the sun for extended periods of time. That was very stressful. I wondered if they were having reactions to the sun, or if something else was going on. I discovered that they were actually allergic to an ingredient in the sunscreen I was using. We put sunscreen on our boys pretty much all of the time, except during the winter months. Truth be told, we should have been doing it then too!

Right away, we switched sunscreens. I found one that I love: Blue Lizard Suncream. It's chemical free because it protects from the sun using an ingredient called titanium dioxide that acts as a physical blocker. You can buy it online for around $10 a bottle.

The key with sunscreen is that you have to reapply it every two hours, all over your baby's body, even under his clothing. You also need to use a lot: a shot-glass size amount on anyone over the age of six months, every two hours.

It's also very important to protect your baby's eyes from the sun. Hats are great, and sunglasses are too. The ultraviolet rays of the sun can damage your baby's eyes just as much as they can damage her skin. It's very important to keep them protected.

When my sons were babies, I always made certain they were wearing sunglasses whenever they were exposed to intensive sunlight.

—Mona Gohara, MD, a mom of four- and two-year-old sons, a dermatologist in private practice, an assistant clinical professor in the department of dermatology at Yale University, and a cofounder of K&J Sunprotective Clothing, in Danbury, CT

Watching Out for Product Recalls

Product recalls used to be as rare as hen's teeth. But these days, there seem to be so many. When a product is recalled, it's for a good reason, and you'll want to know about it to keep your baby safe. One way to be in the loop is to fill out and mail in the product registration forms that you receive with the products you buy.

Another way to be notified of recalls is to sign up for alerts, such as those posted on the Consumer Product Safety Commission's website, CPSC.gov. Also consider joining e-mail lists such as the one for Safe Kids USA. Their enewsletter offers valuable safety information, including the latest recalls.

I downloaded the "Baby Bargains" book and signed up for the updates. The company sends e-mails about product recalls immediately. It's been very reliable.

—Rachel S. Rohde, MD

I've already gotten two e-mails regarding product recalls, but I found that it's really important to pay attention to product serial numbers and the date that I bought the item before I get too excited. Once I checked the serial numbers on the products I had bought, I found that neither of the recalls applied to those items.

—Jennifer Bacani McKenney, MD

As a pediatrician, I keep up with the recalls, and I get mail alerts as well. I'm not sure how my name got on the lists, but I get things in the mail and via e-mail as well. Our pediatric department is very careful to notify parents about recalls. Asking your child's pediatrician is very helpful. Sometimes pediatricians post the recall notices and alerts on their websites or distribute flyers in their offices.

—*Sonia Ng, MD*

༄

I'm a pediatrician and an internal medicine specialist, so I keep on top of all product recalls. I get a lot of questions about recalls from my patients, who are wondering what to do. Especially with medication recalls, you have to carefully check the lot numbers on the package to see if the product that you purchased has been recalled. I find that pharmacists are very helpful answering questions about medication recalls.

For my family, when a brand-name product has been recalled, I simply switch to the store's generic brand. For instance, I might buy Walmart's generic acetaminophen rather than Tylenol.

—*Christy Valentine, MD*

Getting on a Schedule

Sure, babies don't really make appointments, nor do they have to punch a time clock. But you do! Just like routines, schedules, and organization suit most grown-ups, they are helpful for babies too. Perhaps even more so. Because babies can't communicate very well, and especially because they are just learning about their world, predictable routines help them to make sense of what must seem like a very bewildering place.

༄

Routine is one of the most important things for kids. It's the cornerstone of development. A predictable routine should start practically at birth. In the beginning, the routine is probably more important for Mom, but it can also impact the baby from the beginning.

I found that routine was critical to keeping organized. I did my best to have very organized days.

—*Gabriella Cardone, MD, a mom of five-, three-, and one-year-old daughters and a pediatric emergency physician at Texas Children's Hospital, in Houston*

Our twins were born full-term, so they came home from the hospital when they were only three days old. Everyone urges new parents to get on a schedule. One of the challenges of having twins is that you can't feed and diaper two babies at once! So my husband and I created a staggered schedule for the babies, in which one twin was always 10 to 15 minutes behind the other. That way I could feed and burp one baby, and then turn to the other. That worked best, especially if I was taking care of the twins by myself.

—*Brooke Jackson, MD, a mom of 3½-year-old twin girls and a 14-month-old son and a dermatologist and medical director of the Skin Wellness Center of Chicago, in Illinois*

When my twins were first born, I breastfed them on demand. But as they got older and gained weight, I was so tired that I couldn't continue feeding them every 1½ to 2 hours. Instead I put them on a schedule, and if one woke up to eat, I would wake the other one too. We adopted a fairly strict schedule, both with feedings and sleeping.

In some ways, looking back, it was a bit rigid, but it seemed to work well for all of us. As my twins entered toddlerhood, having that foundation actually made them happier, more secure children. Developmentally that makes sense because children in that age group need and thrive on routine.

—*Ann Contrucci, MD*

Getting on a schedule is so helpful for kids so they know what to expect. When I went back to work, I had to have my family on a schedule. The nanny arrived at a certain time each day, and my husband and I came home at a certain time each day. Having a set routine made life so much easier.

However, you don't want to be too structured and regimented. I think it's important to have some flexibility. Otherwise you lose all of those special, spontaneous moments that make parenting such a gift. If you spend too much time focusing on what you should be doing, you aren't as focused on your child, which is the most precious thing.

—*Mona Gohara, MD*

Chapter 3
3rd Month

Your Baby This Month

YOUR BABY'S DEVELOPMENT

As your baby continues to learn and grow, he's doing so at his own rate. All babies are different, unique, and special. The third month is a wonderful time. Babies this age are generally more alert, active, and responsive than newborns.

Around three months, your baby's eyes start working in concert, and he probably no longer looks cross-eyed when he focuses. Also, at this age, his pupils start to shrink in bright light or dilate when he's in the dark. Babies as young as three months can distinguish photos of adult male and female faces. Around this age, your baby might be easily distracted by an interesting sight or sound.

Your baby is still most attracted to bold, black-and-white patterns or contrasting colors, such as dark objects on light walls. You might notice his ability to focus improving, as he studies things like a floral pattern on a couch with great concentration.

Before this time, your baby depended upon others to initiate interaction. But by the end of his third month, your baby will probably start to engage people with facial expressions, sounds, and even gestures. He'll start to squeal with delight, and he might even be able to laugh out loud.

When your baby is around 10 weeks old, he'll start to distinguish night from day—hurrah! By the end of your baby's third month, his number of daytime naps might drop from around four to three, and he'll begin to sleep longer at night. Three-quarters of babies sleep for one long unbroken period during the night by this time. Most three-month-old babies sleep around five hours during the day and around 10 hours at night.

Around now, your baby probably has enough muscle control and strength to lift his head up to 45 degrees. In yoga, this is aptly called the Baby Cobra pose. He might even be able to lift his head up to 90 degrees when he's having tummy time. Some babies can raise their chests, supported by their arms. Your baby might hold his head up for a while and check out his surroundings by rotating his head from side to side.

By now, your baby's hands have loosened, and he begins simple hand play. Your baby's hands are probably his new favorite toy! If you hand your baby a toy now, his fingers will curl around it, and he'll hold it for a while—until he's bored or distracted by something else. Around now, your baby is able to hold onto your fingers, and he will probably do it every chance that he gets, in a wonderful finger "hug."

Your baby likely spends a lot of time reaching out for things. Look out! Hair, eyeglasses, and ties are well within your baby's reach. There's a good chance that your baby's little hands often find their way into his mouth. Your baby might be able to bring his hands together in a joyful baby clap.

Your baby can also communicate his happiness to you now with spontaneous smiles, which no doubt elicit spontaneous smiles from you too. At this age, your baby will begin to identify the behaviors that get your attention. Your baby might be able to make simple vowel sounds now, such as *ooh* and *aah*. He can probably laugh out loud and squeal with delight.

Babies this age generally cry less than they did at two months. At three months, most babies cry around an hour each day. As your baby struggles to understand his world, he looks for predictable patterns. If you stray from his routine, he might act unsettled, even upset.

By this time, you and your baby are becoming better at understanding each other's nonverbal and verbal communication. Different cries are starting to mean different things. This makes communication easier—and more fun.

Taking Care of You
Pace yourself. Parenting is a marathon, not a sprint.

Justification for a Celebration
Your baby's first expressions of joy—first smiles, first claps, first laughs—are certainly cause for celebration.

Reading to Your Baby

Your baby spent nine months inside of you listening to the sound of your voice—his favorite sound. He still loves to listen to you, and one wonderful way to indulge that is by reading to him. (And why not enjoy this now because when he's a teenager, he'll do everything possible to tune you out!)

Reading to your baby offers many benefits, including teaching him about communication; introducing concepts such as stories, numbers, letters, colors, and shapes; building listening skills; and giving him information about the world around him. So what's the answer? Look in a book!

c/o

My babies always enjoyed the Richard Scarry books, but we didn't start reading these books to them until they were about four to six months old.

—*Michelle Storms, MD, a mom of 24- and 20-year-old sons and a 21-year-old daughter, the assistant director of the Marquette Family Medicine Residency Program, in Marquette, MI, and a member of the health professionals board for Intact America*

c/o

Every night after bath, before bed, we read books. It's part of our bedtime routine. I think that structure is so important for kids, so that they have an idea what to expect each day.

Reading is wonderful when kids are small. It's even more fun when your kids get older, and they start reading to you.

—*Mona Gohara, MD, a mom of four- and two-year-old sons, a dermatologist in private practice, an assistant clinical professor in the department of dermatology at Yale University, and a cofounder of K&J Sunprotective Clothing, in Danbury, CT*

c/o

It is great to read to your baby, but choose those books carefully! Once your child gets old enough to recognize the content of the story (which certainly won't happen during the baby's first year), many children beg to hear the same story over and over and over. You can really get tired of a boring story! So make sure that the storybook has enough subtlety and imagination to charm you after 50 readings, or you'll want to pull your hair out. No kidding!

—*Elizabeth Berger, MD, a mom of a 28-year-old son and a 26-year-old daughter, a child psychiatrist, and the author of* Raising Kids with Character, *in New York City*

∽

My husband and I often sit together with our baby and have story time. We usually read in the nursery while I'm nursing the baby or while she is getting ready for a nap. It's kind of funny because so far we've only been reading books that my husband and I read, like *How to Win Friends and Influence People* and *Eat, Pray, Love,* so maybe our baby will end up being self-motivated, but dramatic!

I think that the important thing is that our baby hears our voices and she hears how the language sounds. When she understands a little more of what we're saying, we'll probably have to back it off to *Go, Dog, Go* or some of our other childhood favorites.

—*Jennifer Bacani McKenney, MD, a mom of a two-month-old daughter and a family physician, in Fredonia, KS*

RALLIE'S TIP

When my youngest two children were babies, I was still in my medical residency program, and I had lots of reading to do. While I was holding my sons or nursing them, I would read my medical books and journals out loud. I'm sure they didn't particularly enjoy or understand the content, but they were happy to hear the sound of my voice. Reading the material out loud helped me to learn what I needed to know while still spending time with my babies.

When my sons got older, that little trick didn't work anymore. They still loved having me read to them, but they insisted on The Berenstain Bears *or* Click Clack Moo: Cows That Type.

∽

I started reading to my oldest daughter before she was even born. The very first thing I ever bought for her was a collection of Beatrix Potter stories. I've been reading to my kids ever since.

We don't have a set reading time; we pretty much read anytime, all day, whenever the mood strikes us, whenever we need some quiet time, or if someone isn't feeling well.

—Kristie McNealy, MD, a mom of eight- and five-year-old daughters and three- and one-year-old sons and a blogger at KristieMcNealy.com, in Denver, CO

When my older son was born, I had a babysitter come help me in my home. She had been watching children for decades. On her first day, she arrived at my house bearing a huge bag of books, which I thought was odd because my baby was only four weeks old. The babysitter explained that it's never too early to start reading to your baby. Babies love to see the colors on the page, hear the sound of your voice, and feel the closeness of your body. I watched as the babysitter held my son and read to him. He was fascinated! Ever since, my favorite baby gift to give has been books.

—Cathie Lippman, MD, a mom of 30- and 28-year-old sons and a physician who specializes in environmental and preventive medicine at the Lippman Center for Optimal Health, in Beverly Hills, CA

Every night, our family has a ritual: dinner, bath, books, bed. We started that at the very beginning. I have pictures of me reading to my daughter when she was a baby. Back then, it might have been more important for me than for her to establish that routine. But even at a very young age, babies benefit from hearing your voice, listening to rhyming sounds, and cuddling.

Our kids have received so many books as gifts, and I also love giving books as gifts to other children. I find that because really young kids love to read the same books over and over and over, it doesn't work as well borrowing books from the library. There were some books my kids wanted to hear every single night. Some of their favorite books early on were *Goodnight Moon* and any Maisy book. They're so silly, but kids love them. We all also love books by Mo Willems. He's hilarious.

—Michelle Paley, MD, PA, a mom of two and a psychiatrist and psychotherapist in private practice, in Miami Beach, FL

Leaking Urine

No one told you about this side effect of having a baby? They didn't tell us either. Welcome to the club! Millions of women have this problem.

Urinary incontinence is twice as common in women as in men. Pregnancy, childbirth, and menopause are major reasons why. In pregnancy, babies push down on the bladder, urethra, and pelvic floor muscles. This pressure can weaken the pelvic floor muscles. Labor and vaginal birth can weaken pelvic floor support and damage nerves that control the bladder. Most problems with bladder control during pregnancy and childbirth go away after the muscles have time to heal.

If urinary incontinence is a problem for you, consider talking with your doctor or midwife. They have several tools to help, including medication, exercise therapy, biofeedback, and surgery.

〜

My last pregnancy was a very hard one, and I had complications that affected my pelvic floor. I was also working long shifts and came home to two toddlers afterward, and I didn't get the rehab that I needed. Leaking urine is common. I used every opportunity that I had to strengthen my pelvic floor, and I continue to do so. For example, when I took the girls to school in the stroller, I made an effort to tighten the appropriate muscles and stand up straight, which also worked my abs. When I played with the baby and lifted her in the air, I did the same exercises, and I lifted her up and down a few more times to work my arms too!

Because it's hard to find time to work out with three children, I exercise while I play with my children or while I watch them play. I work my pelvic floor, back, and abs. Whenever I lie on the floor and start exercising, invariably my 18-month-old or my

? When to Call Your Doctor

Urinary incontinence should begin to resolve within a week or two after your baby is born. If it persists past that, talk with your doctor or midwife.

three-year-old hops on top of my belly for a horsey ride. The girls think it's a game and a lot of fun. They also know Mom is exercising, and they try to imitate me. This helps them to understand that exercising is fun and important.

Once you have babies, it's important to continue to strengthen your pelvic floor muscles to keep things where they belong and to help with bladder control.

—*Gabriella Cardone, MD, a mom of five-, three-, and one-year-old daughters and a pediatric emergency physician at Texas Children's Hospital, in Houston*

Thank goodness, I didn't have a problem with leaking urine because I had a C-section. However, the C-section was a problem in and of itself!

—*Christy Valentine, MD, a mom of a five-year-old daughter, a specialist in pediatrics and internal medicine, and the founder of the Valentine Medical Center, in Gretna, LA*

Personally, I didn't have any problems with leaking urine, but I've had many patients with this condition, especially women who delivered big babies after long labors. The bladder can get bruised during labor and delivery, and it needs time to heal. Also, after your baby is born, your estrogen level drops, which makes your bladder more "irritable." Plus, new moms who are breastfeeding are really thirsty, so they drink a lot of extra fluids, which works their bladders even more.

It can help to wear a pad. Sometimes I suggest wearing one or two super tampons to help support the bladder.

—*Melanie Bone, MD, a mom of four, ages 16, 15, 14, and 13, a grandmom of one grandson, a gynecologist, the founder of the Cancer Sensibility Foundation, and the author of the syndicated column Surviving Life and the book* Cancer, What's Next?, *in West Palm Beach, FL*

RALLIE'S TIP

When Nature calls, do her bidding! Babies relieve their bladders and bowels with abandon whenever the need arises, and moms can take a lesson from their little ones. No matter how busy you are, make time to empty your bladder whenever the need arises. Frequently emptying your bladder throughout the day can reduce your risk of getting a urinary tract infection. Heeding the call of Nature also applies to moving your bowels. If you feel the urge to go and you ignore it, you might be inviting abdominal discomfort and constipation.

Most women experience bladder weakness and leakage of urine for a few weeks after delivery, and I was no different. After the births of my first two sons, I tried to remember to do Kegel exercises regularly to improve my bladder control, but I just didn't enjoy doing them.

I found that one of the best ways to improve my bladder control was jumping on a mini trampoline for a few minutes a day. Like Kegels, the exercise forces you to tighten the same muscles you would if you were trying to stop the flow of urine. As soon as my doctor gave me the okay to begin exercising after the birth of my third child, I started using a mini trampoline, and I regained control of my bladder in far less time than I had following the births of my first two children using Kegel exercises alone.

Coping with Colic

The word *colic* strikes fear in the hearts of parents-to-be. Colic is very common. It's estimated that up to 40 percent of babies have it. But knowing this isn't very comforting if your baby has the condition. How can you tell for sure if your baby has colic? When a healthy baby cries for more than three hours per day, more than three days per week, for at least three weeks, it's called colic. Generally, the condition starts between the third and sixth week of life and ends by the time the baby is three months old. Unfortunately, the only cure for colic is time.

⤫

If a baby is crying a great deal due to colic, I think the most important thing is to make him feel comfortable and secure, by holding him and swaddling him. This will help him be less needy as he grows up. Of course, you have to feel confident that your baby has colic and not some condition that needs immediate attention.

—Hana R. Solomon, MD, a mom of four, ages 35 to 19, a

board-certified pediatrician, and the author of Clearing the Air One Nose at a Time: Caring for Your Personal Filter, *in Columbia, MO*

Almost as soon as my milk came in, my daughter screamed constantly throughout the day, except for a half-hour in the morning and a half-hour in the afternoon, when she took brief naps. This was one of the reasons I went back to work a month after delivery, and I found an earth mother with incredible patience to comfort my daughter while she screamed. It was also helpful to have reassurance that this would probably resolve at three months.

> —*Stuart Jeanne Bramhall, MD, a mom of a 30-year-old daughter and a child and adolescent psychiatrist, in New Plymouth, New Zealand*

My twins definitely were colicky babies for their first six to eight weeks. My husband and I tried everything. Car rides, the car seat on top of the dryer, the hair dryer (worked nicely), the snuggie packs, and swings were great! When they were four to six weeks old, the "baby burrito" (aka swaddling) worked wonders. The bonus was they looked awfully cute with just their tiny faces sticking out of the blankets.

> —*Ann Contrucci, MD, a mom of 12-year-old boy-girl twins who works as a pediatric emergency physician, in Atlanta, GA*

My older daughter had colic. One thing I found that seemed to help was using a brand of bottle called Dr. Brown's. I think that this type of bottle helped with her colic because it reduces the amount of air the baby ingests while she's eating. But really, there is no single "cure" for colic. You can try several things and see what works for your baby. Mostly, you just have to survive it, as it can last for several weeks.

> —*Sadaf T. Bhutta, MD, a mom of a five-year-old daughter and three-year-old triplets and an assistant professor and the fellowship director of pediatric radiology at the University of Arkansas for Medical Sciences and Arkansas Children's Hospital, both in Little Rock*

My older daughter had colic. It was awful. I used to joke that if my ob-gyn had a return policy, I might have taken her up on it. It's hard to be joyful with a difficult child.

At the time, my husband and I lived in a tiny one-bedroom apartment in Manhattan. When my daughter screamed, all of the neighbors would hear her. So on top of her keeping *us* up, the whole apartment complex had to know she was up.

My baby had colic in January, so there was nowhere for us to go. I tried everything to calm my daughter down. Mainly, I put her in the Snugli and walked around our apartment for hours and hours and hours.

My daughter's "colic" turned out to be an allergy to breast milk. I was beside myself when a baby nurse told me that. I'm a scientist, so I stopped breastfeeding for a few days. My daughter stopped crying. So I started nursing again. Sure enough, the baby nurse was right. Of course, it took me weeks to convince myself. I was devastated. They say that humans develop antigens to milk because of all of the cow's milk we drink, and that can make it difficult for the baby to tolerate breast milk. Perhaps if I had eliminated dairy products in the weeks before I delivered my baby, I could have nursed her longer.

—*Eva Ritvo, MD, a mom of 20- and 15-year-old daughters, a psychiatrist, and a coauthor of* The Beauty Prescription, *in Miami Beach, FL*

~~~

All *four* of my babies had colic. It defies all logic! My babies all cried for most of their waking hours, until they were each around three months old.

For each of my babies, I was able to find something that did help. One was soothed by the sound of the vacuum. My older son would calm down if I put him in his baby swing, but on his belly. He looked like Superman swinging back and forth. (Certainly don't try this unless you will be within reach of your baby!) Another was pacified by my pacing around with her. For my youngest, a fast-paced ride along the neighborhood sidewalks in an umbrella stroller was helpful.

I wish that I had known then what I know now about probiotics. I would definitely have given my colicky babies probiotics. You can buy infant formulations at health food stores; simply follow the directions on the package label or as per your child's physician.

—*Ann Kulze, MD, a mom of 22- and 15-year-old daughters and 20- and 19-year-old sons; a nationally recognized nutrition expert, motivational speaker, and family physician; and the author of the best-selling book* Eat Right for Life, *in Charleston, SC*

RALLIE'S TIP

Two of my sons were colicky, and I think I tried everything in the world to deal with the condition. One very effective remedy for colic is probiotics, but unfortunately, I didn't know about them when my children were babies. The science supporting the use of probiotics in children and infants is very new.

A study published in the January 2007 issue of the medical journal Pediatrics *demonstrated that daily doses of* Lactobacillus reuteri *significantly reduced symptoms in infants diagnosed with colic. Researchers reported that by the seventh day of treatment, 95 percent of infants receiving probiotics showed an improvement in colic symptoms. Only 7 percent of infants receiving simethicone, a commonly prescribed anti-gas medication, demonstrated a reduction in colic symptoms.*

Although parents of colicky babies might be sorely tempted to take matters into their own hands, it's best to consult with a physician before administering any medications or supplements to infants and children.

Crying is normal baby behavior! The average baby cries up to three hours a day. By definition, colicky babies cry more, sometimes much more. If your baby is crying this much, it can be tremendously helpful to have a friend or family member come over. Having someone else handle even half an hour of that crying can make a big difference.

Lots of new research is being done on swaddling colicky babies. I found that getting the stretchy cotton blankets was best, because the "give" of the blankets made the swaddling stay on better when

I made a "baby burrito." Talking in a low, rumbly voice with your baby tucked next to your chest is also very calming.

My second son seemed to have worse reflux, and he cried a lot. A friend of mine who's a pediatrician would come over to hold him and give me a break. She'd take him upstairs so I couldn't hear him crying, and she joked that he just needed a change in altitude.

New research suggests probiotics might help. I definitely would have tried probiotics if I had known about them then!

*—Amy Baxter, MD, a mom
of 13- and 10-year-old sons
and an 8-year-old daughter,
the CEO of MMJ Labs, and the director of emergency research of
Children's Healthcare of Atlanta at Scottish Rite, in Atlanta, GA*

My eldest cried almost nonstop for four months. I was breastfeeding and eating a very healthy diet. I tried to remove all lactose and soy from my diet. I tried giving her reflux medications and infant massages—just about anything and everything you could imagine.

Ultimately, I tried a hypoallergenic infant formula, and within hours, I *finally* had the happy, smiling baby that everyone else took for granted. When my baby was 11 months old, we had her tested for food allergies, and we found out that she had a severe allergy to egg whites!

In my second pregnancy, I eliminated the 10 most common allergy-producing foods from my diet and tried breastfeeding again. Within two weeks, my infant had bloody diarrhea, and we were in the specialist's office debating the need for a colonoscopy. Having learned from my first baby, I stopped breastfeeding and tried the hypoallergenic formula. The problem resolved within days.

When I became pregnant with my third baby, and my eldest spilled the beans to our pediatrician, my pediatrician looked at me and said, "Please promise me you are not breastfeeding this one!" I now try to support all my new moms whether they decide to breastfeed or bottlefeed, and I share my experience. Breastfeeding is something I think that every mom should attempt, but they should remember that not all babies do better with breast milk!

—*Marra S. Francis, MD, a mom of seven-, six-, and four-year-old daughters and an ob-gyn, in The Woodlands, TX*

My older son screamed all day, every day. It would get so bad that I would have to leave the house. I couldn't tolerate the crying.

Thank goodness for my husband. He would sit in his rocking chair with earplugs in and his hunting headphones on top and rock our son for hours and hours—while he shrieked. Periodically, my husband would ask me, "Is this ever going to end? Will he go to kindergarten yelling like this?"

If you have a baby like that, you have to know where your breaking point is—and act before you reach it. When I was home alone with the baby, if I felt I was nearing my breaking point, I'd put him in his crib, close the door, jump in the shower, and stand there until the hot water ran out. I knew that it didn't matter what I did; my son was going to scream anyway.

My son cried like that until he was around eight months old. Today he's the happiest child you could imagine.

—*Carrie Brown, MD, a mom of seven- and five-year-old sons and a general pediatrician who treats medically complex children and specializes in palliative care at Arkansas Children's Hospital, in Little Rock*

My third child had the worst colic. It always seemed to flare up after dinnertime, and it could go on for hours and hours into the night. He would cry and cry, and there was little that I could do to soothe him. My husband and I would try all of the usual things—changing, feeding, burping, walking, and rocking—all to no avail. It was *very* hard to deal with, especially for my husband.

Maybe it was because he was my third child and I was more relaxed, and maybe because it seemed like a classic case of colic when I looked it up in my Harriet Lane Pediatrics Handbook, but I didn't freak out about it and I just rode it out. My son seemed to have the classic "Rule of Three" conditions—crying for three or more hours per day, at least three times per week, within a three-month period.

I never looked into any medications, herbs, or really changing my diet. I just figured that colic was something that my son would eventually grow out of, and he did at about three months. It might sound weird, but I even looked at this period as almost a special time with my son. He needed me, and I was there for him. I would cuddle him, rock him, sing to him, hold him, and nurse him, and eventually, *eventually*, he would fall asleep.

—*Stacey Weiland, MD, a mom of a 12-year-old daughter and 7- and 5-year-old sons and an internist/gastroenterologist, in Denver, CO*

Stressing Less

New baby, not enough sleep, who wouldn't be stressed?

∽

Even in my son's first year, I continued to make time to ride my horses, which helped me stay balanced.

—*Leigh Andrea DeLair, MD, a mom of a two-year-old son and a family physician, in Danville, KY*

∽

I received this great advice early on: It's impossible to be Superdoc, Supermom, and Superwife all at the same time.

—*Cathie Lippman, MD*

∽

As a mom, it's easy to take everything too seriously. But parenting issues aren't black and white. The recommendations in books are just guidelines. As long as you keep your kids safe and give them lots of love, the rest comes kind of naturally.

—Heather Orman-Lubell, MD, a mom of 10- and six-year-old sons and a pediatrician in private practice at Yardley Pediatrics of St. Christopher's Hospital for Children, in Pennsylvania

I found that if I was stressed, my babies felt it. I don't think it's an accident that a lot of firstborn babies scream all of the time; they're "colicky" babies. Yet a lot of second- and third-born babies are more laid-back. I think it's because the parents have "chilled."

Looking back, I probably didn't do as much to take care of myself that first year as I should have. You sort of lose yourself. I should have taken more time to have someone else watch the babies while I went for a run or went shopping. I didn't do that enough. No question you're a better parent when you have some time away from your children, and you shouldn't feel guilty about that.

—Ann Contrucci, MD

There's so much about parenting that's out of your control. You have to try to let go of any obsessive-compulsive tendencies you might have.

It was hard for me to do this. I had my medical practice for five years before I had kids; my practice was my child. But I quickly learned to back off from my work and focus on my family first. Instead of focusing on that chronic sense of "I can't do it all," I focused on thinking, "I'm doing the best that I can." Really, that's all that you can do.

—Brooke Jackson, MD, a mom of 3½-year-old twin girls and a 14-month-old son and a dermatologist and medical director of the Skin Wellness Center of Chicago, in Illinois

My advice: Don't sweat the small stuff. I used to be the most uptight person, and then I had kids. It changed my life. I don't worry nearly so much now about things like crumbs on the floor. Having kids has even made my work life easier because I don't get upset about insignificant stuff.

My husband says that I walk around with birds chirping around my head because I'm so happy. He'll look at me and say, "Chirp, chirp."
—*Rebecca Reamy, MD, a mom of six- and one-year-old sons and a pediatrician in emergency medicine at Children's Healthcare of Atlanta, in Georgia*

∾⌒∿

One thing I found to help alleviate stress was taking a few minutes for myself on my way home from work. I would just park my car for a few minutes and look at a garden. It's important to block out a little extra time in life to make transitions easier.

Whenever you start to feel exhausted or irritable, take a step back and think, *What have I done lately to take care of myself?* New moms often feel like they're running behind, racing to catch up. It took me some time to realize that I didn't have to crush all of my activities together and leave no time for transitions. Give yourself a little space and time between events in so that you don't always have to rush.

Mommy MD Guides–Recommended Product
Natural Calm

Many Americans adults are deficient in magnesium, which is an essential mineral that helps to offset the negative effects of stress. Magnesium can help boost brainpower, especially in people with memory problems. It's useful in alleviating a number of respiratory symptoms, and it can ease a migraine pronto. It's very soothing to the gastrointestinal tract and has wonderful laxative properties. In people suffering from anxiety or insomnia, magnesium can promote a sense of calm and can facilitate more restful sleep.

An easy, tasty way to get more magnesium is with a supplement called Natural Calm. It's a powder that dissolves easily in water. It comes in several organic flavors, sweetened with organic stevia.

You can buy Natural Calm online and in health food stores for $15 to $16.

—*Nancy Rappaport, MD, a mom of 21- and 16-year-old daughters and an 18-year-old son, an assistant professor of psychiatry at Harvard Medical School, an attending child and adolescent psychiatrist in the Cambridge, MA, public schools, and the author of* In Her Wake: A Child Psychiatrist Explores the Mystery of Her Mother's Suicide

RALLIE'S TIP

You're a whole new person after your baby comes. Consequently, you're not as prepared to deal with the little stressors of life that wouldn't have bothered you before. Before my babies were born, I didn't realize how much I relied on exercising outside to alleviate stress and to make me feel healthy and happy.

After my babies were born, I found that I was spending far more time in the house than I was accustomed to. I had a treadmill in my basement, and I used it regularly when my babies were napping, but it just wasn't the same as taking a jog outside in the fresh air. With the combined stress of adjusting to a new baby and being cooped up inside, I felt like I was on the verge of a meltdown at any moment.

Thankfully, my husband came to the rescue. As soon as he realized that I needed to spend more time in the great outdoors to de-stress and recharge my batteries, he would push me out the door to go for a run while he watched the children. I was always refreshed when I returned, which made life better for me and the whole family.

With my first baby, I was (probably like most new mothers) very concerned about doing everything "by the book." I remember feeling that if I didn't do everything perfectly "right" when my baby was an infant, then somehow I would be messing her up for the rest of her life! That's a lot of pressure.

This was most evident during sleep training. Prior to my daughter's birth, I had read books and talked to friends and decided that it was important for her to have a good sleep routine. From the time my baby was just a few weeks old, I tried to keep her on a feeding and sleeping schedule, but sometimes she got hungry before it was "time" to eat. Or sometimes she wouldn't sleep when she was supposed to. What was I doing wrong?

In my own sleep-deprived state, I was very stressed that my newborn was not sticking to my schedule! It sounds ridiculous to me now. But I cried while she cried. Finally, I called a friend who was also a pediatrician and a parent for advice. Her children seemed to be happy—and good sleepers! I had to know her secret!

My friend said, "Just relax. It will come. Rock that baby to sleep. Hold her. Feed her when she's hungry. The time will come when she can soothe herself and fall asleep on her own, but it's too early for that. So just relax and enjoy this baby!"

After hearing those words, a great sense of peace washed over me, and I took that advice to heart. And, yes, eventually my daughter began to follow a feeding schedule, and eventually she soothed herself back to sleep when she awoke at night. But that took months. And that's okay! I was much more relaxed about all of this with my two younger children, and I was able to enjoy their newborn periods so much more.

—*Lezli Braswell, MD, a mom of a six-year-old daughter and four-and one-year-old sons and a family physician, in Columbus, GA*

Preventing and Treating Acid Reflux

If you've ever had acid reflux, more accurately known as gastro-esophageal reflux but more commonly known as heartburn, you can understand why a baby who has it would cry and cry and cry. It *hurts*.

Acid reflux occurs when the contents of the stomach splash backward into the esophagus. It generally happens after a feeding, but it can happen when your baby cries, coughs, or strains to have a bowel movement.

Generally, infant acid reflux goes away as a baby grows and spends more time sitting up, around 12 to 18 months.

Babies with infant acid reflux sometimes spit up, cough, wheeze, refuse to eat, and cry when placed on their backs, especially right after eating.

One of our twins was a generally peaceful baby, but she cried whenever she was lying down. She would only sleep in her swing.

When she was around four months old, her pediatrician suspected she was having gastrointestinal discomfort and ordered a diagnostic test called a barium swallow. The results of the test showed that my baby had acid reflux. The doctor prescribed an infant dosage of Tagamet, and my daughter got better very quickly. The barium swallow is considered the gold standard in the diagnosis of reflux, and it is much better for the baby to undergo this one test with X-rays than to be in pain.

—*Lillian Schapiro, MD, a mom of 14-year-old twin girls and an eight-year-old daughter and an ob-gyn with Peachtree Women's Specialists, in Atlanta, GA*

One of our twins was diagnosed with acid reflux. Because it was so difficult to get two babies fed and to keep track of who was eating what and how much of it, we switched both girls to the million-dollar-special-reflux formula. It did help with our daughter's reflux, and as soon as she was able to sit up, the reflux pretty much went away.

—*Brooke Jackson, MD*

The muscular sphincter that acts like a valve between the baby's esophagus and stomach is very lax in infants. So all babies have a bit of reflux. It might not be bad enough to cause them to throw up, but it might be plenty to cause them pain.

Here's one trick that helps reduce reflux: When making formula, mix it by gently swirling it instead of shaking it so that you create fewer air bubbles. You can also let the formula sit in the fridge for a few hours to allow the bubbles to settle out.

At bedtime and naptime, it's also helpful to put a pillow under the head of your baby's mattress. This helps to keep the stomach contents in the stomach where they belong, rather than splashing up, or refluxing, into the esophagus. Putting a pillow under the mattress is safer than putting pillows or bedding around your baby's head.

—*Amy Baxter, MD*

When to Call Your Doctor

If you think that your baby has infant acid reflux, or if your baby isn't gaining weight or spits up forcefully, talk with your doctor about it.

If your baby has been diagnosed with infant acid reflux, call your doctor right away if your baby:

- Spits up yellow or green fluid, blood, or material that looks like coffee grounds
- Doesn't want to eat
- Has blood in his stool

My older son was a miserable baby. He vomited after every meal, and he screamed for hours every day. I bawled hysterically—a lot.

My son was diagnosed with acid reflux, and I tried everything to make him feel better. I was breastfeeding, so I tried an elimination diet. I stopped eating one food at a time to see if anything helped my baby. It didn't make a difference.

Even though I really wanted to breastfeed my son, I switched him to a hypoallergenic formula. We even tried giving him medication, but nothing made a difference. My son still vomited and cried all of the time, but at least he was growing. And that's really what it comes down to. There are surgical interventions available for infants with reflux, but there's no reason to resort to that if your baby is growing well. Eventually, my son outgrew his reflux.

As luck would have it, my younger son didn't have reflux at all. He never even threw up as a baby.

—*Carrie Brown, MD*

❧

Both of my babies had horrible acid reflux. That helped to explain why they didn't sleep well. When they were diagnosed with acid reflux, it helped me to cope better with their sleep issues. My husband and I learned, sometimes through trial and error, what worked to make our babies feel better, and we made sure that all of our sons' caregivers and babysitters also knew what to do for them.

My older son's reflux was so bad that when he spit up, the contents of his stomach would hit the other side of the room. It was unbelievable. He was miserable. He wanted to be held all of the time, and I'm sure it was because his stomach hurt when he was lying down. My BabyBjörn was a godsend because it kept my son upright.

Our pediatrician tried a few different medications until he found one that worked for our son. We found that elevating the head of my son's crib also helped. During the first few months of my son's life, he slept mainly in his car seat.

Ironically, my older son still struggles with reflux, especially after he has a stomach bug. My second child followed the norm; he outgrew his reflux by his first birthday.

—*Heather Orman-Lubell, MD*

∽◦

Kids who have reflux are tough—a real test of a mom's endurance. It's a long, tiring road.

My daughter had really bad acid reflux. I'd nurse her, and she'd throw it all up 10 minutes later. Then she'd look at me like, "Do you have any more?"

It was such a struggle because I really wanted to breastfeed. I started expressing my milk and adding rice starch to thicken it so she could keep it down. But it was such a huge ordeal. My pediatrician finally said, "It's okay. You can stop nursing." That was such a relief.

It helped a lot if I kept my baby upright. She spent a lot of time up on people's shoulders. My husband and I even had her sleep lying at a 30-degree angle. They make several products now, such as a Nap Nanny, Tucker Sling, and RES-Q Wedge, to help keep your baby's head elevated.

My daughter's pediatrician put her on medication for reflux, and eventually she got better.

—*Ari Brown, MD, a mom of two, a pediatrician with Capital Pediatric Group, and the author of* Baby 411, *in Austin, TX*

Preventing and Treating Diaper Rash

Diaper rashes can be really alarming. They look angry, red, and irritated. No wonder parents want to do what they can, as quickly as they can, to heal their babies' bottoms. The good news is, diaper rashes usually respond very well to home care and TLC.

Diaper rashes are most common in babies between four and 15 months old. They often begin when a baby starts eating solid food.

You'll find a whole arsenal of creams and lotions designed to prevent and treat diaper rash. Most parents are loyal proponents of the diaper rash cream that worked best for them.

❧

Triple Paste is the best invention ever. It's a little pricey, like liquid gold, but it's worth it. It has no additives, nothing to worry about. It's safe and effective.

—*Heather Orman-Lubell, MD*

❧

I really loved the Aveeno Baby Diaper Rash Cream. It doesn't smell bad, and it works really well. You can buy it online and in stores for around $6 a tube.

—*Melody Derrick, MD, a mom of a 17-month-old daughter and a family physician in private practice with Central DuPage Physician Group, in Winfield, IL*

❧

My one daughter had the most sensitive skin, and she developed horrible diaper rashes within minutes of wetting her diaper. We found that the very best way to prevent rashes (besides very quick diaper changes) was to literally frost her little behind like a cupcake with Desitin.

—*Lesley Burton-Iwinski, MD, a mom of 20- and 18-year-old daughters and a 14-year-old son, a retired family physician, and a parent and teacher educator with Growing Peaceful Families, in Lexington, KY*

❧

For diaper rash cream, I use Desitin Creamy. I'm very anti–diaper rash, so I was zealous about applying the cream. I found out later that it made the diapers leak if I put too much cream on my baby's bottom. It clogged up the absorbent part of the diapers.

You can buy Desitin Creamy pretty much everywhere for around $3.50.

> —*Sonia Ng, MD, a mom of seven- and two-year-old sons, a pediatrician, and a sedation attending physician at the Children's Hospital of Philadelphia Pediatric Care and the University Medical Center at Princeton in Princeton, NJ, and the Pediatric Imaging Center in King of Prussia, PA*

My daughters have sensitive skin, and I had to work my way through diaper rash creams to find what worked. We liked Weleda Calendula Diaper Care. That seemed to work better than anything else.

You can buy Weleda Calendula Diaper Care for around $15 for 2.8 ounces online.

> —*Robyn Liu, MD, a mom of seven- and four-year-old daughters and a family physican with Greeley County Health Services, in Tribune, KS*

My favorite diaper rash ointment is Dr. Smith's. I don't know why, but it always seemed to work better than other brands when my babies had a bad diaper rash—like the kind they got whenever they had diarrhea.

You can buy it online for around $13 for 3 ounces.

> —*Lezli Braswell, MD*

Using cloth diapers instead of disposable diapers went a long way toward preventing diaper rash. But I also put Desitin and A+D Ointment on my babies' bottoms to act as a moisture barrier and keep the irritation down.

> —*Susan Besser, MD, a mom of six grown children, ages 26, 24, 22, 21, 19, and 17, a grandmom of one, a family physician, and the medical director of Doctors Express-Memphis, in Tennessee*

I used Triple Paste on my son both to prevent, and also to treat, diaper rash. (See "Mommy MD Guides–Recommended Product: Triple Paste" on page 174.) But I always monitored diaper rash very carefully. Babies are quite fragile. If a rash doesn't improve in a few days, it might be more than a simple diaper rash. Sometimes babies get yeast infections in their diaper areas. If you suspect it's more than a diaper rash, call your baby's pediatrician.

—*Judith Hellman, MD, a mom of a 13-year-old son, an associate clinical professor of dermatology at Mt. Sinai Hospital, and a dermatologist in private practice, in New York City*

My sons seemed to be most prone to diaper rashes when we were adding new foods to their diet. So when we started solids, for instance, we'd have a rash of diaper rash! I tried to prevent this by using a lot of Desitin Original diaper rash cream. If my babies had the slightest hint of a rash, I'd let their bottoms air out without a diaper for a while, even taking them out in the sun for a bit so their skin could really dry out. We are fortunate to have a room that receives a lot of indirect light. I would hold them in a towel on their tummies and let their bottoms get exposed to the indirect light for 20 to 30 minutes.

My middle son has a condition that requires him to take antibiotics often. That makes him prone to a particular type of diaper rash caused by yeast. This type of rash looks different from regular diaper rash. It has little red dots called satellite lesions. If your baby's rash looks like that, or if his rash doesn't respond to regular treatment such as frequent diaper changes, take him to the pediatrician to make sure it's not a yeast rash. One thing that helps to prevent a yeast rash is to mix two tablespoons of distilled white vinegar into 12 ounces of water and pat that on the skin with a clean makeup sponge. It changes the pH of the skin and may help prevent recurrent yeast diaper rash.

—*Amy Thompson, MD, a mom of four- and two-year-old and nine-month-old sons and an ob-gyn at the University of Cincinnati College of Medicine, in Ohio*

My kids almost never got diaper rash, unless for some reason they had diarrhea during the night and the poop sat next to their skin for longer than necessary. I was careful about cleaning their bottoms with warm water and a washrag and drying the skin well. I'm amazed at all of these contraptions such as wipe warmers and lotions. If your baby gets a diaper rash, the best thing to do is wash it well, dry it completely, and then apply Triple Paste.

—*Hana R. Solomon, MD*

Diaper rash wasn't a huge problem for my children, though it could come and go. Probably the best advice for prevention is frequent diaper changing, with quick changes especially after a bowel movement. We used Desitin primarily, and I would also occasionally apply a little antifungal cream as well, since *Candida* yeast is frequently a cause of diaper rash. I would use Monistat antifungal cream sparingly if my children had severe diaper rashes.

—*Stacey Weiland, MD*

RALLIE'S TIP

Exposure to urine, stool, and soap can remove natural, protective oils from your baby's skin. When my babies were little, I used petroleum jelly or baby oil to protect their skin, but if I had babies now, I would use only products with all-natural ingredients. Smoothing a dab of olive oil over your baby's bottom after a diaper change helps protect his tender skin from the irritants in urine and feces and might help prevent diaper rash.

If your baby has a mild case of diaper rash, the anti-inflammatory and antimicrobial properties of olive oil make it an excellent remedy.

Every baby gets a diaper rash sooner or later. When it happens, the two most important things to do are to expose the rash to air and apply zinc oxide, which is found in products such as Desitin or Butt Paste. Really coat it on.

When you're exposing your baby's bottom to air, you might worry that her legs will get cold. You could simply put on a pair of adult tube socks or try BabyLegs. They're soft leg warmers for babies that were invented by a mom whose baby had really bad diaper rash and had to crawl around for days sans diaper.

You can buy BabyLegs for around $12 at BabyLegs.com.

—Katherine Dee, MD, a mom of six-year-old twin daughters and a four-year-old son and a radiologist at the Seattle Breast Center, in Washington

Mommy MD Guides–Recommended Product
Triple Paste

"Like most babies, my son was prone to diaper rash," says Judith Hellman, MD, a mom of a 13-year-old son, an associate clinical professor of dermatology at Mt. Sinai Hospital, and a dermatologist in private practice, in New York City. "I used a product called Triple Paste, made by Summers Labs. I used it as a preventive measure. That way, the rash didn't come up. Every time I changed my son's diaper, I put a little Triple Paste on.

"Triple Paste is great. It outdoes the other brands 100 to 1. It was my secret weapon against diaper rash, and I've given it to many moms-to-be as gifts. It comes in huge tubs, and it's good for diaper rashes and most types of skin irritation. It's very calming to the skin."

You can buy Triple Paste online and in stores for around $20 for an eight-ounce container.

My babies had a lot of diaper rashes. It was very stressful for me because I felt so guilty, wondering if this would have happened if I was home with them. The rashes seemed so painful for my babies, and it probably tapped into my feeling of guilt for not being there for them. It was so clear to me: I needed to be in both places at the same time, home and work, and I did the best that I could in both places. But there were moments when I felt sad about what I was missing because I was working.

When my eldest got diaper rash, I'd buy 43 tubes of Desitin and send them off with her to her grandparents, since they watched her while I was at work. I felt bad, but in the grand scheme of things, diaper rash is not the end of the world.

—*Siobhan Dolan, MD, a mom of 15- and 12-year-old daughters and a 10-year-old son, a consultant to the March of Dimes, and an associate professor of obstetrics and gynecology and women's health at Albert Einstein College of Medicine/Montefiore Medical Center, in Bronx, NY*

Rallie's Tip

When my babies got diaper rash, I'd use a hair dryer set on low heat to dry their little bottoms thoroughly after a diaper change. What I've learned since my boys were little is that the antibacterial agents in diaper wipes not only kill the bad bacteria, they also kill the beneficial probiotic bacteria on the skin, and this allows yeast organisms to grow out of control. The yeast are often responsible for diaper rash.

Now I tell my patients to take a capsule of probiotics, which you can buy at most health food stores, and sprinkle it on their babies' bottoms after a diaper change. It replenishes the probiotic bacteria on the skin and helps keep the yeast under control. It's a wonderful remedy for preventing and treating diaper rash.

❧

My daughter had persistent diaper rash for three months, which failed to respond to either cortisone ointment or antifungal cream. It turned out to be eczema complicated by a yeast infection. In the end, my daughter had to be treated for one week with the antifungal cream and then for one week with the cortisone ointment. This one I had to figure out by trial and error, because for some reason the pediatrician couldn't diagnose the problem.

—*Stuart Jeanne Bramhall, MD*

Having Your Baby's Hair Cut

Some babies are born with lots of hair, other babies are born with none, and most babies are born somewhere in between. In any event, your baby's first haircut is likely to be a big deal—to you and also to him!

My older daughter had very patchy, mangy hair. It was short in the front, long on the sides, and completely rubbed off on the back. It looked horrible.

My husband is Chinese, and there's an old tradition to shave the baby's head on her 100th day. So it was perfect: We had a party to celebrate our daughter's first 100 days, and then we shaved her head. Her hair grew back in very cute.

My younger daughter was born with a full head of hair. She actually had highlights when she was born. Her hair was dark, with blonde tips. We didn't have her hair cut until she was 2½, when she insisted on it. Now she's four, and she wears her hair in a cute pixie cut.

—*Robyn Liu, MD*

I gave my son his first haircut with a Conair comb that had a hidden razor in it. I combed his hair, and he didn't notice that he was getting a haircut.

Now that my son is older, he gets his hair cut at the same place, and at the same time, as his dad and his older brother. He doesn't complain. He follows everyone else's example.

—*Sonia Ng, MD*

Before having kids, I had no idea that babies hate having their hair cut! When my son has his hair cut, he screams like we're killing him. It's so awful that my husband tries to clip the flyaway loose ends, while I try to distract my son. My husband gets in one or two cuts at a time, and then we laugh because our son's haircut is so crooked!

My husband and I sometimes watch *Live! With Regis and Kelly* in the morning, and I was so grateful that Kelly Ripa said that her kids scream bloody murder when they're having their hair cut. Otherwise I would have thought it was just my kids.

—*Jennifer Gilbert, DO, a mom of 18-month-old twins and an ob-gyn at Paoli Hospital, in Pennsylvania*

Having a haircut can be a traumatic experience for your child, but it doesn't have to be. We grow a lot of hair in my family, so all of my kids definitely needed their first haircut by age one—the boys especially so that people would stop saying, "What a cute little girl you have there!"

I think it is fun to make the experience into an event. We always had our camera with us, and everyone in the family came to the beauty parlor. We always went to a kid-friendly place where the hairdressers have experience with kids. These places also gave the kids a certificate with their name on it and the date of the haircut, and I saved them in their albums with their "before" and "after" photos for them to look at when they got older.

—*Stacey Weiland, MD*

My babies are not very good at growing hair. However, my oldest daughter managed to give herself several haircuts, and so her first "real" haircuts were to salvage the haircuts she gave herself.

Fortunately, none of my kids have ever been afraid of having their hair cut. In summer, I give my older son a buzz cut, and he thinks it's the best thing ever. I think it's because the clippers tickle his head. He doesn't mind going to get his hair cut, probably because his sisters like to go. At their ages, they want their hair cut for style.

—*Kristie McNealy, MD*

I've never had my daughter's hair cut, but she just cut it herself for the first time. She has very long hair, and she took a pair of scissors to it herself when I wasn't looking. Later she told me that she "wanted her hair like Mommy's," and so she cut it.

My daughter didn't really cut off too much hair, and looking back on it now, I can laugh. I figure if a kid cutting her own hair is the worst thing you have to worry about, life is good.

—*Christy Valentine, MD*

Diagnosing Depression

Depression hurts. *Lots of things* can help—exercise, fresh air, a good talk with a friend, healing foods, and if necessary medication. What *doesn't* help is keeping it all in, soldiering on, and toughing it out.

Most new mothers feel a bit of the baby blues in the weeks following pregnancy. But the blues pass in a couple of weeks or so as hormone levels normalize. About 13 percent of new moms develop postpartum depression (PPD), which can hit any time in the year following delivery. When someone is depressed, their depressed, sad, anxious, or empty feelings don't go away, and these feelings interfere with day-to-day life. PPD is serious. For your own health and for the health of your baby, if it's affecting you, get help.

Here's a quick self-test for PPD. If you have had five or more of the following symptoms for the past two weeks, talk with your doctor right away.

- Feeling sad, helpless, overwhelmed, or empty
- Loss of interest in activities you usually enjoy
- Sudden crying spells or crying a lot
- Trouble falling asleep
- Trouble staying asleep
- Lack of energy or motivation
- Eating more than usual or not as much
- Feeling unable to focus or concentrate
- Feeling worthless or guilty
- Having unexplained, persistent headaches, stomach problems, or aches and pains

If you *ever* have any bizarre thoughts, suicidal thoughts, or thoughts of harming your baby, call your doctor immediately.

With my second baby, I had postpartum depression. One day when my daughter was two weeks old, I was sitting at the table after dinner, and hot tears started pouring down my face. I couldn't even say why.

My mom had been staying with us, and she was supposed to go home the next day. Without saying a word, my mother left the kitchen and returned a few minutes later, saying, "I've changed my mind. I'm going to stay two more weeks." I didn't know how to ask for that, but my mom sensed that it wasn't a good time for her to go. I just needed her company and support to make it through those next two weeks.

Now that I'm older, I am better at identifying what I need and knowing how to ask for it. If I don't get the help I need when I ask, I keep on looking. As a mom, you have to take care of yourself so that you can better meet the needs of your children and your family.

—*Lesley Burton-Iwinski, MD*

When to Call Your Doctor

Call 9-1-1 or other emergency help if you think you cannot keep from harming yourself, your baby, or another person. You can also call the national suicide hotline, National Hopeline Network, at 800-784-2433, or the National Child Abuse Hotline at 800-422-4453.

Call your doctor immediately if you have symptoms of postpartum depression, such as depressed mood, loss of pleasure in activities, sleep problems, extreme fatigue, feelings of worthlessness or guilt, or difficulty concentrating.

Also call your doctor immediately if you have hallucinations involving smell, touch, hearing, or sight or if you are having thoughts that might not be based in reality (delusions). Examples of delusions are fears that someone is watching you, stealing from you, or reading your mind.

My daughter was almost two years old when our triplets were born. I knew that I needed help, but it was hard to find. I tried some live-in nannies. The first one was a disaster. The second one left after two weeks. My mom came to help, but she had to go home to Pakistan when the babies were only five weeks old.

I didn't realize it at the time, but I was also battling postpartum depression. I was so exhausted, so overwhelmed. All I remember from my triplets' first seven weeks is darkness.

Two weeks after my mom left, in desperation, my husband and I along with our four babies flew back to Pakistan. It was a trip from hell! But as soon as we got home, it was awesome. My dad, a retired pediatrician, arranged for three pediatric nurses and three hospital workers to help with the babies. That helped me to rest, and almost immediately I felt like a cloud had been lifted off my head. I believe that the change in my environment helped a lot, and having so much help and support from my family was critical.

—*Sadaf T. Bhutta, MD*

I actually did not suffer from the immediate postpartum depression that typically occurs anywhere between one to six months after delivery. For me, it seemed to be delayed. My theory is that my depression was related to breastfeeding.

Although estrogen and progesterone levels undergo a dramatic drop in the immediate postpartum period, even in breastfeeding women, another hormone, called prolactin, does not undergo this immediate drop. (In women who aren't breastfeeding, prolactin levels drop just as dramatically as estrogen and progesterone.) The scientific data regarding the relationship between prolactin levels and postpartum depression in women is not clear. However, I found that I experienced a progressive rise in anxiety, depression, and racing thoughts as I began weaning my children. These feelings peaked when I stopped breastfeeding entirely, and then they gradually improved.

—*Stacey Weiland, MD*

I experienced postpartum depression after the birth of my son. Immediately after he was born, I felt great, and I recovered from my C-section very well. My son and I bonded, and breastfeeding was going well.

About eight weeks after my son was born, I started to worry excessively. I became very concerned about his health and germs, and I feared that he would get sick. My worries were out of proportion, and then I started to become depressed and found myself not enjoying life as much as I normally did.

I overcame the postpartum depression by talking about my symptoms with my friends and family and by seeking the help of a psychologist who specialized in postpartum depression. I continued to breastfeed my baby, and I began taking a medicine to help treat the symptoms of depression. I continued to exercise and talk with loved ones about my experience.

After about one month of treatment, I began to feel much better, and I began to thrive again. I enjoyed my daily activities, stopped worrying so much, and thrilled in the joys of raising my infant son. I found it so odd that as a physician, I did not recognize my symptoms and the diagnosis earlier. But as a new mother, I thought perhaps that the symptoms I was experiencing were par for the course. Looking back, I am thankful I received help as soon as I did, and I am thankful for the love and support of my friends and family during that difficult time.

—*Leigh Andrea DeLair, MD*

Pregnancy, delivery, and motherhood are monumental and transcendent experiences, which shake you to your core. This is true philosophically and also biochemically. It's natural to be overwhelmed and weepy at moments, with emotions that are hard to name.

Our first child's name is Jacob. When he was just born, I used to sing to him the old hymn "We Are Climbing Jacob's Ladder." But I was so overcome with joy and amazement at my baby that I burst into tears before I could get through the first verse, every single time I tried to sing it. I still tear up, today, when I sing that song, which tells you that it isn't "pregnancy hormones" acting on my mood because Jacob is married now and a college teacher.

All the same, the biochemistry of a woman's mood sometimes can get out of harmony after childbirth, and true depression during this time is not uncommon. If you enjoy a good sentimental cry and occasionally feel unusually worked up after having your baby, you can write this off as perfectly ordinary. But feelings of guilt, worry, sadness, lack of energy, hopelessness, and anger shouldn't last more than a few days. More than a week of depressed mood should be a red flag. Talk with your doctor and keep a daily log of your state of mind. For many new moms, exercise and plenty of sunshine or light therapy can help, without adding medications. It is much easier to treat depression before it takes root, so speak up promptly.
　　—*Elizabeth Berger, MD*

Going Back to Work

In 1964, 500,000 American kids were in day care. Today, that number has skyrocketed to 5 million. But that doesn't make the transition any easier.

The reality today is that most families need two incomes to make it—despite the fact that Salary.com estimates that if stay-at-home moms were paid like other laborers, they would earn on average $131,471 a year, which includes $88,009 for overtime.

⁓

I have a solo medical practice, and I was able to back off of my schedule the first two months after my twins were born. My kids were adopted, so I didn't *have* to take much time off, but I did. I only saw patients in my office two or three days a week. My husband and I adjusted our schedules so that one of us was home each day with the twins during their first two months. That worked out well and gave us the opportunity to bond with them.
　　—*Brooke Jackson, MD*

⁓

During my babies' first years, I found it difficult to balance work and home. Frankly, I didn't do it well for the first six years. Then I changed to working part-time, and that made a huge difference.

I was also fortunate to have two very excellent sitters after our third child was born. They came into our home to watch our kids and do housework, and they cared about our kids as much as we did.

—*Michelle Storms, MD*

I went back to work when my baby turned two months old. One thing that helped to ease the transition was to start checking my e-mail and phone messages a few weeks before I went back to work so that I wouldn't be overwhelmed on my first day. I can't imagine how difficult it would have been if I had all of that work waiting for me when I got back!

I work in a practice with my dad, who's been a doctor for 30 years. My sister works in our office too. While I was on maternity leave, my sister brought faxes and mail to me at the end of almost every day. It was like being home sick from school, and having your best friend bring your homework over!

—*Jennifer Bacani McKenney, MD*

The biggest challenge for me during my baby's first year was making the transition from being a stay-at-home mother to a *working* mother. Because my husband was in school, I had to go back to work when my sons were six and eight weeks old.

It was very hard, but I found that it's probably easier to go back to work sooner rather than later. I think if you stay at home with your baby for four to six months, you become really attached to your routine, and you feel rusty when you go back to your job.

—*Lauren Feder, MD, a mom of 17- and 13-year-old sons, a nationally recognized physician who specializes in homeopathic medicine, and the author of* Natural Baby and Childcare *and* The Parents' Concise Guide to Childhood Vaccinations, *in Los Angeles, CA*

My first babies were twins. I spent four months at home with them, but after my first day back at work, my milk was totally dried up.

Six years later, when I had my next baby, I went back to work for only half days the first week after my maternity leave ended. That week I went home to nurse my baby. After that, I had my nanny bring the baby to my office so I could nurse her during my lunch break. If you want to continue breastfeeding after you return to work, it really helps to make the necessary arrangements ahead of time.

—*Lillian Schapiro, MD*

My younger son was a late-in-life surprise. I was 46 when he was born. I didn't get a paid maternity leave at my job, but I was able to stay home with him for two months after he was born. I was lucky that my husband is a stay-at-home dad, and so that helped me to get back to work when I needed to.

—*Rebecca Reamy, MD*

I went back to work 10 days after delivery. I think it's easier to see 40 patients than to take care of a baby. Taking care of a baby is very challenging!

I like to be stylish and wear beautiful clothing. When I first went back to work, my daughter was still breastfeeding. I never knew when my milk was going to let down. I'd be talking with a patient, and suddenly I'd have milk stains on my clothing! But I didn't miss a beat. I simply put my white lab coat on over my clothing and kept talking. I ruined a lot of good clothing, though.

—*Debra Jaliman, MD, a mom of a 19-year-old daughter, a dermatologist in private practice, and an assistant professor of dermatology at Mt. Sinai School of Medicine, in New York City*

RALLIE'S TIP

Before I had children, I had no idea how hard it would be to leave them in the care of someone else to go back to work. While you're pregnant, arranging for child care seems so simple and straightforward, because you're thinking logically rather than emotionally, and you don't yet know your child's personality.

With each of my children, I ended up changing child care arrangements at least once. It wasn't necessarily because the sitters weren't nice people or that the day care centers weren't good places; it was because they weren't right for my child.

My oldest child was happiest in a church day care where he could play with other children, but my youngest son didn't like that setting at all. He did much better staying at home with a sitter until he was older.

The most important thing I did was listen to my gut instincts about whether or not my children were happy and thriving in the environment they were in. When I knew my children were happy and well cared for, I felt good about going back to work.

The hardest thing for me during my baby's first year was trying to coordinate my work schedule so that I could spend as much time as possible with my son. When I was pregnant with my oldest son, I opened up my own medical practice. After my baby was born, I took him to the office with me. I set up a playpen in my private office. I remember talking on the phone or writing notes and breastfeeding at the same time. When I was seeing patients, my secretary would keep an eye on the baby.

I was on staff at a local hospital, and when I went to do rounds and check on patients there, I brought my son along, either in his infant car seat or umbrella stroller. I was blessed that he was a very good baby!

—*Charlene Brock, MD, a mom of 28-, 25 , and 23 year old sons and an 18-year-old daughter and a pediatrician with St. Chris Care at Falls Center, in Philadelphia, PA*

My biggest challenge during my baby's first year was finding the right balance between home and work. It was hard for me to find the number of hours per day, and the number of days per week, that I felt comfortable working. I was fortunate to be essentially self-employed in a medical practice at that time, so I had lots of options about the number of hours I wanted to work. I could work four hours one day, and 12 hours the next.

I ended up going back to work when my daughter was 12 weeks old. That was a huge challenge for me. I hadn't thought it through completely before my daughter was born, and so I had to take a deep breath and figure out what made sense for me as I started my journey as a new mom. I found it helpful to be flexible.

—Ann V. Arthur, MD, a mom of a nine-year-old daughter and a seven-year-old son, a pediatric ophthalmologist in private practice at Park Slope Eye Care Associates, and a blogger at WaterWineTravel.com, in New York City

One of the best tips I received as a new mom came from a senior doctor in the pediatrics department. She told me that as a working mom, when you leave home, don't ever show guilt. You are leaving because you need to do important work. And your work is important no matter what it is that you do. You work because you provide an important service, or need it for your own fulfillment, or so that you can put food on the table.

If you show that you feel guilty about leaving home, your children will feast on that and make you feel terrible! Don't say, "I'm so sorry to leave you." Be confident that you have placed your children in good, capable hands. If you must leave them, do it confidently and without guilt. Remember that you are off to do important work, and that's what your kids will think too!

—Ayala Laufer-Cahana, MD, a mom of 15- and 13-year-old sons and a 12-year-old daughter, a pediatrician, and the founder of Herbal Water Inc., in Wynnewood, PA

My husband is a stay-at-home dad, and that arrangement worked out well for us. As an intern and resident, I worked 100-hour weeks, and my husband was the work-from-home dad. As our son grew, my husband was also the hockey dad, referee, driver of kids, band dad, snack dad, you name it. He was so involved that when I was able to attend one of our son's events, the other moms would look at me and ask, "Who are you?"

I missed a lot of things those early years, but my husband was always there with my son. And to us that was what was most important: That one of us was there.

Even though I missed many practices and games, my son and I had our own very special bond, forged from our own special traditions. Each week on payday, I'd come home from work and say, "Let's sneak out and do something!" It might have been just taking a walk, treating him to a meal or sweet, or taking a trip to the craft store. I took off each year on Martin Luther King Jr.'s birthday, and my son and I would have our special day. We did whatever he wanted. Some years we went to amusement parks; other years we went to the movies. It might have been only one day a year, but that date with Mom meant the world to both of us.

As my son got older, I began working in my private practice, and I had much more free time, so I got to attend many more events. Today my son is in college, and we have the most amazing relationship. We're extremely close, and he's a great kid.

—JJ Levenstein, MD, FAAP, a mom of a 20-year-old son, a pediatrician in private practice who serves on the clinical staff at three hospitals, and a co-creator of Baby Silk, the first personal care line for babies developed by pediatrician-moms, in Encino, CA

My greatest challenge during my baby's first year was going back to work full-time. I started out working part-time for two weeks. During that time, I was so happy, and I was thinking, *This is easy to be a mom and work!* But when I was working full-time again, whoa—a different story!

I felt like I wasn't able to fully focus on either of my jobs as a doctor or as a mom. I felt like I could never finish anything, like laundry or dishes. I'm not the best housekeeper as it is, but it got so bad that I was scared for my daughter to crawl on the floor! I overcame these challenges by focusing on what's most important and letting the other, less important things go. So I don't have the cleanest house in the world, big deal. When my daughter grows up, she's not going to remember me for my clean house; she's going to remember me for the time I spent with her and the things I taught her.

Also, I tried to focus on the "here and now" and stop worrying about what came next. If I could focus on work while I was at work and fully focus on my daughter when I was with her, my life was a lot better! I felt like I could be successful as a mother *and* as a doctor.

—*Melody Derrick, MD*

With my first baby, my biggest sense of trepidation came from thinking about going back to work. When your baby is first born, you don't have the perspective yet that parenting is a long-distance run, not a sprint. There are plenty of opportunities to reconnect with your child.

When a new mom returns to work, there's a mourning period, and you feel that this transition is going to be irreparable. But your baby will remember you after you go to work! Babies don't forget their mothers. Even though you are leaving your baby with another caregiver, you are not being replaced.

That tension of wanting to be present with your kids and also needing to meet your own needs is most difficult in your first year with your first child. Now that I'm an older parent with teens, I'm able to look back with perspective on that time of struggle between work and being a mom. I'm so grateful that even though I was pulled in two directions—being with my kids and going to work—I know that because I've had a gratifying profession, I'm a much better parent to my teenagers.

—*Nancy Rappaport, MD*

Enjoying Sex

If you're reading this thinking, *Ha! Enjoying sex, that's a good one!* you have plenty of company. All things in good time.

I had a C-section, so I didn't expect to have any problems getting back to a normal sex life. Also because I didn't have any vaginal sutures, I didn't expect to have any pain. But let's say my husband and I have had to go back to the pre-intercourse days for a while.

When you have a C-section, you don't have the vaginal

stretching that you would have had with after a vaginal delivery, so it can be difficult resuming intercourse, especially if you're like me and didn't feel very sexy toward the end of pregnancy. I thought that intercourse would be easier after a C-section than after a vaginal birth, but it wasn't for me. You have to go back to the beginning and start slowly.

—*Jennifer Bacani McKenney, MD*

Mommy MD Guides-Recommended Product
Valera Certified Organic Vaginal Lubricant

Hormones, sulfa preservatives, silicone, fragrances, petrochemicals, parabens, glycerin, and synthetics: That's a pretty good list of things you don't want to put inside your body. And that's why you'll find none of them in Valera, which is the world's first USDA-certified organic natural female lubricant that's proven to moisturize the vaginal tissue, improve vaginal dryness, improve vaginal comfort, and improve sexual pleasure and arousal.

What Valera does contain is natural, plant-based organic ingredients, including aloe vera, shea butter, lavender, evening primrose, and coconut oil.

Many women experience vaginal dryness, which can be caused by hormone changes and even by stress. (Honestly, what doesn't stress cause?) Valera was invented by Darlene Gaynor-Krupnick, DO, a mom of five- and two-year-old daughters and a female urologist fellow trained in pelvic reconstruction and neurology, in northern Virginia.

It's important to note that Valera isn't compatible with latex condoms, but it is compatible with polyurethane condoms. Also, Valera isn't a contraceptive or spermicide. So unless you want to skip ahead to the "Thinking about Another Baby" section on page 459, be sure to use some sort of birth control.

You can buy a three-ounce tube of Valera at **MYVALERA.COM** for $24.95.

Sex only happens when the kids are with their grandparents. The baby holds onto me at night, and he won't let go. If I try to slip him off, he wakes up. It's really bizarre. He keeps a hand or a leg on me. Thank God for grandparents!

—*Sonia Ng, MD*

❧

My husband and I were on two different arousal schedules, unfortunately. I was interested in sex when I was pregnant, and he felt kind of weird about it. He then got interested after I delivered. But, first my privates were all torn up. (I had a third-degree tear.) Then it was like the Sahara Desert down there. Not to mention I was tired, stressed out, leaking milk, etc.

Thank goodness for K-Y Jelly, particularly their "warming" formula. It definitely kept our marriage together!

—*Stacey Weiland, MD*

❧

After my daughters were born, I noticed decreased vaginal lubrication, which makes intercourse difficult. I began to use Valera, which is a USDA-certified organic, nonhormonal vaginal lubricant and moisturizer that I developed for my patients who experience vaginal dryness and don't have many options.

—*Darlene Gaynor-Krupnick, DO, a mom of five- and two-year-old daughters, a female urologist fellow trained in pelvic reconstruction and neurology, and the inventor of Valera, a USDA-certified organic vaginal lubricant, in northern Virginia*

RALLIE'S TIP

Before the birth of our baby, my husband and I enjoyed a wonderful intimate relationship that was based entirely on spontaneity. But with a new baby in the house, we found that this plan no longer worked very well. There was just too much to do!

One of the best things we did for our relationship was to plan a date night at least twice a month. We'd hire a babysitter and go out for a few hours on the weekend. Being alone as a couple helped us keep our romance alive.

Mark E. Crawford, PhD, wrote one of the best books I've ever read on this topic, entitled When Two Become Three: Nurturing Your Marriage After Baby Arrives. *I didn't read it until my children were already in school, but I've found Dr. Crawford's advice to be incredibly helpful to parents, regardless of how old their children are.*

❧

I delivered my baby vaginally, and my husband and I had sex within the month. I remember breastfeeding one minute, putting the baby safely down, and then telling my husband, "Okay, let's do this" the next.

The important thing is that you should always feel comfortable about having sex. If you're not comfortable, figure out why you're not. You shouldn't have sex because it's "the right thing" or because you're "supposed to."

—Ilana R. Solomon, MD

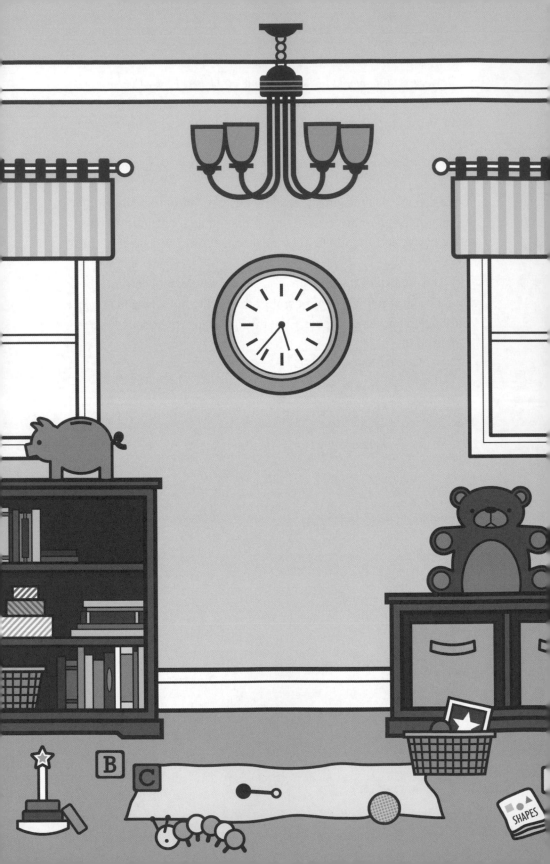

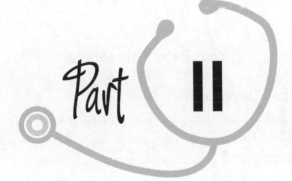

Part **II**

THE SECOND QUARTER

Chapter 4
4th Month

Your Baby This Month

YOUR BABY'S DEVELOPMENT

Although each baby develops differently, in your baby's fourth month, she's likely becoming more alert and more mobile with every passing day.

At around four months, your baby's optic nerves can now transmit the information from her eyes to her brain, allowing her vision to develop dramatically. She's starting to fuse the images from each eye, and so she can perceive depth. Suddenly, the world is in 3D! This new skill is called binocular vision. Your baby's ability to track objects is also developing. If you move your hand from side to side in front of her face, she'll follow it with her eyes from side to side, a full 180 degrees.

Your baby's eyes are also developed so that she sees her world in a rainbow of colors. Before now, your baby's preferences were black and white, but at this age, babies begin to show a preference for natural, bright, primary colors such as reds and yellows. Interestingly, they still usually shun pastels.

You won't see your baby's teeth for a few more months, but your baby might be *feeling* them. Your baby might be drooling more and chomping on things with her gums. Another reason babies drool so much is that they have immature nervous systems. They don't have as much motor control of their mouths as older kids and adults do.

What a wonderful sound: If your baby hasn't yet, by around four months old, she has gained enough control over her vocal cords to laugh. Her larynx is small and floppy, so her laugh might sound more like a high-pitched, dolphin-like squeak, but it will still be music to your ears. Your baby's laughs are a wonderful sign of socialization.

Another sound that you might be hearing around now is raspberries. Between four and six months, about three-quarters of babies figure out how to make wet razzing sounds, and they delight in doing it over and over. This is actually part of learning how to talk, as your baby experiments with moving her lips and tongue.

Got sleep? By around this time, most babies are developmentally ready to start sleeping through the night. Though not all babies are with that same program!

By four months, your baby is able to recognize you and other familiar caregivers. She's learning to make connections now, such as your face with warmth, a bottle with food. Your baby's memory is increasing now.

Your baby can probably lift her head up 90 degrees when she's on her belly. At around four months, most babies start to roll over by themselves. Most babies first roll from tummy to back, before rolling from back to tummy. When you gently and slowly pull your baby from lying on her back to sitting up, she might be able to keep her head level with her body.

Your baby can probably now sit up with the support of your hands or pillows. She's probably reaching out for objects now, and she can grasp an object in her hands. When your baby puts this new skill together with her new binocular vision, she can reach for something and actually grab it—most of the time. She still does this with both hands, though, rather than only one hand, as if she's embracing the toy and gathering it to herself. Your baby's arms and legs wriggle with a purpose now.

At four months, babies start to become picky about the company they keep. They show a marked preference for familiar faces, and they withdraw around unfamiliar ones.

When your baby cries now, it's more deliberate. She might even pause and wait for your response. When your baby is happy, she probably laughs out loud with abandon. She might be able to say simple vowel-consonant combos, such as "ah-goo." At this age, babies *recognize* all of the sounds of human speech, and before you know it, your body will be making them too!

Taking Care of *You*
See your doctor for a checkup. These days, your baby goes to the doctor for plenty of well visits. It's important for you to have a checkup too!

Justification for a Celebration
Watching your baby delight in rolling over—again and again and again—is wonderful!

Safely Taking Your Baby Swimming

Lazy days at the beach, fun times at the pool—swimming is a wonderful part of life for most people. Sand, surf, and sun are great, but with a baby these elements of nature have to be enjoyed with safety in mind.

It's a sobering fact that drowning is the second-leading cause of injury death for children ages one to 19. Babies are even more at risk because they can drown in less than two inches of water. So you'll want your little one to be within sight—actually within *reach*—anytime you're near the water. That's not just the beach, but also the pool, hot tubs, fountains, buckets, and even deep puddles filled with rainwater.

Children over age four should learn how to swim, and babies as young as one can benefit from "little splashers" mommy-and-me classes—not so much to learn to swim but to have fun with you in the water. The American Academy of Pediatrics (AAP) doesn't recommend children take swimming lessons until they are age four. Until then, children aren't developmentally ready to learn to swim.

All children need supervision in the water, even if they know how to swim. And before age one, you need to provide touch supervision—*every single second*.

Take a walk around your neighborhood to identify all of the water hazards. You might be surprised by what you find. Who has a fish pond? Where does water collect? Is there a creek or stream nearby?

If you have a pool, pond, or hot tub, it is an enormous responsibility. To protect your baby, and other people's babies, a fence is essential. In fact, the AAP stresses that pool covers and alarms are not effective in preventing very young children from drowning. The AAP emphasizes that fences are the best measure of protection. And, of course, you have to remember to close and lock the gate, each and every time.

According to the Consumer Product Safety Commission, fences must be at least four feet high, with no foot or handrails for climbing, with slats less than four inches apart, and with self-closing and self-latching gates. The latches should be out of kids' reach. You should keep all toys and furniture far from the fence so kids can't use them as step stools.

Another critical piece of safety equipment near water is a phone. Keep your cell phone or a landline handy in case you need to call 9-1-1.

Keep all toys out of the pool when they aren't being played with; they are child magnets. Most important: If a baby is ever missing, check the water first. Seconds are critical.

Two other water worries for babies are diseases that can be transmitted in water and chemicals in the pool. It sounds silly, but be sure to rinse off your baby after she swims. Wash her well with clean water and baby soap. Also, dry your baby's ears carefully with a towel to help prevent swimmer's ear.

Whenever your baby is in the water, monitor the water temperature very carefully. Babies can lose body heat quickly, and if your baby looks cold, shivers, or has blue lips, get her dry and warm immediately. On the flip side, hot tubs can be too hot for a little one. Babies can get overheated quickly.

Babies *themselves* can actually be hazards in the pool—due to leaky diapers. A leaky bowel movement can unleash bacteria, viruses, and parasites into the water. One parasite in particular, called *Cryptosporidium*, can cause severe diarrhea, nausea, and vomiting if it's swallowed by other people. The chlorine in a pool isn't strong enough to fight it.

Babies must wear swim diapers. You can buy disposable swim diapers or washable cloth ones. Disposable "swimmies" cost around $1 per diaper, and the washable ones cost between $5 and $20 each. Both are available in stores and online. Most pools and parks prefer the fabric kind; some even *require* them. Swimsuits that have built-in diapers aren't as effective.

Watery poop can leak out of even the sturdiest swim diaper, so if your baby has had diarrhea in the past two weeks, she should stay out of the pool entirely.

When buying a swim diaper, be sure that it fits snugly around your baby's waist and legs. It shouldn't have any gaps between your baby's skin and the diaper. If your baby has a bowel movement, get her out of the pool and changed ASAP! Your baby's swimming companions' health and happiness depend on it!

❧

We have a pool, and so it was critical that we babyproofed it. We have alarms on all of the doors and windows of our house so if any of them are opened, a loud buzzer sounds. That way, we'll know if one of the kids might be going outside and heading for the swimming pool.

My kids also started swimming lessons when they were six months old. Because we can swim year-round in Arizona, my kids took swimming lessons throughout the year, not just in the summer. I don't think they can remember those skills for any length of time until they're around five or six years old. They're especially likely to forget how to swim if they fall into water unexpectedly or if the water is very cold.

As a safety precaution, we had a rule in our home that we could only get in the pool if there was one adult with each child under age five. So if my husband was at work, we simply didn't swim.

—Lisa Dado, MD, *a mom of three children, ages 21 to 16, a pediatric anesthesiologist with Valley Anesthesiology Consultants, and a cofounder and CEO of the Center for Human Living, which teaches life skills and martial arts training, in Phoenix, AZ*

❧

I took my daughter swimming when she was a baby. You have to watch babies near the water every single second. They love the water, and they have no fear. From a very early age, my daughter has had the belief that she can swim, and of course she can't.

This summer, my daughter is taking formal swimming lessons so that she really will learn how to swim. It's so very important for children to know how to swim.

—Christy Valentine, MD, *a mom of a five-year-old daughter, a specialist in pediatrics and internal medicine, and the founder of the Valentine Medical Center, in Gretna, LA*

When my oldest son was about six months old, we signed him up for swimming classes at a big sports club nearby. It had a splash pool for the babies, and they taught parents basic things like how to get your baby used to the water by blowing bubbles and then gently dunking their heads.

I also used bath time to help our kids get used to the water. When I gave them a bath, I'd sit in the tub with them. I'd turn on the shower and let the water splash over our faces. Sometimes I'd hold them tight and count "1, 2, 3" while I moved their heads gently through the spray. They thought it was great! My kids have never been afraid of the water.

—*Amy Thompson, MD, a mom of four- and two-year-old and nine-month-old sons and an ob-gyn at the University of Cincinnati College of Medicine, in Ohio*

My husband and I started to take our babies to the pool when they were around four months old, and when they were around six months old, we took Mommy-and-me classes.

My husband and I also started to take our babies to the beach at very early ages. We watched the kids every single second that we were near the water. We'd grab them anytime they started to crawl toward it. We would let them sit and put their hands and feet in the ocean, but we were careful not to hold the babies while we stood in the water. If a strong wave knocked us down, we could all go under.

When my son was seven months old, we went to Hawaii. It was a lot of fun—but tiring. My kids are both beach bums now, and I have so many great memories of being at the beach with them.

—*Alanna Kramer, MD, a mom of an eight-year-old son and a six-year-old daughter and a pediatrician with St. Christopher's Hospital for Children, in Philadelphia, PA*

Taking your baby swimming can be a fun experience for the whole family. Several important measures should be considered, however, before embarking on your first family swim trip.

First, safety is number one! Babies should *never* be left un-attended anywhere near water. Drowning has been known to occur even in only a few *inches* of water!

I was always *extremely* paranoid when my children were near water, whether it was in a pool or even the bathtub, probably until they were at least four or five years of age. I cannot tell you how many times I have made a major save of my children even when they were just sitting next to me on the step of the pool, or when they just lost their footing and got into a slightly deeper part of the water.

Babies have large heads, and they tend to be top-heavy. So even if they are sitting nicely on a step, if they lose their balance, they always go down headfirst. *Never* take your eyes off of your little children around water even if it means missing out on a conversation with your friends or missing a call on your cell phone. If you have to use the bathroom, it is better to pull your child out of the pool screaming and wet into the ladies room rather than let him unattended for *one second*.

There are several flotation devices available, and we always used a device that was a combination of an inner tube and seat such as the My Baby Float Raft Intex Tube. These devices are nice because they have a little backrest that keeps your baby upright while her legs dangle in the water. Even with these devices, an adult always needs to be *in the water* with the baby, preferably with at least one hand on the inner tube or the baby.

Protection from the sun is also a must because a baby's skin is very sensitive to burning. Getting a sunburn at an early age puts a child at a much higher risk of skin cancers when she is an adult. The American Academy of Pediatrics actually recommends that children be kept in the shade until the age of six months!

My husband and I tried several different brands of sunscreen with our children. Our daughter especially had very sensitive skin and developed a rash with several products. She did do well with Coppertone Water Babies SPF 50.

Another must is the swim diaper. Most pools will not even let you put your un-potty-trained child into the water without one. We generally used Huggies brand disposable swim diapers. I've also seen some mothers put washable swim pants and then a bathing suit over their babies' diapers. The swim diapers work fairly well containing an accident involving number two, preventing what my husband and I liked to call a "Code Brown" in the water. Code Browns generally cause a huge uproar and require the entire pool to be evacuated. The happy pool staff is then required to get out the Hazmat chemicals to clean it up. (Anyone remember *Caddyshack*?) Unfortunately, there's nothing grosser than changing a number two swim diaper, and generally, once this happened, my husband and I felt it was time to leave the pool anyway.

—*Stacey Weiland, MD, a mom of a 12-year-old daughter and 7- and 5-year-old sons and an internist/gastroenterologist, in Denver, CO*

Molluscum (a wart virus) is a common skin condition that can be contracted through water contaminated by people with molluscum. To minimize the chance of contracting molluscum, don't share other peoples' belongings (towels, kickboards, etc.) at the swimming pool or beach.

—*Amy J. Derick, MD, a mom of two-year-old and nine-month-old sons and a dermatologist in private practice at Derick Dermatology, in Barrington, IL*

Transitioning to the Stroller

Around 1733, William Kent, an English architect, designed the first baby carriage. It was shaped like a scallop shell and pulled by a goat.

Strollers have come a long way since that, baby. Today you'll find a dizzying array of stroller options—everything from no-frills umbrella strollers to strollers for multiples costing more than $1,000. Several websites focus exclusively on strollers. They're great resources to compare and contrast brands, options, and prices. Many of the sites include stroller reviews too, such as Strollers.com and TotalBabyStrollers.com.

You'll also find lots of stroller accessories. A few to consider are stroller sun shades, rain covers, bug netting, buntings, cup holders, and organizers and tote bags to help you haul all of your baby's essentials. (No, you don't look like a Sherpa, really.) You can buy seat liners to change the look of your stroller—or more practically to protect it from stains and spills. They sell handle extenders for tall folks to push, and toys that dangle off handles for babies to play with.

Before strapping your baby into her stroller, it's important to consider stroller safety.

- Beware of hand-me-down strollers. The ASTM (formerly known as the American Society for Testing and Materials) published new stroller standards in 2007, so older strollers might not meet current safety guidelines.
- Watch out for little fingers. When you open and close the stroller, make sure that your baby is a safe distance away. Those stroller hinges are powerful, and they can severely pinch and injure a child's fingers or hands.
- Buckle up. When your baby gets older, it might be tempting not to use the safety straps. That's risky business. If you hit a bump, your baby could fall out, or she could wriggle out of the stroller or become trapped between the seat and the tray.

- Take a brake. Putting on the stroller's brakes every time you stop is a good habit to get into, even if you're stopped on level ground.
- Don't leave your baby unattended. A stroller might seem very safe, but if your baby wakes up and doesn't see you, she might panic, try to climb out, and tip the stroller over.
- Don't overload it. It sure is tempting to hang things off the handles, but your baby weighs only a few pounds, not enough to offset the "damage" from a shopping trip to the mall. Bags could cause the stroller to tip over backward.

Mommy MD Guides–Recommended Product
StrollAway Stroller Hanger

You've managed to fit three kids into a two-bedroom apartment. You've found a way for your Philippe Starck to live with their Fisher-Price, your Noguchi with their Noggin.

Through clever storage and cool new modern designs in children's gear, you finally have a place where your children and your style can happily coexist—except for that stroller! It's huge, it cost you a fortune, and it's a necessity. But where do you put it? The neighbors scowl if you leave it in the hallway. ("Illegal," they say! "A fire hazard!")

The stroller folds, but the fact that it's on wheels makes it impossible for it to stay upright in a closet, and at about $1,000 a square foot in your city, it's costing you a fortune in lost space!

Mommy entrepreneur Mary Ann Malone created the Stroll-Away, an over-the-door stroller storage system. Because the Stroll-Away hangs over the door, it doesn't damage the wall or door with screws.

You can buy StrollAway stroller hangers on **MommyMD Guides.com** for $39.99.

- Check the size recommendations. Some strollers aren't safe to use until a baby is a few months old, for instance.

Happy strolling! Mr. Kent would be shocked to see how far his little invention has come. And there's not a goat in sight!

❧

When my twins were infants, I took them for walks in the old-fashioned pram that my mother had saved from my childhood. It was great because my babies could lie flat. Plus, it had gigantic wheels and springs so it gave them a nice, smooth ride.

—*Lillian Schapiro, MD, a mom of 14-year-old twin girls and an eight-year-old daughter and an ob-gyn with Peachtree Women's Specialists, in Atlanta, GA*

❧

When my sons were being walked outside in their strollers, my simple rule was to extend the strollers' physical sun screen to block the sun.

—*Amy J. Derick, MD*

❧

We live in Minnesota, and so the cover that fit over our infant car seat was really helpful. I put my daughter into her car seat, bundled her up, and then popped the seat into her stroller. I could walk and talk to my friends on my cell phone's headset for an hour and a half. It was critical for my sanity!

The jogging stroller was very important because it allowed me to bump the stroller up and over snow banks.

—*Katja Rowell, MD, a mom of a five-year-old daughter, a family physician, and a childhood feeding specialist with FamilyFeedingDynamics.com, in St. Paul, MN*

❧

I'd inherited a stroller/car seat combo, which was fine when my son was tiny, but it didn't handle well on uneven terrain. Cheri, who was my mommy mentor and also equally frugal friend, told me that it was worth spending a little money to have a good stroller and recommended the Baby Jogger City Mini. I got lucky and found the stroller on sale, but it was worth paying full price. It handles so well that I can steer it with one finger! This stroller can go *anywhere*.

I'm a wimp about sun, so I bought a sunshade for my stroller. My friends call it the "Baby Burqa," but I love being able to take my son for long walks without having to worry about too much sun exposure.

—*Lennox McNeary, MD, a mom of a two-year-old son, a specialist in physical medicine and rehabilitation at Carilion Clinic, and a cofounder of the Mommy Doctors Bakery (makers of Milkin' Cookies), in Roanoke, VA*

RALLIE'S TIP

When my second son was born, my in-laws bought us a beautiful stroller. It was a really big, sturdy stroller with plush upholstery and a canopy, and I couldn't wait to use it. As it turned out, I ended up using that stroller only a couple of times. I carried my son in my arms or in his baby carrier—my husband and I called it the "baby bucket"—for the first few months.

The first time I tried to use that enormous stroller by myself, it took me about 20 minutes to lug it out of the car and figure out how in the world to unfold it. My son cried the whole time, and my milk let down and soaked my shirt. I had to fold the stroller back up, put it back in the car, and go back home.

After that, I bought a lightweight umbrella stroller for less than $20. I could pull it out of the car, snap it open with one hand, and strap in my son in about two minutes, before he even knew what hit him. If it weren't for that umbrella stroller, I might have never left the house!

I did not use a stroller or a carriage—or a play pen, changing table, or diaper bags for that matter. My husband and I had many of these things as hand-me-downs, but our children did not like them the first time we tried them out, and so we quit using them.

—*Elizabeth Berger, MD, a mom of a 28-year-old son and a 26-year-old daughter, a child psychiatrist, and the author of* Raising Kids with Character, *in New York City*

Feeding Your Baby Cereals

The official American Academy of Pediatrics stance is not to feed babies solid food until they are six months old. But when your baby turns around four months old, she might be showing signs of readiness to eat solid foods. The one person who's probably more excited about this than her is *you*!

Transitioning to solid foods is a big step. Here are a few questions to ask yourself before picking up that spoon. The more "yes" answers you have, the more likely it is that your baby is ready for solids.

- Can your baby sit by herself—without support?
- Can your baby hold her head in a steady upright position?
- Has your baby doubled her birth weight?
- Does your baby drink at least 32 ounces of breast milk or formula each day?
- Does your baby frequently put things into her mouth?
- Is your baby interested in solid food, watching you eat and even opening her mouth like a baby bird?
- Did your baby's doctor give you the green light to introduce solids?

As you introduce solids, continue giving your baby breast milk or formula. That will continue to be her primary source of nutrition until she's a year old. You might find it helpful to separate nursing/bottlefeeding and meals from the very beginning, giving your baby her solid food when you and your family eat. Choose a time of day when your baby is alert and in good spirits. Certainly it would help if your baby is hungry, but you don't want to go to the other extreme, waiting until she's overly hungry and fussy.

A good place to start is cereal. Some babies will love this from the beginning—others not so much. You might want to get your camera, or even your video camera, ready for this adventure.

Carefully strap your baby into her high chair. This is important for her safety, and sitting down to eat is also an important health habit for life. (Who spoons mac 'n cheese out of the pot standing over the stove?) Put a bib on your baby to protect her clothing. Don't wear your Sunday best either! This is going to be messy. It's best to use a small, babysize spoon.

Most doctors recommend beginning with rice cereal. Why is rice so nice? It's a single grain, gentle on the stomach, and has a smooth, fine texture that's easy for babies to eat. You can buy it in grocery stores, in the baby food section. Mix one tablespoon of cereal with four to five tablespoons of breast milk, formula, or water. It's a good idea not to warm it; babies like things at room temperature. Yes, it looks like a soupy mess. But no, don't put it

Mommy MD Guides–Recommended Product
Baby Dipper

Most moms remember giving their babies their first solid food like it was yesterday, probably because it was such a huge mess! Moms quickly learn that feeding a baby requires four hands: one to hang on to the bowl, a second to hold the spoon, a third to entertain the baby, and a fourth to clean up the mess.

So with no free hand to contain the mess, it quickly goes everywhere—on the baby, on the high chair (a gigantic drip catcher with dozens of nooks and crannies), on the floor, and on Mom.

A new feeding bowl makes this whole process a lot easier— and neater. With the Baby Dipper bowl, you can feed your baby with one hand. The bowl is triangular-shaped and stays where you put it. You can use your free hand to clean or entertain your baby, or to keep your baby's hands out of the bowl. Toddlers can see through the transparent sides of the bowl, and so they concentrate on getting the food onto their spoons and into their mouths. The Baby Dipper feeding set prevents the frustrations of chasing the food around the bowl and the bowl around the table!

You can buy the Baby Dipper bowl, spoon, and fork set at **BABYDIPPER.COM** for $12.95.

in a bottle. Serve it to your baby from a bowl with a spoon. As your baby gets the hang of eating the cereal, gradually reduce the amount of breast milk, formula, or water that you mix into it.

You'll want to choose a baby cereal that's fortified with iron. Around this time, a baby's iron stores decrease, and so she needs to begin getting this essential mineral from her diet. Iron is critical for growth and development. It also helps to prevent iron deficiency anemia, and it's part of the hemoglobin that transports oxygen in the blood from your baby's lungs to every single one of her precious cells.

Some baby cereals are organic. (See "Switching to Organics" on page 409.)

If your baby doesn't want the food, don't push it. She'll let you know if she doesn't want it by turning away, leaning backward, or refusing to open her mouth. Give it a few days, or even a week, and then try, try again.

Wait about three days after introducing rice cereal before trying the next food. Keep an eye out for signs of allergy, such as rash, diarrhea, or vomiting. After your baby has adjusted to rice cereal, most doctors suggest trying oatmeal baby cereal or barley.

❧

When my sons were four months old, we started them on rice cereal mixed with breast milk or formula. When they first started eating, it was all over the place. They smeared themselves with it.

—*Jill Wireman, MD, a mom of 14- and 11-year-old sons and a pediatrician in private practice at Johnson City Pediatrics, in Tennessee*

❧

Once I was feeding my twins, with a spoon in each hand. Across from me, a friend of mine was sitting, feeding her third baby. She had such wonderful calmness about her. Whether it was me watching my friend, or my babies watching her baby, that was the turning point when both my twins and I realized this feeding process was not a big deal after all.

—*Lillian Schapiro, MD*

When to Call Your Doctor

As you introduce each new food to your baby, keep an eye out for allergies. Signs and symptoms include a rash, diarrhea, or vomiting. If any of these occur, call your baby's doctor the next business day.

If your baby has trouble breathing, it could signal a severe allergy. Call 9-1-1.

When we first gave our babies cereal, we diluted it with a lot of formula. They took to it easily. We didn't have any problems, except it was very messy!

—*Penny Noyce, MD, a mom of 23- and 21-year-old daughters, two 21-year-old sons, and a 13-year-old son, the author of the preteen novel* Lost in Lexicon, *and an internal medicine specialist, in Weston, MA*

One of the first foods we gave my son was oatmeal. He would only eat it when it was thick. He still pushes it away if it isn't thick enough.

—*Sonia Ng, MD, a mom of seven- and two-year-old sons, a pediatrician, and a sedation attending physician at the Children's Hospital of Philadelphia Pediatric Care and the University Medical Center at Princeton in Princeton, NJ, and the Pediatric Imaging Center in King of Prussia, PA*

I started all of my babies on rice cereal first. I mixed it with water so that we didn't get confused between using breast milk and formula.

—*Susan Besser, MD, a mom of six grown children, ages 26, 24, 22, 21, 19, and 17, a grandmom of one, a family physician, and the medical director of Doctors Express-Memphis, in Tennessee*

The pediatrician was extremely helpful with feeding, and he had me add solids according to the age at which infants develop the enzymes to digest them. When it was time to start my daughter on solid foods, I started to feed her rice cereal, mixed with bananas to sweeten it.

—*Stuart Jeanne Bramhall, MD, a mom of a 30-year-old daughter and a child and adolescent psychiatrist, in New Plymouth, New Zealand*

My younger daughter took about two months to adjust to eating solids. She didn't sleep well, and I was desperate to get her to eat in the hopes that it would help her sleep better at night. My daughter, however, didn't think that eating solid food was a good idea. She just wanted to nurse. I just kept offering her solids every day. I mashed up fruits and vegetables. My daughter thought that pears were the most horrible thing she'd ever tasted. My husband and I kept thinking, *If she gets hungry enough, she'll eat it.* In hindsight, her reluctance to take solid foods was probably more about her eating when she was ready to eat.

My husband and I kept at it, and our persistence paid off. By about eight months, our daughter was eating solids fairly consistently.

—*Cheri Wiggins, MD, a mom of four- and two-year-old daughters, a specialist in physical medicine and rehabilitation at St. Luke's Magic Valley, and a cofounder of the Mommy Doctors Bakery (makers of Milkin' Cookies), in Twin Falls, ID*

I think it's important to introduce kids to a great variety of foods from the very beginning. I'm Egyptian, and my husband is Indian, and both cultures have very unique tastes in food. A lot of people might say, "Don't give your baby that. It'll upset his stomach," but our pediatrician really encouraged us to expose our boys to a lot of different foods early on.

With my older son, I followed the traditional schedule of introducing foods in the order that pediatricians recommend. With my second son, my husband and I really broke the "rules." We gave him pureed Indian food very early on, which is largely vegetarian, such as chickpeas and spinach.

Our pediatrician emphasized that it's helpful to expose kids early and often to different foods for two reasons. First, you want them to eat what you eat. Second, it helps them to develop a diverse palate.

—*Mona Gohara, MD, a mom of four- and two-year-old sons, a dermatologist in private practice, an assistant clinical professor in the department of dermatology at Yale University, and a cofounder of K&J Sunprotective Clothing, in Danbury, CT*

When my son was a baby, he didn't want to eat at all. He was a tiny baby, 5th percentile for weight. Feeding him for his first year and a half was a total nightmare.

I asked our babysitter to write down every bite that our son took to make sure he ate a certain amount of food each day. I even bought a series of videos, called Baby's First Impressions, and I'd play them while I fed him, hoping that would help him to eat more. It didn't help my son eat any better, but at least he learned his ABCs and how to spell at a very young age!

Eating was a struggle for many years, but then suddenly when my son was around seven years old, he began to eat more, and his weight jumped from the 5th percentile to the 80th percentile! I don't believe that kids' development progresses in a smooth, upward slope. Rather I think they have developmental leaps, or jumps.

—*Judith Hellman, MD, a mom of a 13-year-old son, an associate clinical professor of dermatology at Mt. Sinai Hospital, and a dermatologist in private practice, in New York City*

I think that many parents transition to solid foods before their babies are physically ready. We get a lot of pressure from other parents, including *our* parents, to do this.

I waited to introduce solid foods until my daughter could sit up in her high chair without support, open her mouth in anticipation of the food, close her lips around the spoon, and not thrust her tongue out at the food, which is a reflex that most babies lose around four to six months of age. My husband and I started pulling our daughter's high chair up to our table when she was around four months old. We often fed her while we ate. When our daughter was around five months old, we gave her some rice cereal. She was ready for it, and it was a very positive experience.

—*Katja Rowell, MD*

With my older son, I followed the standard way of introducing foods. I made all of my own food, even cereal and yogurt, from scratch!

But with my younger son, I've tried something different: baby-led weaning, which is not the same thing as child-led weaning (letting the child choose when to stop nursing). Baby-led weaning eliminates all of the work of baby food. One key to this approach is understanding that when babies are learning to eat solid food, they are still getting most of their nutrition from breast milk or formula. With baby-led weaning, you wait until the baby reaches the developmental milestone of being able to sit unassisted, which is typically at six months. Then instead of starting with pureed food, you start with soft finger foods. It's awesome!

During my son's first week of this program, he got almost no food into his mouth, but then he started to learn how to feed himself. I gave him cut-up avocado and bananas. With baby-led weaning, you don't feed your baby until he's sitting up well, so he's not likely to choke. If he picks up a piece of food that's too big, he's likely to spit it out.

My baby was cheerfully eating quesadillas when he was 6½ months old. He ate plenty of fruits and vegetables, anything he could pick up from his high chair tray. This past Thanksgiving was a joy. We put turkey and stuffing on his tray, and he ate it.

Baby-led weaning requires no extra prep work for parents. I simply give my son pieces of the food we're eating. We can go anywhere and give him just about anything we eat. It was funny, we recently went to lunch with my aunt, and she said, "That's what we used to do!" Somehow we've created this whole baby food industry, which dictates that you have to introduce foods in these regimented steps. Baby-led weaning is much easier. And it's fun.

—*Rebecca Reamy, MD, a mom of six- and one-year-old sons and a pediatrician in emergency medicine at Children's Healthcare of Atlanta, in Georgia*

One of the most indispensable items during the first year of life is a light portable seat that allows a baby to sit at any table, such as a Sassy seat. The chair has sturdy arms that tightly grasp the edge of the table.

—*Elizabeth Berger, MD*

My son had a milk allergy, so feeding him solid food the first year was very tricky. Many baby food items contain dairy ingredients.

I became very good at reading labels carefully, looking not only for milk as an ingredient but also learning some of the by-products of milk such as whey, which would also produce an allergic reaction in my son. I also learned that it was not necessary to spend a fortune at health food stores. Many grocery stores carry dairy-free baby-friendly foods, such as soy and rice milk products, including yogurts, cheeses, and ice cream.

—*Saundra Dalton-Smith, MD, a mom of six- and four-year-old sons, an internal medicine specialist, and the author of* Set Free to Live Free: Breaking Through the 7 Lies Women Tell Themselves, *in Anniston, AL*

Tackling Teething Pain

A few babies are actually born with teeth, but they are in the minority. This is nothing to worry about.

Most babies get their first tooth between four and seven months. The first teeth to break through the gums are usually the bottom two front teeth. A month or two later, the four front

Mommy MD Guides-Recommended Product
Hyland's Teething Gel

By the time we're old enough to be able to remember teething, it's long over. So it's hard for adults to judge just how much teething hurts. But logic says that a very sharp, pointy thing pushing up and through soft tissues is going to cause some pain!

If your baby seems irritable or cranky due to teething pain, a safe, gentle, effective remedy is Hyland's Teething Gel. Follow the directions carefully and remember that more isn't always better.

You can buy Hyland's Teething Gel online and in health food stores for around $6.50. (Talk with your doctor before giving your baby this or any medication.)

upper teeth break through. Next are the first molars, and finally the eyeteeth. Most children will have their primary teeth, all 20 of them, by their third birthdays.

You might suspect that your baby is teething if she begins drooling more than usual and wants to chew on everything in sight. If you give your baby a teething ring, never tie it around her neck. It could get caught on something and become a strangling hazard.

Pointy teeth poking through tender gums can make some babies cranky or irritable. If your baby seems to be in pain, give her an appropriate dose of acetaminophen (Tylenol). (Talk with your doctor before giving your baby this or any medication.) Older folks might recommend putting an aspirin on the gum or even a bit of whiskey! Just say no: Don't even consider it!

Some lucky babies seem to sail right through teething. Hopefully yours will be one of them!

⌒⌒

One of my favorite firsts during my son's first year was his first tooth. But it didn't come without some challenges. Keeping teething rings chilled in the refrigerator seemed to help soothe those sore gums better than anything else, and it beats gumming dirty little fingers.

—*Saundra Dalton-Smith, MD*

⌒⌒

My son got his first tooth at nine months. He's a year old now, and he still doesn't have all of his baby teeth. When he started teething,

> ### ? When to Call Your Doctor
>
> If your baby seems to be very uncomfortable teething, talk with her doctor. It's commonly believed that teething causes high fevers or diarrhea, but that's not usually the case. If your baby has a fever (any fever in a baby younger than three months old or a fever of 101°F or higher in a baby three months old or older) or diarrhea, it's likely caused by something else and warrants a call to your doctor.

he liked to chew on frozen bagels. Frozen bagels are great for older babies who are able to chew and swallow well. For teething babies who are younger, I would stick to baby teething rings because there's no danger of choking on them.

—*Sonia Ng, MD*

సౌ

For my babies, the biggest problem with teething was the drooling. I put bibs on my babies nonstop, especially when they were around three months old and they really had the drool going on. I had a very large collection of absorbent bibs, and my babies were never without one.

—*Robyn Liu, MD, a mom of seven- and four-year-old daughters and a family physician with Greeley County Health Services, in Tribune, KS*

సౌ

When babies begin teething, they often drool. Drool can cause skin to become raw and irritated. To prevent raw and irritated skin on baby's face, I simply applied Vaseline around my sons' mouths and chins prior to feeding to prevent drool from contacting their skin.

—*Amy J. Derick, MD*

Preventing and Treating Plagiocephaly

It's actually normal for a baby's head to have a bit of a pointy or elongated shape after being pushed through the birth canal. That should go away in a few days or weeks after birth. More worrisome, though, is when a baby is born with, or develops, a flattened spot on the back or side of the head.

Because an infant's head is soft to allow for the incredible brain growth that occurs in her first year of life, it is susceptible to being molded. Technically, the word *plagiocephaly* means "a malformation of the head marked by an oblique slant to the main axis of the skull." But more recently, the term has come to mean any condition characterized by a persistent flattened spot on the back or side of the head. It's also known as *flat head syndrome*.

A generation ago, babies were placed on their bellies to sleep, and back then, moms didn't have bouncer seats, infant carriers, and swings to rest their babies in. Their babies spent a lot more time being held, or at least not lying flat on their backs. It's a safe bet that most moms in the 1970s and 1980s had never heard of plagiocephaly.

Today, the American Academy of Pediatrics (AAP) strongly urges parents to put their babies "back to sleep," and a huge industry now produces baby seats in which to plop your little one. Not surprisingly, flat head syndrome is becoming more and more common. The number of positional plagiocephaly cases increased sixfold from 1992 to 1994, occurring in 33 out of every 10,000 babies.

Don't be tempted to put your baby to sleep on her belly to prevent plagiocephaly. In fact, the AAP recommends putting babies on their backs to sleep even once they can roll over. But allow your baby to roll over if she wishes, and don't feel that you have to run into her room and reposition her on her back.

As babies grow and develop, their risk of developing a flattened head decreases. Most cases of flattened head actually correct themselves by the time a baby celebrates her first birthday. Plagiocephaly is usually easy to treat, such as with specially designed helmets, and the earlier it's spotted, the better.

∽

When my babies were newborns, I took them to a specialist to have craniosacral therapy and osteopathy to make sure their necks, heads, and spines were aligned. This was just a preventive measure, to make sure everything was all right.

—*Lauren Feder, MD, a mom of 17- and 13-year-old sons, a nationally recognized physician who specializes in homeopathic medicine, and the author of* Natural Baby and Childcare *and* The Parents' Concise Guide to Childhood Vaccinations, *in Los Angeles, CA*

∽

One of my good friends had a baby with the flattest head I've ever seen, and so I make a point to give my daughter lots of tummy time to prevent plagiocephaly. Also because she's our first baby, we hold her a lot. Her head is looking nice and perfect!

—*Jennifer Bacani McKenney, MD, a mom of a two-month-old daughter and a family physician, in Fredonia, KS*

∽

Both of my kids had a little flattening of their heads. I simply turned them around in their cribs because they both slept facing the door. This way, they'd turn their heads the opposite way. Both of them are perfectly normal now.

—*Michelle Hephner, DO, a mom of a two-year-old son and eight-month-old daughter and a family physician in private practice with Central DuPage Physician Group, in Winfield, IL*

∽

My second child was critically ill when he was born, and he spent six weeks in the NICU. For at least the first three weeks of his life, he was lying on his back 24/7. He developed a flattened spot and a bedsore on the back of his head. He still has a scar there, but it's now covered up by his hair.

I really wasn't too worried about plagiocephaly, and it didn't change the way that I positioned my two younger kids.

—*Ann Kulze, MD, a mom of 22- and 15-year-old daughters and 20- and 19-year-old sons; a nationally recognized nutrition expert, motivational speaker, and family physician; and the author of the book* Eat Right for Life, *in Charleston, SC*

RALLIE'S TIP

As soon as my sons were strong enough to support themselves reasonably well, I started putting them on their tummies to play. I'd just spread a blanket on the floor, and I'd put them on their bellies with a few toys so they could wriggle around and get some exercise for two or three minutes.

At the time, I thought it was a great way to tire them out so they'd sleep better, but as it turns out, it's important for infants and babies to get plenty of tummy time to help them develop necessary learning and behavioral skills. A study conducted by the American Physical Therapy Association found a significant increase in motor delays among infants who spend too much time on their backs while they're awake, especially when they're strapped into strollers, car seats, and infant carriers. Ideally, babies should be placed on their tummies for brief periods of time, starting with one to two minutes, after every nap, diaper change, and feeding.

Preventing and Treating Rashes

Rashes are common in babies, and some babies even have rashes of rashes. (We couldn't resist!) Red, itchy rashes can be caused by viruses, and they appear suddenly after a baby has been sick. Heat often makes rashes worse, and so parents often notice them while giving their babies baths in warm water.

About one in 10 babies develops a particular type of rash called eczema. It's actually an umbrella term that refers to a number of skin conditions in which the skin is red and irritated and sometimes has small, fluid-filled bumps that become moist and ooze. Typically, eczema appears in a baby's first few months, and if it's going to start, it almost always happens before age five. More than half of kids who have eczema outgrow it by their teenage years, just in time for acne.

Eczema often starts as itchy, dry, red skin and small bumps on a baby's cheeks, forehead, or scalp. Then it might spread to the arms, legs, and trunk. Baby eczema generally occurs when a baby is exposed to irritating substances, such as the chemicals in some lotions or bubble baths.

⁓

My son had bad eczema, which is a chronic skin disorder marked by itchy, scaly rashes. We used a product called Theraplex Clear Lotion.

? When to Call Your Doctor

If your baby suddenly develops an unexplained rash, especially if she also has a fever (any fever in a baby younger than three months old or a fever of 101°F or higher in a baby three months old or older), call her doctor. Also contact the doctor if the rash covers a large area of her body, or if her skin appears to be infected, indicated by increasing redness, swelling, or the presence of pus.

We smeared it all over him throughout his early childhood. You can buy it online for around $16 for 8 ounces.

—*Penny Noyce, MD*

⤬

My second child, who is currently six months old, suffers from severe eczema. It was hard to watch; he would scratch himself until he bled. I didn't want to use topical steroids on his skin long term, so I only bathed him about twice a week instead of giving him daily baths. I also found Aveeno products to be very helpful for soothing his skin.

—*Bola Oyeyipo, MD, a mom of three-year-old and six-month-old sons, a family physician in private practice, and the owner of SlimyBookWorm.com, in Highland, CA*

⤬

My older daughter had eczema as a baby. I had to be very careful about the kind of laundry detergent I used to wash her clothing. Her skin didn't get along with Dreft. Through trial and error, I discovered that Tide Free, which is fragrance and dye free, worked. Woolite also worked well.

I also had to be careful what soaps and lotions I used on her. I found the California Baby Super Sensitive brand has worked quite well. It's natural and fragrance free. We still use it, and my daughter is seven years old.

You can buy California Baby products at CaliforniaBaby.com.

—*Robyn Liu, MD*

My younger son has terrible eczema. He is such an easy, happy baby, but we have to keep him lubed up in hydrocortisone cream.

My son actually loves having us put the cream on him because he knows that it will stop his skin from itching. In wintertime, his eczema gets a lot worse because everything is so dry. We have found that bathing less frequently helps a lot. We use a washcloth to clean his face and hands, but we try to limit baths to twice a week because they dry him out so much.

—*Rebecca Reamy, MD*

Like many babies with allergies, my son suffered with eczema. I found that it was extremely important to keep his skin moist at all times. I used a rich, emollient hypoallergenic lotion twice a day on his whole body and especially after any baths. My favorite is Aveeno Baby Soothing Relief Moisture Cream. I would reapply it to his face during the day, because his face was most prone to irritation. You can buy a tube for around $6 online and in stores.

Despite all of our moisturizing, in the winter I had to begin using a mild prescription steroid cream on his cheeks for a week to control the increasing redness and swelling of the skin in this area. I found that using a humidifier during the winter helped to prevent future drying of his delicate skin.

—*Saundra Dalton-Smith, MD*

Eczema produces dry skin and is common in infants. Both of my sons had eczema. Normally, I apply Aquaphor Baby ointment after my sons bathe, but during the eczema phase, I applied Vaseline immediately to damp skin after towel-drying my sons.

An eczema remedy that is becoming increasingly popular is to wash your baby in very dilute bleach water. The bleach solution decreases bacteria on the skin—a contributor to eczema.

Here are bathing directions: Fill a baby bathtub with a gallon of warm water and mix in one teaspoon of bleach. Yes, the very same bleach you use in your clothes washer. Soak your baby for five to ten minutes, and then thoroughly rinse your baby with clean water. This technique might sound odd, but it is analogous to why chlorine is added to swimming pools. *Caution:* Keep the bleach water away from your baby's face—especially your baby's eyes and mouth.

—*Amy J. Derick, MD*

My younger son had roseola, which is a common condition in babies that causes a high fever and a rash. After my son had a fever for about three days, I took him to the doctor to find out what was going on. While we were at the doctor's office, the rash finally made its appearance. At that point I knew that roseola was causing my son's fever, but because I was already in the office, I stayed for the visit.

Because roseola is caused by a virus, rather than bacteria, antibiotics don't help. It pretty much just has to run its course. I kept my son comfortable by trying to keep him cool.

—*Sonia Ng, MD*

One day, my son had a high fever but no other symptoms. Then suddenly he broke out in a rash. It was roseola. We didn't take him to the pediatrician because I knew what it was. He was perfectly comfortable, and he was back to his normal self as soon as the fever broke and the rash developed.

—*Michelle Hephner, DO*

Out of nowhere, when my oldest son was about four months old, he developed a purplish, blotchy rash, similar to hives. It looked so terrible that we even took pictures of it. It was a little scary when it first appeared, but I was pretty certain what was causing it.

I took my son to the pediatrician, who confirmed what I had thought: It was an uncommon rash called erythema multiforme, usually caused by a reaction to a virus or an antibiotic. What was unusual was that he wasn't on any medication and hadn't been sick at all. There's no treatment for erythema multiforme. It just takes time for it to go away. Fortunately, the rash didn't seem to bother my son at all, and it went away in a few days.

—Charlene Brock, MD, a mom of 28-, 25-, and 23-year-old sons and an 18-year-old daughter and a pediatrician with St. Chris Care at Falls Center, in Philadelphia, PA

Getting Baby Stains out of Clothes

Babies might not be playing in the mud or working on construction sites, but they sure do have a knack for getting stains on clothes. One of the most frustrating things is that a lot of times clothes look clean, but after you've put them away for a few weeks, the baby spit-up stains magically reappear. We didn't believe it either, until we saw it with our own eyes!

✎

I learned this tip while my younger daughter was in the NICU: If something is badly stained with spit-up, which seems to reappear over time like magic, make a paste of powdered Biz detergent and water. Spread the paste on the stain, let it sit for an hour or two, then wash. If that doesn't work, soak the clothing in a mixture of Biz

Mommy MD Guides–Recommended Product
Fels-Naptha Soap

It's a very good bet that the absolute number one best stain remover out there was in your Grandma's laundry room—and that you've never heard of it.

Fels-Naptha Soap is a mustard-yellow colored bar of laundry soap. It's excellent for pretreating stains, especially greasy, oily stains and baby formula.

For more than 100 years, Fels-Naptha laundry bar has been a time-tested stain remover and pre-treater. Fels-Naptha works on oil-based stains, like perspiration and ring-around-the-collar, and also helps to remove chocolate, baby formula, and make-up. Usually priced around $1, this golden bar is a great value.

and water in a bucket—kept far out of your baby's reach, of course. Those tricks got enough stains from my super-puker-uppers' clothes that I was able to resell some of them!

—*Kristie McNealy, MD, a mom of eight- and five-year-old daughters and three- and one-year-old sons and a blogger at KristieMcNealy.com, in Denver, CO*

∽

I pretreated stains on baby clothing with Resolve. That worked pretty well, and even though my one daughter has very sensitive skin, it never seemed to cause her any problems.

A larger problem was getting stains out of *my* clothes. There are plenty of items that I can now only wear under a sweater or that I'll never be able to wear again.

—*Robyn Liu, MD*

∽

Babies get stains on clothing so often, and despite my best efforts, I couldn't always get those stains out. I received a lot of baby clothes as gifts, and I didn't want someone to be disappointed because my baby wasn't wearing the outfit they had given her. So the first time my baby wore a gift outfit, I took a picture of her! That way I could show my friends or family members the photo of my daughter wearing the cute outfit they had given her.

—*Jeannette Gonzalez Simon, MD, a mom of a two-year-old daughter who's expecting another baby and a pediatric gastroenterologist in private practice, in Staten Island, NY*

∽

Unless an outfit was a gift, all of my children's clothing came from Walmart or Target. So I didn't feel bad about throwing away anything that was badly stained. You have to figure, what is your time worth? I'd rather spend 15 minutes playing with my sons than scrubbing stains out of a $2 pair of shorts. If a shirt or a pair of pants got thrown up on or pooped on, it generally went into the trash.

—*Carrie Brown, MD, a mom of seven- and five-year-old sons and a general pediatrician who treats medically complex children and specializes in palliative care at Arkansas Children's Hospital, in Little Rock*

Babyproofing

It might seem hard to believe, but very soon your baby is going to be crawling, walking, even running. The trick of putting things out of her reach isn't going to work anymore; you've got to up your game. Some parents babyproof their houses practically from front door to back. Other parents take a more laissez-faire approach. You have to find your own comfort level.

Here's your room-by-room guide to babyproofing.

NURSERY

- The only things that should be in your baby's crib are the mattress pad, a tight-fitting crib sheet, and your baby— no stuffed animals, bumpers, pillows, blankets, or toys.
- Make sure your baby's crib is far away from furniture she could use to climb out and curtains and miniblinds she could grab.
- When your baby is able to push up on her hands and knees, if you have a mobile, remove it from her crib.
- Keep all of your diaper-changing supplies—diapers, wipes, diaper rash cream, diaper pail—within easy reach of the changing table so you can keep your hands on your baby at all times. If you're worried your baby might roll over on the changing table and fall, simply change her diaper on the floor.

KITCHEN

- Never drink or carry hot beverages and foods while holding or carrying your baby.
- Whenever you're carrying hot foods or beverages, know where your baby is so you don't trip over her or spill the hot food or drink on her.
- When cooking, use the back burners of the stove and turn pot handles toward the back of the stove.
- When you set hot food or beverages on the table, put them near the center of the table to prevent them from

spilling on your baby. Or serve hot food from the stove or countertop instead.

- If you use tablecloths, consider switching to placemats, which your baby is less likely to grab on to.
- Never hold your baby while cooking. Put her in a safe place so you can keep an eye on what you're cooking. It's helpful to set a kitchen timer when you're cooking so you don't forget something on the stove. Unattended cooking is the number one cause of cooking fires.
- Consider installing an oven lock so your baby can't grab ahold of the oven bar and pull the oven open. They're available online for around $5.

BATHROOM

- Place nonslip mats in the bathtub and on the floor next to the tub.
- Don't allow your baby nearby when hot appliances, such as curling irons, are plugged in and turned on. Even an infant might be able to grab a cord and pull the appliance down onto herself.
- Make sure your appliances such as hair dryers have large, rectangular plugs. Inside them are circuits that sense water and shut off the power to the appliance.
- Never give your baby medication in the dark. Read the dosage on the label each and every time in milliseconds.
- Install a whiteboard in your bathroom (or kitchen) on which to record when you gave your baby medication so you, or someone else, doesn't accidentally give her another dose too soon.
- Always keep the toilet seat down, and consider installing a toilet lock.

LIVING ROOM

- If your baby naps or sleeps in a Pack 'n Play, when she is sleeping, the only things that should be in the Pack 'n

Play are the mattress pad, a tight-fitting crib sheet, and your baby. No stuffed animals, bumpers, pillows, blankets, or toys.

- Always keep the sides of the Pack 'n Play locked. Otherwise the play yard could collapse or the baby could roll into the space between the mattress and the loose mesh sides and suffocate.

- Never place a bouncer seat, car seat, or Bumbo chair on a counter or table. Even very young babies can lean forward or sideways, tip over a seat, and topple to the floor.

ALL AROUND THE HOUSE

- If you haven't already, install smoke alarms and carbon monoxide detectors, at least one on every floor of your home and outside of each bedroom. Test your smoke alarms monthly. Replace the batteries at least once a year; a good time is when you change your clocks for Daylight Savings Time in October.

- Also if you haven't done so already, talk with your partner about a fire escape plan and establish a meeting place outside. As your baby gets older, talk with her about fire safety and hold fire drills several times each year.

- Post emergency numbers by each phone, including emergency services (9-1-1 or the equivalent in your community), your baby's pediatrician, your cell phone number, your husband's cell phone number, poison control (800-222-1222 will connect you to your local center), the closest hospital, and a neighbor or two.

- Install locks on cabinet doors. Better yet, move anything dangerous to higher cabinets and then lock those cabinet doors.

- Bolt heavy furniture such as TV cabinets and bookcases to the wall and/or floor.

- Move heavy items, such as TVs, back away from the front of shelves.

- Consider padding sharp edges of furniture, or removing furniture such as coffee tables temporarily from the room.
- Make sure window curtains, miniblinds, and strings are safely out of your baby's reach.
- Move plants out of your baby's reach.
- Think twice about buying used baby gear. Older products might have broken or missing parts or not meet current safety guidelines.
- Keep your home clutter free. When you're carrying your baby, you don't want to trip and fall. Clean up spills quickly for the same reason.
- Get into the habit of scanning rooms for small items that might have fallen to the floor, such as coins, beads, and plant leaves. You want to beat your baby to them.
- Make your home a no-smoking area!

When my son was a baby, choking was a great concern of mine. An easy rule of thumb that I followed is that if an object, such as a toy, is small enough to fit inside a cardboard toilet paper roll, it's small enough for a baby to choke on.

—*Sharon Giese, MD, a mom of a two-year-old son and a cosmetic plastic surgeon in private practice, in New York City*

My daughter puts absolutely everything into her mouth. She's not mobile yet, so for now it's pretty easy to keep small things away from her. Once she gets more mobile, it will be a challenge to keep her away from her brother's small toys. I think we'll just have to move them all to higher ground.

—*Michelle Hephner, DO*

The house we moved into was already babyproofed because the prior owners had twins. I checked all of the products we bought for recalls before we had the baby.

I also covered all of the electrical plates in the house, and I made sure that all of the wiring was hidden. Working in the emergency room, I've seen several kids who got electrical burns from chewing on wires.

—*Sonia Ng, MD*

Pretty early on, my husband and I bought gray bumpers from One Step Ahead and affixed them to furniture with sharp corners in our house, such as the kitchen table. The bumpers were very good quality, and I recommend using them on items along a baby's "running paths," such as on coffee tables that the baby could bump into or fall on.

One thing we didn't buy is a toilet lock. That was never an issue for us, but I could see that it would be very important for parents with very inquisitive kids.

—*Katja Rowell, MD*

My husband and I did a lot of babyproofing for our first son. We installed gates at the top and bottom of stairs. We put plugs in every outlet, pads around the fireplace, and protective cushioning around the hard edges.

We were a little more relaxed with our second son. Ironically, he really didn't end up having more bumps and bruises than our first son did.

—*Carrie Brown, MD*

We live in a center-hall Colonial, and our family room is in the front of our house. We made that the "baby safe" room, and that's where we keep most of the kids' toys. We gated off both entrances to that room and took out all of the pictures and anything else that could hurt the kids. We put protective cushions around the edge of the fireplace and on the corners of the TV cabinet. We replaced our coffee table, which had heavy wrought iron legs, with a soft ottoman. I was nervous about the babies crashing into those hard legs. I know that some people bolt their TVs down so they can't topple onto the babies, but we haven't done that yet.

I'm trying to strike a balance between the family room being comfortable for my husband and me to relax in, yet making it safe for the kids.

—*Jennifer Gilbert, DO, a mom of 18-month-old twins and an ob-gyn at Paoli Hospital, in Pennsylvania*

～

It's very challenging to babyproof when you have older children. It's very hard to keep the small pieces that are appropriate for an almost-five-year-old away from the baby. For instance, my oldest son got a Lego dragon for Christmas, which is full of teeny tiny pieces. We let him work on that in the basement, and if the dragon isn't actively being played with, it stays on a high shelf.

We were surprised that we had to babyproof different areas for each child and keep watching for new hazards as our children matured. For our oldest, it was obvious: stairs, electrical outlets, cleaning products, medications, stove knobs, and exterior door knobs. Our second child loved to hang on the oven door handle. We had to remove the handle completely! When we purchased a new stove, we were able to find one with a manual lock button on the control panel.

—*Amy Thompson, MD*

～

It's a good idea for new parents to take a first aid class. But we didn't. My husband is an emergency medicine physician, so he didn't need it. I looked into it, and most hospitals (including ours) offer the course for a small fee, but I didn't take it because I was overwhelmed at home. I found many great videos on the web teaching infant first aid and CPR and watched them instead.

—*Rachel S. Rohde, MD, a mom of a five-month-old daughter, an assistant professor of orthopaedic surgery at the Oakland University William Beaumont School of Medicine, and an orthopaedic upper-extremity surgeon with Michigan Orthopaedic Institute, P.C., in Southfield, MI*

Making Time to Exercise

The phrase "use it or lose it" takes on new meaning after having a baby. That's great reason to get moving—today!

I took prenatal yoga classes during my pregnancy, and I continued to do yoga with my sons after they were born. It was a lot easier to do yoga with them while I was still pregnant though!

—*Lauren Feder, MD*

I have been using Wii and Wii Fit now more than ever! My daughter plays in her exersaucer and watches Mommy "Just Dance!"

—*Rachel S. Rohde, MD*

Give Stroller Strides a Try

Having a new baby is a great *excuse* not to exercise, but it's not a good *reason* not to exercise. Moms whose babies are at least six weeks old can join Stroller Strides, which is a 10-year-old organization that offers fitness classes for moms. Stroller Strides is a total fitness program that moms can do with their babies.

Generally, moms exercise with their babies while the babies are in their strollers. Once the babies are too old to stay in the strollers, Stroller Strides offers free LUNA Mom's Clubs playgroups.

Stroller Strides workouts are generally an hour long. Each class begins with a five-minute warm-up followed by a 45-minute Power Walk with the stroller. The Power Walk includes body toning stations, and during the last 10 minutes, moms do abdominal work and stretching.

To keep the babies entertained, Stroller Strides instructors weave songs and activities into the routine. During class, if despite the instructor's best efforts, a baby gets fussy, the mom is encouraged to "tend to your baby first." The instructors stop every few minutes for body toning, so moms can always catch up with the group if they fall behind.

Stroller Strides offers more than 1,200 locations in 44 states. A single class costs from $10 to $15. Visit **STROLLER STRIDES.COM** to learn more.

When my older son was a baby, I used to carry him in his BabyBjörn while I walked (slowly!) on the treadmill. I think the motion was soothing to him.

—*Heather Orman-Lubell, MD, a mom of 10- and six-year-old sons and a pediatrician in private practice at Yardley Pediatrics of St. Christopher's Hospital for Children, in Pennsylvania*

When my daughter was a baby, I needed to exercise, but I felt very guilty not paying attention to her. So I put on an exercise video, but with the volume off. Then I played one of her children's CDs and put her in her bouncy seat or on a mat. She would listen to her music and watch me exercise. I think she thought I was dancing for her!

—*Lauren Hyman, MD, a mom of an eight-year-old daughter and an ob-gyn at West Hills Hospital and Medical Center, in West Hills, CA*

I decided to start yoga after my third baby was born, and it was great for mind and body after baby. Finding time wasn't always easy, but calling in "favors" from friends and family members for an hour away to exercise was well worth it! Unfortunately, life gets crazy with three busy kids, so finding time now is actually harder than when they were babies.

—*Marra S. Francis, MD, a mom of seven-, six-, and four-year-old daughters and an ob-gyn, in The Woodlands, TX*

In my baby's first years, we walked in the park almost daily. We live near the water, so we would also often walk along the bay with the stroller. The walks were great exercise for me, and also so very peaceful.

—*Michelle Paley, MD, PA, a mom of two and a psychiatrist and psychotherapist in private practice, in Miami Beach, FL*

When my twins were young, I didn't need to make time to exercise. I got plenty of exercise carrying them around!

It's a good thing too. Once I tried to go play tennis while I left my daughter at the tennis club's child care center. She just couldn't tolerate it. They paged me off the courts and asked me to take her back!

—*Penny Noyce, MD*

◎╱◎

I don't go to spas or anything, and I don't have a gym membership. In the summer, when my baby was old enough, I strapped him in a baby bike seat, and he loved it. We do a lot of hiking, but the baby wants to walk by himself, so we have to hold onto him. We have pictures of him hiking trails at the Grand Canyon.

—*Sonia Ng, MD*

◎╱◎

I had a babysitter who came to our house to watch my babies while I worked. One day, I had an epiphany: If she came a half-hour earlier, I could go to the gym! That was wonderful because exercising helped me clear my head, and it helped me to lose the baby weight too.

—*Ann V. Arthur, MD, a mom of a nine-year-old daughter and a seven-year-old son, a pediatric ophthalmologist in private practice at Park Slope Eye Care Associates, and a blogger at WaterWineTravel.com, in New York City*

◎╱◎

When my youngest baby was born, my older daughters were in school. It's a 10-minute walk to my daughter's school, and on days when the weather is nice, I put my baby in the stroller, and we walk to school. That has helped me to strengthen my pelvic floor and get my legs back in shape. It's also helped me to regain my energy. Before that, I was totally worn out.

I take every opportunity I have to incorporate exercise into my daily life. It takes more time to get my three children into their car seats than it does to get the stroller and grab the tricycles and walk to school. Also when things are out of control and everyone is losing it, getting the kids out of the house for a bit of exercise is lifesaving for all!

—*Gabriella Cardone, MD, a mom of five-, three-, and one-year-old daughters and a pediatric emergency physician at Texas Children's Hospital, in Houston*

With a new baby, it's very hard to get to the gym. One of the great things about New York City is that you can walk everywhere. When my daughter was a baby, a friend and I walked around the reservoir twice each day (3.2 miles). She kept track of the total number of miles we walked; it ended up being in the thousands!

I also took my daughter for walks in her stroller. I used a collapsible stroller. That way, if I got tired of walking, I could collapse it and catch a cab home!

—Debra Jaliman, MD, a mom of a 19-year-old daughter, a dermatologist in private practice, and an assistant professor of dermatology at Mt. Sinai School of Medicine, in New York City

RALLIE'S TIP

One of the very best baby items I ever bought was a jogging stroller. I bought it secondhand at a yard sale, and I loved it. I had been a runner before the birth of my second son, and after he was born, I couldn't always find someone to watch him for an hour while I went out for a jog. When I got the jogging stroller, I felt a whole new sense of freedom and joy. I could take my baby with me for a run!

I loved running with my baby so much that when my third child was born the following year, I bought a double jogging stroller. Those strollers made it possible for me to exercise when my babies were young, and that helped make me a happier and more relaxed mother.

❧

For me, the biggest obstacle to exercising is giving myself the "permission" to take the time to do it. It's been hard to get over the guilt. I've gone back to work, and when I get home, I feel like I should be playing with the boys. The easiest thing is for me to take them on a walk with me. That way we can spend time together and get to exercise.

Some people are good at squeezing exercise into their days in small chunks. They can just plop down and do a few push-ups here, a few sit-ups there. I'm not one of those people. I need to set aside time to focus on exercise, or I won't do it.

One type of exercise I've found that I enjoy is kickboxing. That was new for me, and I really like it. My older son does karate, and we go to the same studio. We use real targets and learn kicks and punches. It's a lot of fun.

—*Rebecca Reamy, MD*

✿

During my baby's first year, I got a lot less exercise than I did before she was born. I tried to make up for it by eating healthy foods.

—*Kathleen Moline, DO, a mom of a 20-month-old daughter and a family physician in private practice with Central DuPage Physician Group, in Winfield, IL*

Connecting with Your Partner

A baby's first year can be stressful for Mom and Dad, and on their relationship. Too much to do, too little time, and far too little sleep can all add up to too much frustration, anger, and resentment. Here's just one example. A study found that more than half of dads stay asleep (or play possum) when their babies cry during the night. Another 22 percent of dads only get up after Mom is already up. The same study found that 60 percent of new mothers feel resentful toward their partners. Eighty-six percent of new mothers said they prefer sleep to sex. It's far too easy to become ships passing in the night, drifting farther and farther apart. Don't let your marriage become a wreck.

✿

It's important to *like* your partner and forgive each other. When a baby comes and you're not getting any sleep, you don't take it out on your child, you naturally take it out on each other. You have to be able to wake up the next morning, laugh, and move on. Having a baby is a stressful time.

—*Ellen McDonald, MD, a mom of four sons and an internist in private practice, in Pasadena, CA*

✿

For fun, my husband and I always have a "date night" at least every other week.

—*Darlene Gaynor-Krupnick, DO, a mom of five- and two-*

year-old daughters, a female urologist fellow trained in pelvic reconstruction and neurology, and the inventor of Valera, a USDA-certified organic vaginal lubricant, in northern Virginia

❧

My husband and I each had a baby backpack when our first two kids were small. We'd go hiking, each carrying a baby. That was a saving grace for me, and it was a great way for us to spend time together.

—Nancy Rappaport, MD, a mom of 21- and 16-year-old daughters and an 18-year-old son, an assistant professor of psychiatry at Harvard Medical School, an attending child and adolescent psychiatrist in the Cambridge, MA, public schools, and the author of In Her Wake: A Child Psychiatrist Explores the Mystery of Her Mother's Suicide

❧

That first year of parenting is the hardest transition you will ever go through. I found it was much easier to go from being single to married than to go from being a couple to a family. It was helpful for me to remember that parenting is a marathon, not a sprint. I tried to take care of myself as best I could. Now as a therapist, I always recommend that couples continue date nights to keep their love alive during this big transition.

—Eva Ritvo, MD, a mom of 20- and 15-year-old daughters, a psychiatrist, and a coauthor of The Beauty Prescription, *in Miami Beach, FL*

❧

Our daughter was born just a few months before our first wedding anniversary. We were getting used to being married and quickly had to shift gears to figure out how to be parents as well. I think the most important part of getting through the very emotional and exhausting first few months of our baby's life was being patient with each other and realizing that neither of us had all of the answers.

—Rachel S. Rohde, MD

❧

During our baby's first year, I had difficulty finding time for my husband and me. It's very important for me to have a good marriage, and so this was really upsetting to me.

My husband and I set date nights three or four times a month. We don't always make the date if other things are going on, but it's always on the calendar: Thursday night is date night. It helps us to focus on our relationship and to have some adult time together.

—*Melody Derrick, MD, a mom of a 17-month-old daughter and a family physician in private practice with Central DuPage Physician Group, in Winfield, IL*

RALLIE'S TIP

When my baby was about six weeks old, I was ready to enjoy a night out with my husband. On my first attempt, I asked our trusted sitter to arrive about a half hour before we were scheduled to leave on our date, which was a mistake. My husband wanted to take a shower, and I wanted to wash my hair and put on makeup, but our son wanted to be held, which made it difficult to concentrate on primping and even more challenging to relax.

The next time date night rolled around, I asked my sitter to arrive an hour and a half before we left, so my husband and I wouldn't feel so harried and rushed. When we scheduled a little quiet time for ourselves beforehand, we had a much more enjoyable and relaxing evening.

I think It's most important for new moms and dads to remember to talk to each other. As new parents, you get so busy that it's easy to go on autopilot, almost living separate lives. My husband and I would walk past each other all day long. There were times when he'd tell me something, and I'd ask, "Really? Is that how you feel? I had no idea." I tried to make a point of talking to him as often as possible.

Also, my husband and I learned at our premarital counseling sessions with our pastor the importance of speaking politely to your spouse. Be nice and be courteous. Don't allow familiarity to breed contempt.

We also sit down together as a family for supper each night. That's how we make the time to talk to each other.

—*Robyn Liu, MD*

Chapter 5
5th Month

Your Baby This Month

YOUR BABY'S DEVELOPMENT

All babies grow on their own schedules, but by the time your baby is five months old, he has probably doubled his birth weight.

Your baby's hearing has been excellent since birth. Around this time, your baby will likely start to consistently respond to his name.

We're all born with sweet teeth, and around now your baby develops an appreciation for salty tastes too. Speaking of teeth, on average, babies get their first teeth when they are between four and seven months old.

Around five months old, many babies find their feet, that is, they are able to put their cute little baby toes into their mouths. Not all babies do this, and those who do don't do it for long, so enjoy this cute phase while it lasts.

Your five-month-old baby should be able to hold his head steady when you hold him upright. He can probably roll over, one way anyway. By five months, your baby can probably bear his full body weight on his legs without standing on his tiptoes.

Your baby might be able to sit like a tripod, up on one arm. This month, some babies can even sit without support. More likely though, at this age, babies still slump over to topple sideways, although at least they're no longer falling forward onto their noses. Your baby's back muscles grow stronger every day, and soon they will be able to support him sitting up.

Your baby might start to use a raking motion to pull objects close. Also, at this age, your baby starts to perfect the one-handed reach. At first, your baby will probably use his whole hand to grab an object, trapping it between all of his fingers and the palm of his hand. Once your baby gets a desired object in hand, watch as it goes straight to his mouth!

By five or six months, your baby starts to understand the concept of putting things in and out. Also babies start to enjoy playing with blocks at about five months. They begin to play more purposefully, such as rattling things that make noise. Also, if you play peek-a-boo now, your baby will smile when he sees your face. That's because he gets the joke: He understands that you still exist even when he can't see you.

You might start to notice changes in inflection or tone as your baby babbles and coos. Babies make a major speech break-through around five months when they discover that they can change the sounds they make by adjusting the shape of their tongues and mouths. What a wonderful development on your baby's path toward talking!

TAKING CARE OF YOU
See your dentist for a cleaning. Your baby is just getting his teeth, which is a great reminder to take good care of yours

JUSTIFICATION FOR A CELEBRATION
Your baby is able to put his toes into his mouth. When else would you want to celebrate that?

Planning Playdates

When we were kids, our moms said, "Go outside and play!" All of our neighbor moms said the same thing. And that was as close to a playdate as it got.

Today, babies' calendars rival the President's with playdates, classes, and appointments galore. But playdates can be fun, and rewarding, for both moms and babies.

༄

When my twins were very young, I started an adoptive family playgroup with some friends and their adopted children. I wanted my kids to understand that adoption is normal and that they aren't the only ones who were adopted. The playgroup is a great way for them to get to know other adopted kids.

—*Brooke Jackson, MD, a mom of 3½-year-old twin girls and a 14-month-old son and a dermatologist and medical director of the Skin Wellness Center of Chicago, in Illinois*

༄

When my sons were babies, we went to Mommy-and-me classes. It was very helpful for me to meet other mothers and to hear how they managed their own difficult situations. I'm still friends with a woman I met there!

—*Cathie Lippman, MD, a mom of 30- and 28-year-old sons and a physician who specializes in environmental and preventive medicine at the Lippman Center for Optimal Health, in Beverly Hills, CA*

༄

I was never that organized around playdates at all, and I never really liked organized play classes. I took my children to the playground now and then. But that was about it for structured play activities.

—*Nancy Rappaport, MD, a mom of 21- and 16-year-old daughters and an 18-year-old son, an assistant professor of psychiatry at Harvard Medical School, an attending child and adolescent psychiatrist in the Cambridge, MA, public schools, and the author of* In Her Wake: A Child Psychiatrist Explores the Mystery of Her Mother's Suicide

Rallie's Tip

When my two youngest sons were born, we lived on a farm in a rural area in Tennessee. Because we didn't have any close neighbors, I had to schedule playdates in order for my boys to make friends and to learn to interact in a civilized manner with other children. Those playdates were a lot of work! I always felt that I had to clean my house, bathe my boys, and make tasty, nutritious snacks ahead of time. By the time our guests arrived, I'd be ready for a nap.

In retrospect, I should have just relaxed and focused on having fun with the children. My friends and I found that it worked better to schedule playdates at a playground or a park. We could pack a lunch, load up the kids, and leave the housework behind. The kids had fun playing wherever they were, and the other moms and I could relax and enjoy ourselves.

Dealing with Your Parents—And In-Laws

Sometimes new moms discover that their relationships with their own parents, in particular their own mothers, dramatically improve after the birth of their babies. Unfortunately, the flip side is true for other new moms. Our mothers (and even our mothers-in-law) can be our biggest fans as well as our harshest critics. With a little luck, you will be drawn closer by the love that you all share for your new baby.

When my kids were three to five months old, we sleep trained them. It was critical for us to formulate a plan on exactly how we were going to do this, and to share that plan with our parents and any other caregivers so that we'd all be on the same page. This really helped the process go more smoothly.

—*Katherine Dee, MD, a mom of six-year-old twin daughters and a four-year-old son and a radiologist at the Seattle Breast Center, in Washington*

People make new moms so neurotic. There was always so much for me to feel guilty about. My mother really made me nuts. For instance, she told me that you have to run a fan in the baby's room. So I went out and bought a fan. I probably ran it 10 times, and then I started to worry that maybe I'm running this fan too much. What if it catches on fire? It's funny the things you worry about as a mom!

—Jennifer Gilbert, DO, a mom of 18-month-old twins and an ob-gyn at Paoli Hospital, in Pennsylvania

Our families live out of state. When our son was a baby and our moms came to visit, they offered to stay up all night with him so my husband and I could get some sleep. They would bring my baby to me to nurse, and then they'd change his diaper and put him back to sleep. "This will be our time together," they assured me.

That was a tremendous gift. I tried really hard not to feel guilty about it!

—Michelle Hephner, DO, a mom of a two-year-old son and eight-month-old daughter and a family physician in private practice with Central DuPage Physician Group, in Winfield, IL

My first challenge with my new baby was having my mom stay with me for a month. We had a difficult relationship, but I remember thinking that while she was with me, I was just going to let her be right. She usually was, but that didn't make her insistence on it any less annoying. I was able to see her joy of being with her first granddaughter, and as a result of my decision to let go of my own need to be "right," our relationship blossomed and moved into a positive place for the first time in many years.

—Lesley Burton-Iwinski, MD, a mom of 20- and 18-year-old daughters and a 14-year-old son, a retired family physician, and a parent and teacher educator with Growing Peaceful Families, in Lexington, KY

A few weeks after my twins were born, my mother-in-law came to stay for the summer. She rented a house nearby. The twins needed to eat every three hours, and my mother-in-law slept during the day and came over to feed the babies each night.

The only challenging part was that my mother-in-law didn't like to be thanked. She said, "We're family. What will my friends think when you say 'thank you'?" My husband is Chinese-American, so I asked him if this was a cultural thing. He didn't know, but he urged me to go along. So whenever I felt like saying "thank you," I just smiled and bit my tongue.

—*Penny Noyce, MD, a mom of 23- and 21-year-old daughters, two 21-year-old sons, and a 13-year-old son, the author of the preteen novel* Lost in Lexicon, *and an internal medicine specialist, in Weston, MA*

With my second son, my mother really harped that I didn't bathe him enough. But the truth was, I bathed him plenty often, and his skin looked fantastic.

I knew that my mom was really upset about more than just bathing frequency. I thought about it, and I realized that what she was really saying was that my second son wasn't getting as much of me as my first son did. I explained to my mom that I understood, and that I even agreed with her. However, he did get enough of me, just in a different way, and he also got his brother too.

I've found that when people give advice, it's best to take the information and make a change if you wish. No one does this mothering thing all right. We're all just doing our best.

—*Wendy Sue Swanson, MD, FAAP, a mom of four- and two-year-old sons, a board-certified pediatrician, and a blogger for Seattle Children's Hospital, in Washington*

When my daughters were born, I was working really hard as an ob-gyn resident, so their first years are a bit of a blur to me. My husband and I were fortunate that our parents helped us. They each lived about a half hour away from us, and they each had full nurseries set up in their homes. Our kids were very comfortable there. Both sets of grandparents also had car seats in their cars for our kids. We didn't have identical things in each house, though, and I think that helped our kids develop flexibility.

It gave me tremendous peace of mind knowing that my babies were being so well cared for. I trusted my parents and my in-laws to care for my kids, and so I didn't micromanage their day-to-day decisions, such as what the kids ate or what type of laundry soap they used if they washed the baby's clothes. For me, knowing that my kids were so well cared for overrode any feelings I might have had of wanting things done a particular way. To this day, my daughters have very close relationships with their grandparents.

—*Siobhan Dolan, MD, a mom of 15- and 12-year-old daughters and a 10-year-old son, a consultant to the March of Dimes, and an associate professor of obstetrics and gynecology and women's health at Albert Einstein College of Medicine/Montefiore Medical Center, in Bronx, NY*

Keeping Up with Housework

Like so many things with a baby, laundry, dishes, and dust bunnies are multiplied, not divided. Luckily, your love for your baby is also multiplied, not divided, so that makes all of the extra housework a lot easier to bear.

❧

One product I found indispensable was the baby swing. When I needed to do anything that wouldn't allow me to hold my son, I put him in his swing.

—*Sonia Ng, MD, a mom of seven- and two-year-old sons, a pediatrician, and a sedation attending physician at the Children's Hospital of Philadelphia Pediatric Care and the University Medical Center at Princeton in Princeton, NJ, and the Pediatric Imaging Center in King of Prussia, PA*

❧

If my baby wasn't sleeping in her crib and I needed to do something around the house, like wash dishes, I put her into her BabyBjörn. That way I had both hands free.

Another thing that helped was the baby swing. My daughter loved it, and that swing was my best friend. I don't know what I would have done without it. My daughter was chubby, so the batteries didn't last long, and sometimes my husband would resort to pushing it himself! I put my daughter in it while I did things around the house or when I took a shower. My husband and I carried the swing from room to room. We actually also had a portable swing, but our daughter didn't like that one as much as the regular swing.

—*Jeannette Gonzalez Simon, MD, a mom of a two-year-old daughter who's expecting another baby and a pediatric gastroenterologist in private practice, in Staten Island, NY*

I was a big lover of the baby swing. My husband and I called it "sleep therapy." We put our daughter in the swing, and she'd be out like a light. We kept the swing in our main living area, and so I could be in the kitchen preparing a meal, relaxing watching TV, or at my desk doing paperwork and still keep a close eye on her. I loved holding my baby, and so the swing was also a way for me to loosen my grip a little bit.

When my daughter was 10 months old, she figured out how to turn the swing off. I think she was determined not to fall asleep!

—*Ann V. Arthur, MD, a mom of a nine-year-old daughter and a seven-year-old son, a pediatric ophthalmologist in private practice at Park Slope Eye Care Associates, and a blogger at WaterWineTravel.com, in New York City*

We had a stationary exersaucer when my boys were small. It had toys for them to play with, and it even swiveled a bit. It was perfect when they were learning to stand up, at around six months. I moved it all over the house, from the kitchen, to the living room, wherever I was going. It kept my sons totally entertained, while also being totally safe. Because it didn't move, I didn't have to worry about the baby rolling down the steps. Plus that gave me the chance to get some chores done.

—*Jill Wireman, MD, a mom of 14- and 11-year-old sons and a pediatrician in private practice at Johnson City Pediatrics, in Tennessee*

The keys to keeping up with chores around the house are to be patient and organized—kind of like how you have to be with kids in general!

Mommy guilt is a very powerful thing. I try to tell myself every day that it's okay to let one thing go. For example, I don't try to make it to the grocery store every single day. Once every three days is plenty. I'll say to myself, *Things really are flowing okay!*

Mommy MD Guides-Recommended Product
Fisher-Price Zen Collection Cradle Swing

"The baby swing was magical," says Rachel S. Rohde, MD, a mom of a five-month-old daughter, an assistant professor of orthopaedic surgery at the Oakland University William Beaumont School of Medicine, and an orthopaedic upper-extremity surgeon with Michigan Orthopaedic Institute, P.C., in Southfield, MI.

"We received one from my brother and sister-in-law, who had used it for their little girls. My baby loved it so much that we bought another one to put upstairs. My daughter likes the swing with the rotating birds, the music, and the mirror in the mobile above her head. Unfortunately, that one runs on batteries, so we have used a lot of batteries.

"The swing that we bought was the Fisher-Price Zen Collection Cradle Swing. It can be plugged into the power outlet, and the seat is removable, so it can be used as a portable seat as well. The mobile above the seat is not as amusing as the one on the other swing we have, but my baby still likes to chat with the little animals.

"The sounds are a little more soothing (even for us) than those of most of the swings, but the swing makes a noise somewhat like a metronome, which likely lulls the baby, but not so much the parents, to sleep!"

"I would put my baby in the swing when I was showering or doing chores and sometimes when she needed a nap but didn't seem to realize it. The swings kept her calm and entertained like nothing else—until the exersaucer."

You can buy the Zen Collection Cradle Swing for around $145 online.

Rather than using up energy beating myself up about things, I try to use that energy to get things done. Worrying doesn't accomplish anything.

    —Gabriella Cardone, MD, a mom of five-, three-, and one-year-old daughters and a pediatric emergency physician at Texas Children's Hospital, in Houston

When I get home from work, I'm tired and ready to just play with my kids and spend time with my husband before going to bed myself. The dishes fill up in the sink occasionally, and when we need spoons, we wash them. It can cause me stress, but you can only do what you can.

    I find that making a list of the household chores that need to be done helps me to set reasonable goals for cleaning. Then as I cross things off my list, I feel a sense of accomplishment—even if it was just to fold some clothes.

    My mom comes over and reassures me that the house looks fine. But I know where all of the dust bunnies are hiding.

    —Michelle Hephner, DO

When my boys were babies, I tried really hard not to push myself to do too much too soon. I accepted help around the house as often as I could, for instance letting my mom come and help me with the laundry. I tried to adopt the attitude of, *It's not going to be done today, but maybe we'll get it done tonight.* For those times that I couldn't keep the house up to the standards we were used to, I hired a cleaning lady.

    —Heather Orman-Lubell, MD, a mom of 10- and six-year-old sons and a pediatrician in private practice at Yardley Pediatrics of St. Christopher's Hospital for Children, in Pennsylvania

To clean my house, I use Shaklee products. They are very clean and green, and they don't harm the environment. But distilled white vinegar goes a long way to clean a house. These days it's easy to find excellent nontoxic cleaning products in health food stores.

    —Cathie Lippman, MD

One thing that helps me around the house is ordering my groceries at Peapod.com and having them delivered. I never loved going to the supermarket, and this saves me a lot of time.

People might think it costs a lot more money to order groceries online than to go to the store, but the delivery fee is reasonable, and I think their prices are comparable to stores' prices. Also because my groceries are being delivered, it's easier to buy in bulk, which saves money. It's wonderful when they pull their big truck up to my garage and unload the groceries.

—*Siobhan Dolan, MD*

﹏

If I started dinner each night when I got home from work at six, there's no chance that my family could wait that long to eat. So when my babies were born, on the weekends I started to do marathon cooking sessions. I put together six or seven meals. I put one in the fridge and the others in the freezer. That way all I have to do is heat something up, and I can have dinner ready in 15 minutes.

I make a lot of Pakistani dishes because they contain mainly meats and vegetables, and they freeze really well. I find that things with potatoes don't freeze well, so if I make a dish with potatoes, we eat that the first night or two so it doesn't have to be frozen.

—*Sadaf T. Bhutta, MD, a mom of a five-year-old daughter and three-year-old triplets and an assistant professor and the fellowship director of pediatric radiology at the University of Arkansas for Medical Sciences and Arkansas Children's Hospital, both in Little Rock*

RALLIE'S TIP

There's a lot of pressure on moms to keep a pristine and super-organized house, thanks in part to popular reality TV shows, such as Clean House *and* Hoarders. *In addition, you might have grown up in a home that was in a perpetual state of readiness for the white glove test, especially if your mother was a stay-at-home mom who kept her housekeeping skills sharply honed. The good news is that you're the mom in charge now, and you get to set the standards for your own home.*

During the first years of my babies' lives, the clutter was almost overwhelming. Babies need so much stuff! It's not just little things, like diapers and wipes, bottles and pacifiers, blankets and toys, but babies need so many really big things, like strollers and high chairs and car seats and swings. I found it impossible to confine my babies' stuff to just one or two rooms. I had baby stuff strewn from one end of my house to the other.

I think it's safe to say that general cleanliness is important for the health and well-being of your family, but a little mess and clutter never hurt anyone. My approach was to keep my house as clean as I could, but to let the clutter go. I tried to deal with the kitchen at least once a day, putting the dishes in the dishwasher and cleaning the counters. I also tried to advance the laundry on a daily basis so that it didn't get completely out of control. That might mean putting a load of clothes in the washer or taking the clothes out of the dryer and folding them.

If I had any time or energy left over, I'd try to tackle one small additional housekeeping project, such as cleaning a bathtub or toilet. I'd also ask my husband to help out by doing one small task each day, such as vacuuming the living room or taking a basket of clothes upstairs. On most days, I probably spent less than an hour a day doing housework. It was enough to keep my sanity intact and my house reasonably clean, if not clutter free.

As a mom, I feel that it's far more important to spend time enjoying and interacting with my children than it is to have a perfectly organized house. As much as I would love to have a place for everything and everything in its place, I realize that this probably won't happen as long as I have children at home. I've made my peace with that. I believe that home should be a warm and welcoming place where kids and their parents can kick back, relax, connect with each other, and enjoy life together.

Preventing and Treating Bellyaches

Few things will tear your heart out more than watching your baby throw up. Most of the time, vomiting in children is caused by gastroenteritis, which is usually due to a virus. It's commonly called the stomach flu, though it's not really a flu at all. It can also cause stomachaches and diarrhea. Once your baby starts eating table food, it can be caused by food poisoning, but that's unlikely at this age.

Vomiting and diarrhea can be dangerous for babies because they can cause a baby to lose too much body fluid and become dehydrated. To prevent dehydration, continue to breastfeed your baby, or if you give formula, your doctor might advise switching to a lactose-free one, which is easier for your baby to digest. Also talk with your doctor about giving your baby an oral rehydrating solution, such as Pedialyte.

The good news is that stomach bugs are called 24-hour bugs for a reason. They usually come and go quickly. Here's hoping your baby doesn't share the bug with you!

◦∽◦

When my babies had upset bellies and vomited, I put them on the BRAT diet: bananas, rice, applesauce, and toast. It really didn't happen that often. We have a joke in our family that *I'm* the one who catches all of those bugs.

—*Nancy Rappaport, MD*

When my twins were very young, they caught rotavirus. That was a nightmare. They were very sick, and we were afraid they'd need to go to the hospital for IV fluids. To keep my twins from getting dehydrated, we kept giving them Pedialyte and monitored their urine output and level of activity. Babies can get dehydrated very easily, so it is always a good idea to have your doctor evaluate your baby if there is a concern for that.

—*Ann Contrucci, MD, a mom of 12-year-old boy-girl twins who works as a pediatric emergency physician, in Atlanta, GA*

I remember one of the worst nights of my twins' first year. It was when they both had rotavirus. One twin started throwing up, and then the other one started. My husband was out of town, and I ended up sleeping on the nursery floor because I was concerned that one of the babies would choke. By the time you've changed their pajamas and bed sheets

? When to Call Your Doctor

If your baby is younger than six months old and is vomiting or has diarrhea, call your doctor. If your baby is six months or older and is vomiting or has diarrhea, call your doctor or take your baby to the closest emergency department if he also has any of the following signs and symptoms.

- Fever (any fever in a baby younger than three months old or a fever of 101°F or higher in a baby three months old or older)
- Signs of dehydration, including dry mouth, fewer than four wet diapers per day, going four to six hours without urinating, or if the soft spot on your baby's head looks sunken or flatter than usual
- Blood in the stool or vomit
- Stiff neck, which could be a sign of meningitis
- Listlessness or unusual sleepiness

Also call your doctor if your baby has been vomiting for longer than eight hours or vomits with great force.

for the third time, there's nothing you can do but laugh! Fortunately, stomach viruses come and go quickly. It lasted just 24 hours, but these things do tend to happen when the husband is out of town!

—*Brooke Jackson, MD*

∽

When my son was five months old, we took a trip to France. All of a sudden after lunch one day, he had projectile vomiting, then diarrhea.

I placed a panicked call to my son's pediatrician, and we determined that most likely my son had caught a virus on the plane that had caused his gastrointestinal upset. The pediatrician recommended I give my son Pedialyte and keep him well hydrated.

—*Sharon Giese, MD, a mom of a two-year-old son and a cosmetic plastic surgeon in private practice, in New York City*

∽

After medical school, some doctors are extremely anxious about germs and have a fear of getting sick. Other doctors, like me, develop a more laissez-faire attitude. I'm confident that our immune systems can take care of most things. I believe in the five-second rule, and I'd let my kids put things back into their mouths that have fallen briefly on the ground.

My kids were almost never sick, and I wasn't the type of parent who ran around sterilizing everything. I think that the more sterile the environment, the more likely kids are to develop allergies. My kids have great immune systems, and I believe it's partly because of all of the things they were exposed to. Vaccinate against the really bad actors, and then don't worry too much about germs.

—*Amy Baxter, MD, a mom of 13- and 10-year-old sons and an 8-year-old daughter, the CEO of MMJ Labs, and the director of emergency research of Children's Healthcare of Atlanta at Scottish Rite, in Atlanta, GA*

RALLIE'S TIP

Since my children were little, I've given them slippery elm bark for bellyaches. Because slippery elm bark is very mucilaginous, it coats and soothes the tissues of the digestive tract. It's also very nutritious.

At Valley Forge, George Washington's troops reportedly sustained themselves through a long, cold winter by eating gruel made of the bark of the slippery elm tree. I'm perfectly happy when a mother tells me she plans to give her older baby a half-teaspoon of high-quality powdered slippery elm bark for a simple upset stomach. It works very well!

Watching for Signs of Asthma

"I feel like a fish out of water." That's how one boy described asthma.

Nearly five million kids under the age of 18 know *exactly* what he was talking about. Asthma is becoming more common in the United States, and experts are puzzled why. Most babies who will develop asthma do so by the time they're six months old.

Asthma is a chronic disease of the lungs that causes the airways to swell, tighten, and produce excess mucus. This causes a baby to feel short of breath and have difficulty breathing. This causes a *mom* to have major worry. Doctors sometimes describe asthma as having "twitchy airways." Signs of asthma in a baby include noisy breathing, wheezing, panting, difficulty sucking or eating, and a softer, different-sounding cry.

Around half of all children with asthma outgrow it by their teen years. Sometimes as children's airways mature, they're better able to handle airway inflammation and irritants, so their symptoms decrease.

My daughter had her first breathing challenge when she was nine months old. I remember sitting at home with her, and she was getting wheezy and coughing. It was a cold night, and so I bundled her up and took her to the emergency room. By the time we got there, she was breathing well, smiling, giggling, and doing just fine. I think the night air helped her to breathe. The doctor diagnosed pneumonia.

Now I'm careful to watch my daughter for signs of asthma. It most commonly flares up after she's had a cold.

—*Robyn Liu, MD, a mom of seven- and four-year-old daughters and a family physician with Greeley County Health Services, in Tribune, KS*

My younger son had a rocky delivery, and his lungs took a bit of a hit. He might have inhaled some meconium.

The nurses in the hospital monitored my son's breathing very carefully. During his first four weeks, he didn't have asthma, and I wasn't too worried about it at first. But when my son was a month old, my husband caught the flu, and then the baby caught it too. It caused him to start wheezing. We took him to the pediatrician, and we were given a nebulizer and medicine. After that, we took the nebulizer and medicine with us even on trips, and we were careful to get his treatments in.

Often my son would cry and cry when we gave him his treatment with the nebulizer. But I didn't mind a bit because I knew the more he cried, the more of that beneficial medicine he sucked in!

—*Leena Shrivastava Dev, MD, a mom of 14- and 10-year-old sons, an assistant professor of medicine at Drexel University College of Medicine, and a general pediatrician, in Philadelphia, PA*

My younger daughter has asthma. I recognized it quickly because I completed a pediatrics internship. When babies have asthma, it sometimes looks like their breathing is very labored, and they're really sucking in air.

My daughter's asthma was especially scary when we were traveling. I would think, *I'm in Jamaica. If something happens to her, I won't be able to get good hospital care here.*

If you have a child with respiratory difficulties, clearly you don't want her to get to a place where it's an emergency situation. It's important to maintain your own calm and to have physical contact with your baby, because that can be very reassuring.

Even though it was scary that my daughter had asthma, it probably was a little easier for me because she's my third child.

—*Nancy Rappaport, MD*

I have a family history of asthma, and during my daughter's first year, she was diagnosed with asthma too. She didn't have wheezing like you might expect. Instead, she had an almost nonstop dry, hacking cough. Sometimes she'd cough so much she'd regurgitate her food. I always kept a change of clothes for her in my diaper bag.

Being away from home could be especially stressful. We always took my daughter's nebulizer with us so we could give her treatments if necessary. We were careful to pack the nebulizer and the medicine in a very accessible place. Once we needed to pull into a rest stop on the highway to give her a treatment. And we certainly always carried it onto planes, never checking it with the baggage. We got some odd looks when the nebulizer went through the X-ray machine at the airport!

It was helpful to learn what my daughter's asthma triggers were. For example, a change in season, being exposed to animals, or just being in a new environment could set off an asthma attack.
—*Ann V. Arthur, MD*

Brushing Your Baby's Teeth and Gums

Baby teeth seem somewhat disposable, but actually your baby will have those teeth until he's at least five to seven years old.

Baby teeth are also sometimes called primary teeth. They start to make their appearance when a baby is between four and seven months. Most kids have all 20 of their baby teeth by their third birthdays. Baby teeth serve several important roles: They help your baby to speak and chew, of course, but they also hold space in the jaws for your baby's permanent teeth, which are growing under his gums.

? When to Call Your Doctor

If your baby is very cranky and unable to eat due to teething pain, call your doctor or dentist. Also see "Tackling Teething Pain" on page 214.

If you are concerned that your baby's teeth are not coming in properly or on time, contact your dentist.

The American Dental Association (ADA) recommends your baby have his first trip to the dentist within six months after his first tooth appears, and certainly by his first birthday. You can think of these visits as "well baby checkups."

The ADA recommends beginning to clean your baby's mouth the first few days after he's born. If that ship has already sailed, the ADA urges parents to begin cleaning teeth as soon as they erupt to remove plaque and prevent tooth decay.

❧

When my kids were babies, I used a washcloth and a bit of baby toothpaste to clean their teeth. The American Dental Association accepts this method for cleaning an infant's teeth. I found that

Mommy MD Guides–Recommended Product
Orajel Tooth and Gum Cleanser

Baby toothpaste might seem like an extra, unnecessary cost, not to mention one more thing to cram into the already overfull medicine cabinet. But actually babies should not use adult toothpaste. Most toothpaste that's made for adults contains fluoride, which is a mineral that prevents cavities.

Fluoride is one of medicine's greatest success stories. It's dental science's main weapon against tooth decay. But as with so many things in life, you *can* have too much of a good thing. Here's the story.

Back in 1901, a young dental school graduate named Frederick McKay opened a dental practice in Colorado Springs, CO. McKay made a startling observation: Many of his patients had permanent brown stains on their teeth, some as dark as chocolate. The locals blamed the stains on eating too much pork or drinking bad milk. But they were wrong. It was actually something in the water . . .

The patients might not have liked how their teeth *looked*, but at least they kept their teeth for a long while. Their teeth were sur-

using a washcloth was easier than using a toothbrush.

—*Ann Kulze, MD, a mom of 22- and 15-year-old daughters and 20- and 19-year-old sons; a nationally recognized nutrition expert, motivational speaker, and family physician; and the author of the best-selling book* Eat Right for Life, *in Charleston, SC*

⤞⤝

My baby doesn't have teeth yet, but I do use a washcloth to clean her gums to get her used to having her mouth cleaned. Also I wash away the milkiness on her tongue. That's all we've gotten to so far.

—*Jennifer Bacani McKenney, MD, a mom of a two-month-old daughter and a family physician, in Fredonia, KS*

prisingly resistant to decay. After some study, McKay and his colleagues discovered that the stains—and also the decay resistance—were caused by high levels of fluoride in the water, which was unique to that area of Colorado Springs.

After careful study, scientists determined the ideal amount of fluoride in water—not too much but not too little, just the right amount to protect teeth from decay without altering their color. Today, more than 200 million Americans benefit from fluoridated water. Because your baby is likely exposed to fluoride in water, you don't want him to also be exposed with his toothpaste because that might lead to discoloration of his permanent teeth.

That's why babies under age two should use special infant toothpaste that contains no fluoride, such as Orajel Tooth and Gum Cleanser. You can buy it in stores and online for around $4 a tube. It contains a special ingredient to remove plaque for cleaner teeth and gums. Plus it's safe if swallowed when used as directed.

I started to brush my babies' gums very early, when they started to eat solid foods, with a finger toothbrush. I brushed their gums before they went to sleep.

As soon as my daughters had teeth that were touching, I started to floss them with dental floss picks. They're easy to use because you can hold the pick with one hand and the baby with your other hand.

—*Robyn Liu, MD*

                                                      ∽

I must admit, I never brushed my baby's gums. I had enough to do let alone brush nonexistent teeth!

But when my babies were a few months old, I let them start playing with the baby toothbrush. Once their teeth began to pop through, then I started to brush them.

—*Kristie McNealy, MD, a mom of eight- and five-year-old daughters and three- and one-year-old sons and a blogger at KristieMcNealy.com, in Denver, CO*

∽

I am supposed to be brushing my babies' teeth on a regular basis, but it is quite a challenge. I find it to be really difficult, and I probably do it three times a week, at bath time.

When my babies were really small, they had major aversions to toothbrushes. I washed their gums with a soft washcloth instead, and that went much easier. I use the mimicking technique. I say, "Open your mouth," then I open my mouth. Sometimes they open their mouths, and I quickly dart in with the washcloth.

—*Jennifer Gilbert, DO*

Clipping Fingernails and Toenails

In the category of who-knew-this-would-be-so-hard, clipping baby's fingernails and toenails can be a real challenge. Coming at your baby with a pointy object is just not fun, for you or for him.

It's not your imagination that toenails do seem to grow slower than fingernails. Don't worry too much about ingrown nails because they are rarely a problem in babies.

I've had the easiest time clipping my baby's fingernails while I'm nursing her or when she's on her changing table because those are both times when she is calmest. I have to clip her fingernails almost every other day to keep her from scratching her face. We keep mittens on her a lot of the time to keep her from scratching herself.

—*Jennifer Bacani McKenney, MD*

Have a Mani-Pedi

Why not reward yourself for the challenge of having to cut your baby's fingernails and toenails with having your own nails pampered? A manicure and pedicure is a great treat. It's a joy to have someone taking care of *you* for a change.

RALLIE'S TIP

My youngest son was a wiggle worm from the moment he was born. As soon as he was able, he would try to slither away from me whenever I tried to change his diaper or dress him. There was no way he was going to sit still long enough to have all of his fingernails and toenails trimmed!

I finally figured out that if I waited till he was sound asleep, I could clip his nails without the slightest bit of resistance. I used that trick until he was three or four years old.

My kids hate to have their nails cut. What I have finally started to do is to sit them on my lap in front of the TV! I cut their nails when there's a show on that really captures their attention, like *Yo Gabba Gabba*. I also give them an extra set of clippers to play with so they're not trying to grab mine.

I must admit, I get far behind on their toenails. I just pray no one looks at their feet!

—*Jennifer Gilbert, DO*

I had often heard that you should cut your baby's fingernails and toenails while she's sleeping. My babies never slept much, so I certainly wasn't going to risk waking them up by clipping their nails!

When my babies were really little, I found that instead of clipping them, it was easier to file them. That way I didn't worry about accidentally cutting their skin.

—*Kristie McNealy, MD*

Nail trimming is a surprisingly challenging experience. Babies tend to curl their fingers inward for the first several months. Further, their nails are tiny and very soft. My husband seemed better able to handle this job than I did. (I actually cut off at least one layer of skin on at least two of my kids when I tried to do it!)

Baby nail clippers are available, which are smaller in size and better suited for little fingers. Sometimes it's easier to have two adults working at once: one holding out the finger and the other doing the cutting.

—*Stacey Weiland, MD, a mom of a 12-year-old daughter and 7- and 5-year-old sons and an internist/gastroenterologist, in Denver, CO*

Giving Your Baby Vitamins

Even though you can buy vitamins everywhere over the counter, it's best to think of them as drugs when it comes to your baby. Early on, it's a great idea to check with your pediatrician to get her specific recommendation for your baby. Generally, doctors don't recommend giving breastfed babies any supplemental vitamins because breast milk typically offers all of the nutrients a baby needs. Along the same lines, formula offers all that a baby needs. When babies grow into toddlers, they sometimes develop erratic eating habits, and then you might want to revisit this topic with your doctor.

I gave my children supplements from an early age. A good combination remedy is called IntraKid by Drucker Labs. It's a liquid, raspberry flavor, and most of the children I've given it to like it. Yes, it is okay for babies. They just take less: one teaspoon for starters. The company also makes IntraMax, which is great for parents. You can buy it online.

—*Cathie Lippman, MD*

When my daughters were babies, we were living in Portland, OR, where there was no fluoride in the water. I gave them a fluoride supplement called Poly-Vi-Flor from an early age. It's a liquid multivitamin with fluoride. It tastes nasty, but my daughters got used to it. When my daughters turned two years old, I switched them to a halved chewable vitamin.

—*Robyn Liu, MD*

I gave my babies the prescription infant multivitamins my pediatrician recommended. At the time, we were living in Germany. Their water doesn't contain fluoride, and so we used a vitamin that also had fluoride.

One thing to watch out for with those infant liquid vitamins is that they stain terribly. To prevent it from getting on my babies' clothes, I gave them their vitamins in the tub during bath time.

—*Ann Kulze, MD*

My kids are fairly good eaters, and so I've never given them vitamins. I'm supposed to be giving them fluoride treatments, but I haven't been able to fill the prescription yet!

—*Jennifer Gilbert, DO*

I haven't started to give my baby vitamins yet. But soon, I'm going to talk to her family physician about it. I think at some point I need to begin supplementing her diet with vitamin D and iron. I know it's coming.

—*Jennifer Bacani McKenney, MD*

Going to the Park or Playground

Pushing a baby on a swing with the wind in his hair, catching him at the bottom of the slide—these are some of the greatest joys in life.

When I take my sons to the park or playground, I protect their skin (physically or with sunscreen) from the sun's harmful rays.

—*Amy J. Derick, MD, a mom of two-year-old and nine-month-old sons and a dermatologist in private practice at Derick Dermatology, in Barrington, IL*

MomMy TIME

Take a Breather

Even though you'll have your baby with you at the park or playground, it's still possible to get some me time while you're there.

If even for only a few seconds, close your eyes and tip your face to the sun. Breathe in the smells of nature, let your shoulders relax, and smile. Take a few deep breaths. You'll be amazed how different the world looks when you open your eyes again.

As soon as my babies could sit up, I started taking them to the park. We live in Florida, so we can go to the park year-round, except in the summer when it's really hot, and we do water activities instead. Both the kids and I have met a number of friends there. We made even more friends once they started preschool. At that point, your social life changes dramatically.

—*Michelle Paley, MD, PA, a mom of two and a psychiatrist and psychotherapist in private practice, in Miami Beach, FL*

It's amazing the difference in parenting a second child. I'm so much more relaxed now. For example, when we go to the park, I let my son crawl around on the ground. I don't overly protect him nearly as much as I did my older son. My baby has a couple more bumps and scrapes to go with that, but he's a little tougher too. He's really been fun.

—*Rebecca Reamy, MD, a mom of six- and one-year-old sons and a pediatrician in emergency medicine at Children's Healthcare of Atlanta, in Georgia*

My kids move nonstop. I have three boys who are pretty close in age, and when they were young, our house was right across the street from a park. It was like our big front yard.

If you go to a playground, make sure that the play equipment your children use is age appropriate. Never leave a baby unattended in a swing. Be sure to bring sunscreen and extra drinks if it's a hot day.

—*Charlene Brock, MD, a mom of 28-, 25-, and 23-year-old sons and an 18-year-old daughter and a pediatrician with St. Chris Care at Falls Center, in Philadelphia, PA*

One of the most indispensable items I used during my children's first years was the playpen. I mean the full-size, fold-in-the-middle, bulky playpen. The German nanny who cared for my oldest child (and three other little ones) while I was at work thought nothing of taking the playpen outside. She taught me that it is wonderful to think of it as something portable, and not just something to keep in the family room. There were naps in the shade of the trees, playing safely while I planted flowers, listening to the birds while I was hanging out the laundry. Sometimes, I could even read while they played safely and comfortably beside me. It was well worth the effort of moving it around.

—*Lesley Burton-Iwinski, MD*

Chapter 6
6th Month

Your Baby This Month

YOUR BABY'S DEVELOPMENT

When your baby reaches the halfway mark of her first year, her growth slows down a bit. Before this, she probably gained half an ounce a day, and that slows for the next six months—for the rest of her life actually!

Around six months, your baby's permanent eye color is starting to set in. What color are they? Your baby's vision has now improved so that she can see you from clear across a room. She can now track a moving object.

By around six months, your baby will start to predictably turn to the sound of your voice. She recognizes where sounds are coming from now. Around this time, she will be able to distinguish the syllables of her name.

By six months, your baby can pick up on her previous experiences. So for example, if you show her how pressing a button on a toy makes a sound, she might remember that and start to press the button all on her own. Patience is a virtue, though, because at this age, your baby might need to hear or see something dozens of times before she'll remember it.

Your baby is probably starting to sleep more at night now than during the day. At this age, most babies sleep around 10 hours at night and around four hours, split between two naps, during the day.

The major development of the sixth month is sitting up. This is a huge milestone for your baby, and it's also a milestone for you. When a baby can sit without needing to use her hands for balance, she can use her hands to communicate her wishes and needs, and she can also use her hands to entertain herself. So your baby is less likely to want to be held and carried every second of every day. This is bound to be bittersweet for you!

By now, when your baby is lying on the floor during tummy time, she can raise herself up almost to her belly button. Watch her do baby push-ups! This amazing development allows your baby to do lots of new things: She can use her arms to steer and pivot herself around on her abdomen, allowing her more freedom than ever before. She can probably now roll over both ways.

Your baby can probably bear some weight on her legs when you hold her hands. She might even be able to stand while holding onto someone or something.

Your baby can start to transfer things from hand to hand. If you try to take a toy away, she'll likely protest like crazy. You are probably trying to prevent her from putting it into her mouth, after all!

Speaking of hands, it might seem like your baby favors one hand over the other. But actually, true handedness isn't usually determined until the toddler years.

At this age, your baby will figure out that dropping something is just as much fun as picking it up, maybe even more so. This quickly becomes the how-often-will-Mommy-pick-this-spoon-up-when-I-drop-it game.

As your baby's tongue thrust reflex goes away, she's starting to be able to eat soft solid foods. She might be able to feed herself some finger foods, such as a cracker.

Separation anxiety often begins at this stage. It often coincides with a baby's learning to crawl. Interestingly, at this age, babies recognize their names. They pay more attention to words following their names than to words spoken after someone else's name.

Your baby is starting to babble, imitating speech in tone and pattern. Beginning baby babble consists of long strings of syllables, such as ba-ba. Amazingly, this is language specific, so an American baby's wah-wah sounds different from a French baby's oui-oui.

TAKING CARE OF YOU
If you smoke, quit! You've never had a better reason to do so.

JUSTIFICATION FOR A CELEBRATION
Your baby is half of a year old! Proudly looking at your baby proudly sitting up—*all by herself*—is cause for a celebration!

Going Shopping with Your Baby

The average shopper visits the grocery store 2.3 times per week. She usually spends 10 to 60 minutes per shopping visit. No one knows how many of those minutes are spent saying, "Stop touching that!"

∽

I have triplets, and I haven't seen the inside of a grocery store in a couple of years! My husband does all of the grocery shopping for me on weekends. During the week, if I notice we need something, I let him know. My husband doesn't bother making a grocery list. Thankfully, he's got a good memory!

—*Sadaf T. Bhutta, MD, a mom of a five-year-old daughter and three-year-old triplets and an assistant professor and the fellowship director of pediatric radiology at the University of Arkansas for Medical Sciences and Arkansas Children's Hospital, both in Little Rock*

∽

All four of my infants had colic. It was so bad that I couldn't take them to the grocery store. I waited until my husband got home from work to watch the kids, and then I went to the store by myself. I shopped at pretty odd hours of the night sometimes.

—*Ann Kulze, MD, a mom of 22- and 15-year-old daughters and 20- and 19-year-old sons; a nationally recognized nutrition expert, motivational speaker, and family physician; and the author of the best-selling book* Eat Right for Life, *in Charleston, SC*

∽

With twins, grocery shopping is a two-parent event. My husband and I each take a cart, and we put one baby in each cart. Inevitably, I end up opening a box of crackers in the store to keep them happy, and then of course we pay for the crackers at the register! I try to get as far as I can before doing that though. We usually get through the store without a whole lot of screaming. But when we don't, we get a lot of "looks." Those people must not have kids.

When I have to take both twins to the store by myself, I put one in the baby seat and the other in the cart, and I push the cart *very* slowly. You do what you have to do!

—*Jennifer Gilbert, DO, a mom of 18-month-old twins and an ob-gyn at Paoli Hospital, in Pennsylvania*

Although I think grocery cart covers can be a wonderful idea, putting that cover onto my grocery cart was one step I just wasn't able to take. As long as my baby was otherwise healthy and doing well, the cart cover made more work for my husband and me. So we let that go.

—*Katja Rowell, MD, a mom of a five-year-old daughter, a family physician, and a childhood feeding specialist with FamilyFeedingDynamics.com, in St. Paul, MN*

When I was thinking about having a third baby, the thought of taking my kids grocery shopping scared me half to death. *Where am I going to put all of these kids and still have a place for groceries?* I wondered.

When my babies were really small, I carried them in the store in a front carrier to keep them comfortable and sleeping—and to free up some space in the grocery cart.

Now that I have four children, I put my baby in the infant seat in one part of the cart. My older son sits in the "kid" seat at the front of the cart, and my younger daughter sits in the main basket of the cart. Then I get a second cart, which my older daughter pushes. That's where we put the food.

Where my college roommate lives, one of the grocery stores has a day care! She says it's more expensive to shop there, but I wouldn't care!

—*Kristie McNealy, MD, a mom of eight- and five-year-old daughters and three- and one-year-old sons and a blogger at KristieMcNealy.com, in Denver, CO*

My babies were pretty good when we had to go to the grocery store. When they were very small, I carried them in front carriers, and when they were bigger, I buckled them into the kid basket in the front of the shopping cart. I don't recommend attaching the infant car seat to the shopping cart. It's dangerous.

Sometimes if I didn't need a lot of groceries, I'd just put my baby into an umbrella stroller. Then I'd tuck the groceries in the basket behind the stroller, rather than getting a shopping cart.

The only time my babies tended to get upset in the store was while we were in the checkout line. That's when they'd scream! I generally would just take them out of the cart and hold them, which usually calmed them down. But sometimes, nothing helped. They'd just scream until we left the store. Today, when I see moms in that situation, I have a lot of empathy. I so clearly remember those days.

—*Charlene Brock, MD, a mom of 28-, 25-, and 23-year-old sons and an 18-year-old daughter and a pediatrician with St. Chris Care at Falls Center, in Philadelphia, PA*

When my older son was a baby, we lived in Charleston. There's a great outdoor mall there, and I would put my baby into the BabyBjörn. I could browse for two to three hours with him happy as can be.

—*Rebecca Reamy, MD, a mom of six- and one-year-old sons and a pediatrician in emergency medicine at Children's Healthcare of Atlanta, in Georgia*

I really loved visiting the toy stores in Dallas. My daughter (who was two at the time) would always enjoy our visits, and she would never fuss when we left.

If I noticed my daughter playing with something that I decided I would like to buy, I would work with the salespeople to buy it surreptitiously. It was pretty easy to sneak the bag under the stroller or in my purse. Then some days later at home, I would bring the toy out and we would enjoy playing with it. She didn't associate being in the store and wanting something with getting it, so she never whined and pitched a fit about getting something. And she still got some wonderful, special toys that held her interest.

—*Lesley Burton-Iwinski, MD, a mom of 20- and 18-year-old daughters and a 14-year-old son, a retired family physician, and a parent and teacher educator with* Growing Peaceful Families, *in Lexington, KY*

If you're breastfeeding, taking your baby shopping can be challenging. Where and how do you do that? With my first baby, I stole away in privacy and covered myself up modestly and hid from the world to nurse.

Then one day in a shoe store in a huge fancy shopping mall in Dallas, TX, I came upon a mother sitting amongst the shoe try-ons nursing her infant without any trouble or embarrassment. She and her baby looked lovely and elegant and perfectly comfortable, with people trying on shoes all around them. She inspired me. I will never forget her.

I nursed my next baby all over the place—in stores and parking lots and even in restaurants. Occasionally people winked at us kindly. This was in a large city in the South almost 30 years ago, and I cannot say that every public culture and personal circumstance is the same, so each mother has to decide for herself what is best for her and her child.

—*Elizabeth Berger, MD, a mom of a 28-year-old son and a 26-year-old daughter, a child psychiatrist, and the author of* Raising Kids with Character, *in New York City*

Finding a Nanny, Babysitter, or Day Care

Finding a nanny, babysitter, or day care for your baby is a very important task. This might have been a choice you made many months ago, or perhaps you're just beginning your search or you need to make a change.

❧

It's funny, when people have extra work to do at the office, they think nothing of hiring extra help. But as mothers, we're not supposed to do that. Before my daughter was born, I had hired a baby nurse to live with us during my daughter's first few weeks. The nurse I chose was a hard-core, military-like nurse. She was older than me, and I prefer that. I'm humble; I want someone who is in that role to know more than I do! I feel the same way about nannies.

> —*Dina Strachan, MD, a mom of a five-year-old daughter, a dermatologist and director of Aglow Dermatology, and an assistant clinical professor in the department of dermatology at Columbia University College of Physicians and Surgeons, in New York City*

❧

It's critical when you work away from home to find reliable, good child care. I was very lucky that I didn't have to rely on family members on a day-to-day basis. I believe that family members take care of a baby the way they want to. But a hired caregiver will care for the baby the way you direct them.

> —*Sandra Carson, MD, a mom of two grown sons and the director of the Center for Reproduction and Infertility of Women and Infants Hospital, in Providence, RI*

❧

When our babies were about 2½ months old, my husband and I hired a night nanny because we were both working. Having a solo medical practice means that you don't really get maternity leave because there is no coverage and your patients want to see you. Our night nanny would arrive at 10 p.m. and leave at 6 a.m., which allowed my husband and me to get a full night of sleep—priceless!

Because we would still both be in the house, we felt comfortable hiring a younger person, a grad student actually. They're up all night studying anyway! She would study or sleep on the couch in the nursery and take care of the twins when they woke up in the middle of the night.

   —*Brooke Jackson, MD, a mom of 3½-year-old twin girls and a 14-month-old son and a dermatologist and medical director of the Skin Wellness Center of Chicago, in Illinois*

When I went back to work, it was very hard to drive off and see my little one being excited to experience the world with someone who wasn't me. I was blessed to find a terrific nanny who really became part of our family. That took the edge off of the separation.

   We chose to find a nanny instead of a day care so our boys could stay in their home environment. Our nanny was recommended to me by a classmate in my prenatal yoga class.

   —*Lauren Feder, MD, a mom of 17- and 13-year-old sons, a nationally recognized physician who specializes in homeopathic medicine, and the author of* Natural Baby and Childcare *and* The Parents' Concise Guide to Childhood Vaccinations, *in Los Angeles, CA*

Initially, I had planned to put my daughter in day care, but there are very few day cares in New York City that take infants.

   Instead, I ended up hiring a nanny to come to my home. That takes a big leap of faith. You have to do a lot of interviewing, and trust your gut. If a situation doesn't feel right, it probably isn't.

   —*Ann V. Arthur, MD, a mom of a nine-year-old daughter and a seven-year-old son, a pediatric ophthalmologist in private practice at Park Slope Eye Care Associates, and a blogger at WaterWineTravel.com, in New York City*

Because many of us in this country are not given more than six to 12 weeks off work when we have our babies, my husband and I felt it was important to find a reliable and loving nanny. We went through a nanny referral service and found a responsible, loving woman we could rely on and occasionally have babysit on weekends.

Remember to check the nanny's references and the quality of those references as well. Don't rely solely on the information provided by the nanny referral service for such an important employee.

—*Darlene Gaynor-Krupnick, DO, a mom of five- and two-year-old daughters, a female urologist fellow trained in pelvic reconstruction and neurology, and the inventor of Valera, a USDA-certified organic vaginal lubricant, in northern Virginia*

My husband and I waited to have children until we could afford to have a nanny come to our house. But finding a nanny was quite the learning process.

It was a different world 22 years ago, and we simply put an ad in the paper. I started interviewing nannies in my third trimester so that the nanny could start working before our baby was born and so we'd have a seamless transfer.

We chose a nanny who was 19 or 20 years old, figuring she'd have more energy than an older lady. She lasted six weeks. After that, we hired a nanny who was in her early to mid-thirties, and she worked out great.

Years later, when we needed to find another nanny, we used a nanny referral service. It's expensive, but it's much easier and safer than trying to find one yourself.

—*Lisa Dado, MD, a mom of three children, ages 21 to 16, a pediatric anesthesiologist with Valley Anesthesiology Consultants, and a cofounder and CEO of the Center for Human Living, which teaches life skills and martial arts training, in Phoenix, AZ*

When my daughter was born 45 years ago, I went back to work a few days later and then worked nonstop. That's the way it was back then.

I worked very hard to find a good babysitter. I interviewed quite a few people until I found the right one. I found a marvelous babysitter who was the wife of a doctor. She was very good to my daughter. She and her husband had three children of their own. Their youngest was five years old, and she loved playing with my daughter.

My daughter liked it there so much that she cried sometimes

when it was time to go home! I think part of it was because at the babysitter's house, she had "siblings."

A few years later, the family moved, and I had to revisit my search for a babysitter. I found another woman nearby who watched kids in her home. It seemed like an ideal situation, partly because the babysitter picked my daughter up from school and took her to her home each day. But one day, I picked my daughter up from the babysitter's house, and I could tell she wasn't happy there. Things weren't quite as they had been presented to me, and the woman was watching more kids than she said she was. I pulled my daughter out of that situation immediately. Fortunately, she hadn't been going there long.

After that, I found a lady a block away from my home who was taking care of two other girls. They were the same age as my daughter, and they all went to the same school. The three girls were all only children, and they became so close that they were like sisters. That was a great situation!

—*Shirley M. Mueller, MD, a mom of a grown daughter and a grandmother of two, a board-certified neurologist and psychiatrist, and the CEO and president of MyMoneyMD.com, in Indianapolis, IN*

RALLIE'S TIP

Before the birth of my second baby, I searched long and hard for a nanny to keep my son at home while my husband and I were working. My neighbor recommended a woman who had been her school-age children's nanny for five or six years, and I was very excited to find her. My husband and I interviewed her and checked her references, and we were confident that she would be the perfect nanny for our new baby. A few weeks after I brought my son home from the hospital, I wanted to introduce him to the woman that I thought would be his new nanny. When I put my tiny newborn in her arms, I could tell she was very uncomfortable. Her arms were stiff, and she spoke to him in a loud voice. She didn't seem to think that he was precious at all! When she handed him back to me, she didn't know how to support his head. Although she had cared for babies years ago, she seemed to have forgotten everything she knew.

I felt terrible, but there was no way I could leave my baby with her when I went back to work. My husband and I had to tell her that we were so sorry, but we had changed our minds. We gave her two weeks' pay and wished her well. I found a new nanny in about a month, and it's amazing how my requirements had changed! Most of all, I wanted my son's nanny to be a kind and gentle person who would love him almost as much as I did. Our new nanny was just that, and she was a very important part of our family's life for the next five years.

I needed to return to work after I had all three of my children. I think that one of my *biggest* regrets is that I couldn't stay at home with them longer. I had six weeks off with my daughter (although it really turned into only 4½ weeks because she came 10 days late), and three months off with my boys.

When I had my daughter, I was a first-year gastroenterology fellow, and my husband was a fourth-year medical student. (He had worked for several years before going back to medical school.) We didn't have much money. We initially asked his mom if she could help us out, but at the time, she was living up in Vail, which was about a two-hour drive from where we were living in Denver. Much to our surprise, she said no!

Looking back now, I think that it was probably better for me that she did not start helping us out daily (she and my father-in-law are, however, a *huge* help!), because particularly with our daughter, I experienced tremendous feelings of insecurity. On the other hand, after going through day care and then a nanny, I think that if you can get a grandma to be the babysitter, it is best for the baby. I remember reading something in *The Girlfriends' Guide to Pregnancy* about how your mother-in-law will love your child so much that if you were in a burning building, she would push *you* out of the way to save your child!

Because we didn't have my mother-in-law as an option, we had to look around. The best advice I can give here is that you *absolutely* need to take your time. It was unbelievably amazing what variability existed! And, for us, the places that we *thought* should have been the best definitely *weren't* the best!

The first place we looked at was a child care center affiliated with the University Hospital, because we both worked there, and a lot of other doctors and nurses sent their kids there. The waiting list was phenomenal. You basically had to put your name down when you were just considering becoming pregnant! Sounds like a great place, right?

Well, all child care institutions, even those in private homes, have documented public records regarding their qualifications, inspections, and complaints. When we researched this place, the complaint list was like a mile long: children with broken arms, recurrent violations, kids getting sent out to buy cigarettes! We were completely floored!

Next, we went to a few church-run facilities. Again we were disappointed. The places just didn't seem sanitary. Children were coming up to us with grimy faces, asking us to take them home with us!

We had our daughter in a private home day care for I think two days or so. The thing that bothered us there was the age mix. The poor lady running the day care was caring for babies and school-age children. We were concerned about their safety, and we worried about how much attention our daughter would receive.

Then we looked at a national day care institution—KinderCare. The children were separated by age, and the facility had the appropriate ratio of caregivers to children. They had daily "lesson plans" (for infants!) and daily progress reports. Most importantly, when we looked up their public records, there were almost no complaints! Unfortunately, when we decided to go with them, they had no spots.

So, we were in a jam. But, I have the *very* best husband. He had just finished up his fourth year of medical school, and instead of going right into an internship, he actually took a year off to be with our daughter. It was definitely the best outcome for our baby, and it was a great bonding experience for them.

Our daughter did get into KinderCare after a few months, and in the meantime, my husband did some research in the radiology department and got himself published, which is always a good thing for the résumé.

The only one who began to have a problem with the whole arrangement, unfortunately, was *me*. It's not that I was unhappy with my husband's care of our daughter—quite the contrary. It's the fact that he was *so good at it!* I felt like I wasn't needed—that *my* baby didn't need me! And, in fact, there were times when she'd want him and *not ME!* "Daddy do it!"—when it was bath time, diaper-changing time, buckling in the car seat, etc. It was a *killer!*

Nursing was the only time when I was the only one, and I *loved* it! But when that ended, and even when my husband started his residency training, our daughter remained a *Daddy's girl*. It has taken me a *long* time to get over that.

> —*Stacey Weiland, MD, a mom of a 12-year-old daughter and 7- and 5-year-old sons and an internist/gastroenterologist, in Denver, CO*

Sitting Up

Look who's sitting pretty! The average baby sits up at six or seven months. This exciting development sets the stage for many more, such as reaching and grabbing for objects. It's a major milestone.

∽

When my babies reached major motor development milestones like sitting, I felt so joyful. I can remember propping my babies up with pillows behind them for support to help them to sit up.

> *Ann Kulze, MD*

∽

My older daughter loved her Bumbo seat. She always wanted to see what was going on. We moved the Bumbo seat from room to room, wherever we were going to be. For example, if my husband and I were washing dishes in the kitchen, we'd place her Bumbo chair on the floor and give her a dish towel and some plastic bowls to play with.

> —*Cheri Wiggins, MD, a mom of four- and two-year-old daughters, a specialist in physical medicine and rehabilitation at St. Luke's Magic Valley, and a cofounder of the Mommy Doctors Bakery (makers of Milkin' Cookies), in Twin Falls, ID*

I never had a Bumbo chair. They came out after my first two kids were born, and I figured I'd lived without one for that long, why get it now?

Instead, I used my Boppy nursing pillow. I put it behind my babies when they were sitting on the floor during that stage when they wanted to sit up more than they really could.

—*Kristie McNealy, MD*

Sitting up is just one milestone among many that new mothers and fathers dutifully track. For our second born, my husband and I were more relaxed, knowing that each child is different, and each child will reach his or her milestone when ready.

—*Amy J. Derick, MD, a mom of two-year-old and nine-month-old sons and a dermatologist in private practice at Derick Dermatology, in Barrington, IL*

Kids don't meet milestones on the clock. If your baby doesn't sit up on schedule, don't stress out over it. I learned early on that my son did everything at his own pace, but when he did things, he did them better than everyone else. For example, he talked somewhat later than most

Mommy MD Guides-Recommended Product
Bumbo Seat

"One product I used often was the Bumbo seat," says Kathleen Moline, DO, a mom of a 20-month-old daughter and a family physician in private practice with Central DuPage Physician Group, in Winfield, IL. "I put my daughter in it to help her to sit up and also sometimes when I was feeding her."

One important safety caution: Never, ever place a Bumbo seat—or any other baby device such as a bouncer seat—onto an elevated surface, such as a sofa, bed, table, or countertop. Even a small baby could get the chair off-balance and topple onto the floor, with serious consequences.

You can buy Bumbo seats online and in stores for around $40.

babies, but today he writes poetry and music, and those are some of his strongest skills.

When a kid turns 18, it doesn't matter at what age he first talked or sat on the potty. People pressure you and try to make these milestones into a competition. But as long as you support your child, you're doing great.

—Judith Hellman, MD, a mom of a 13-year-old son, an associate clinical professor of dermatology at Mt. Sinai Hospital, and a dermatologist in private practice, in New York City

 ⟳

When you have to go back to work, you're going to miss some things. You might not be there when your baby sits up for the first time, or when he first crawls or walks. You can't beat yourself up about it. It's not important the first time they do it; what matters is the first time you see them do it!

This was great advice I got in medical school, and I still use it today when I feel I missed something amazing taking place with my boys because I wasn't around to see it.

—Leena Shrivastava Dev, MD, a mom of 14- and 10-year-old sons, an assistant professor of medicine at Drexel University College of Medicine, and a general pediatrician, in Philadelphia, PA

Considering Sleep Training

On the TV show *Mad about You*, Paul and Jamie Buckman Ferberized their baby, Mabel. Interestingly, the episode was shot in one continuous take, as the characters debated the psychological and moral implications of letting a baby cry herself to sleep.

The term *Ferberize* has actually become pretty well known. But many people might not know that it's named for Dr. Richard Ferber, director of the Center for Pediatric Sleep Disorders at Children's Hospital Boston. Dr. Ferber wrote at length on training children to self-soothe by allowing them to cry for a predetermined amount of time before receiving external comfort.

Sleep training is a hot-button issue in parenting, with parents divided over how much, or how little, a baby should be allowed to cry. This can be difficult waters for new parents to navigate because there's not much middle ground: Either you sleep train or you don't. Plus, most parents who are even *considering* sleep training are tremendously sleep deprived and might not be thinking all that clearly.

❧

My son was four months old and still not sleeping through the night. My husband and I decided to start sleep training him. One night, my husband got up and turned off the monitor.

"What are you doing?" I asked.

"If you're not going to go in to get him, listen to your own advice," he told me gently.

I drifted off to sleep. A while later, I woke up and turned the monitor back on. All was quiet; my son had fallen asleep too.

—*Ari Brown, MD, a mom of two, a pediatrician with Capital Pediatric Group, and the author of* Baby 411, *in Austin, TX*

🎯 Mommy MD Guides-Recommended Product
Summer Infant Day and Night Video Monitor

If you're considering sleep training, no doubt you've braced yourself for some rough times. One thing that might make it more bearable is to buy a video monitor. No, you don't want to watch your baby crying every second, but at least you can check on her to make sure that she is okay.

One monitor that's very well reviewed is the Summer Infant Day and Night Video Monitor. You can hear your baby and also see her clearly on a five-inch square monitor. The camera has night vision, so you can even see her in a dark room. It costs around $95 online and in stores.

Or consider the more portable Day and Night Handheld Video Color Monitor for $180.

It's a very personal decision, but my husband and I were okay with letting our daughter cry for short periods of time when she was falling asleep. She cried for only around four minutes, and it seemed like she needed to do that to put herself to sleep. I think it's important for little ones to be able to settle themselves, and they sometimes fuss as they go into and out of sleep cycles. Our daughter woke from each nap and each morning with a huge smile on her face, so we didn't worry too much about a little crying.

—*Katja Rowell, MD*

When our twins were four months old, we started sleep training. We read the book *Healthy Sleep Habits, Happy Child*, and we followed it to the letter. Mark Weissbluth is a genius! Both girls were sleep trained in about eight days.

I must admit that I was the softy and my husband was the rock. The first night I went out and walked the dogs for a long time because the girls screamed for almost an hour. But the next night, they cried for only 42 minutes, then 35 minutes the next. By eight days, it was over with.

It's hard to sleep train, but once your baby is on a schedule, you function better. As a bonus, after my husband and I put our twins to bed, we could actually have a conversation!

—*Brooke Jackson, MD*

I didn't want to do it, but I had to sleep train my twins when they were 11 months old. After almost a year of terrible sleep, I could hardly function and barely felt human at times.

I'm a huge believer in sleep training because it worked for my baby. It took five nights, but we stuck with it because we could see that it was working. It goes back to teaching a baby self-soothing techniques. It's much easier to do it sooner rather than later because those first few nights of listening to my baby cry and scream were hard. I was really wishing we had done it sooner.

Sleep was good for all of us! Sleep issues will come back to haunt you at another point in childhood if they're not addressed early on. In fact, when I was in private practice, questions about sleep issues were some of the most frequently asked by the parents of my pediatric patients.

—Ann Contrucci, MD, a mom of 12-year-old boy-girl twins who works as a pediatric emergency physician, in Atlanta, GA

The number one thing I recommend to my pregnant friends and patients is to read *Secrets of the Baby Whisperer* by Tracy Hogg while they're still pregnant and they have time to really think about it. If they're really geeky like me, they should read it with their partners and discuss a plan for sleep training before the kids arrive.

With twins, I knew I had to get them to sleep, or I would go insane. I returned to work 12 weeks after they were born, and I needed to be able to function as a doctor and a mom. Even though my three babies were very different from each other in personality and size, all three were sleeping 12 hours at night by the time they were three to five months old.

Once we got to the point where our babies were only getting up once each night, around 2 a.m. to eat a little and then fall back to sleep, we Ferberized them. At that point, my husband and I knew in our hearts that they weren't waking because they needed something, but more out of habit. We knew that our babies needed to learn how to fall back to sleep by themselves.

Sleep training totally worked. I've heard that it takes about a day for each month of the baby's age to work. So, for instance, if a baby is three months old, it would take three nights of crying herself to sleep before she'd start to fall asleep without crying. That's exactly what happened for our babies. We did it when our twins were three months, and it took three days. Our son wasn't ready until he was five months, and it took five days.

If you wait until your baby is older to start sleep training, it will take longer, and it will be more painful to go through—for the baby and for you. I think it's better to make an attempt at three months. Then it's not that bad.

—Katherine Dee, MD, a mom of six-year-old twin daughters and a four-year-old son and a radiologist at the Seattle Breast Center, in Washington

A big challenge for me was getting my babies to sleep through the night. The problem is that babies can't tell you why they're crying in the middle of the night. Are they bored? Hungry? Wanting to play? It's really challenging to figure out what's going on.

I breastfed all of my babies, so I had to be there every time they wanted something. But I was lucky that my husband got up in the night with me to share the joy.

When my oldest son was six months old and eating solid food, I knew that he could make it through the night without eating. One night, after an especially rough bout of crying, my husband and I decided enough was enough. We checked to make sure our son was clean and dry and not wrapped up in the crib sheet. Then we walked out of his room and shut the door.

My husband sat on one side of the door, and I sat on the other, and we listened to our son cry for 3 hours and 15 minutes. Any time my husband or I looked like we might get up and check on our son, the other one would say, "Sit down. He'll be fine."

The next night, our son slept clear through the night and slept through the night from then on. With our other babies, we did this a little earlier because we knew it was safe and that we could get away with it.

—*Susan Besser, MD, a mom of six grown children, ages 26, 24, 22, 21, 19, and 17, a grandmom of one, a family physician, and the medical director of Doctors Express-Memphis, in Tennessee*

For me, the biggest challenge of my babies' first years was the sleep schedule and transitioning the babies from my bed to their cribs. I co-slept for the first four to five months, and then I transitioned them to their cribs. Those first few nights were pure torture: going in and comforting them every 15 to 20 minutes all night long until they fell asleep, trying to make sure the baby didn't wake up the other children, and trying not to cry myself to sleep as well.

However, I now have the most amazing sleepers, and they can sleep anywhere. I find that the most stressed-out moms that I see are the ones who never get a night of uninterrupted sleep. I try to remind them that sleep deprivation is a form of torture! I think that the sooner you get a baby on a good sleep cycle, the happier the whole family is!

—*Marra S. Francis, MD, a mom of seven-, six-, and four-year-old daughters and an ob-gyn, in The Woodlands, TX*

I didn't sleep train my babies. If they cried, I would go get them and bring them in bed with me, and they'd fall back to sleep. Interestingly, when I was working in the hospital all night, my husband always reported that the babies all slept through the night. As an obstetrician, my primary goal during the nights I spent at home was to get as much sleep as possible.

—*Lillian Schapiro, MD, a mom of 14-year-old twin girls and an eight-year-old daughter and an ob-gyn with Peachtree Women's Specialists, in Atlanta, GA*

Sleeping, for both my baby and for my husband and me, was the biggest challenge my baby's first year. All of our friends who are parents recommended we Ferberize him. But because my husband and I worked so much, we felt guilty doing that. We felt that we weren't there for him during the day, and we felt awful not being there for him at night too.

When we did try to sleep train our son, it failed because he'd cry and throw up, and we'd give in. It wasn't a good scene.

When our son was around 1½, he finally slept through the night. But I don't think that was the way to go.

Our pediatrician had great advice. He said that teaching your baby to sleep is just like teaching him to read. It's a necessity. The key is that you have to *teach* babies how to sleep through the night. It's not something they know how to do instinctively.

Recently I went to a sleep seminar, and I learned that there is no such thing as a "good" or a "bad" sleeper. Everyone wakes up multiple times each night. Some people know how to soothe themselves back to sleep. Those are the people we call "good" sleepers. Babies need to learn how to soothe themselves back to sleep.

Sleep is critical for good health, especially for kids. So much of their mental and physical growth happens while they sleep.

—Mona Gohara, MD, a mom of four- and two-year-old sons, a dermatologist in private practice, an assistant clinical professor in the department of dermatology at Yale University, and a cofounder of K&J Sunprotective Clothing, in Danbury, CT

Preventing and Treating Colds and Flu

There's good reason we call it the "common cold." In the first year of life, most babies have up to seven colds, which means that you are likely to have up to seven colds this year as well.

Babies' immune systems aren't mature yet, plus most babies spend a lot of time in the company of other babies and kids, who aren't always so good about washing their hands.

A cold is simply an infection of the upper respiratory tract, including your nose and throat. Colds are caused by viruses. In babies, the most common signs of a cold are a runny nose and nasal congestion.

Stuffy noses can make it hard for babies to nurse or drink from a bottle, so watch your baby closely for signs of dehydration, including dry mouth, crying with few or no tears, fewer than four wet diapers per day, going four to six hours without urinating, or if the soft spot on your baby's head looks sunken or flatter than usual.

Flu is more than just a supercharged cold. It's caused by different viruses and is much more severe. Doctors recommend babies older than six months get a flu shot to protect them against this very contagious illness. If there is flu in your area, it's best to keep your baby away from crowds.

⤳

When a baby catches a cold, all you can do is wait it out.

—Nancy Rappaport, MD, a mom of 21- and 16-year-old daughters and an 18-year-old son, an assistant professor of psychiatry at Harvard Medical School, an attending child and adolescent psychiatrist in the Cambridge, MA, public schools, and the author of In Her Wake: A Child Psychiatrist Explores the Mystery of Her Mother's Suicide

Babies really differ in terms of what comforts them when they're not feeling well.

For example, my daughters both liked to be rocked and sung to if they were sick. My son, on the other hand, needed quiet. If I tried to sing

When to Call Your Doctor

If your baby is less than three months old, call your doctor at the first sign of a cold. Babies are at increased risk of complications from a common cold, such as pneumonia.

If your baby is three months old or older and catches a cold, call your doctor if he or she has any of the following signs or symptoms.

- Signs of dehydration, including dry mouth, fewer than four wet diapers per day, going four to six hours without urinating, or if the soft spot on your baby's head looks sunken or flatter than usual
- Fever (any fever in a baby younger than three months old or a fever of 101°F or higher in a baby three months old or older)
- Pulling on ears
- A cough that lasts longer than a week
- Thick, green nasal discharge

Take your baby to the emergency room or call 9-1-1 if she refuses to nurse or drink, coughs hard enough to vomit, coughs up blood-tinged sputum, has difficulty breathing, or turns bluish around her mouth.

If your baby has signs of flu, call your doctor right away. These signs include the following.

- Sudden-onset fever (any fever in a baby younger than three months old or a fever of 101°F or higher in a baby three months old or older)
- Shaking chills
- Less activity than normal
- Dry cough

to him, he'd put his hands over his ears and say, "No sing, Mommy."
—*Lisa Dado, MD*

When my babies got colds, I ran humidifiers in their rooms to make it easier for them to breathe.
—*Mona Gohara, MD*

When my babies had a cold, I just used a lot of bulb suctioning of their poor little noses. There's not much else you can do besides giving lots of extra love—and hand-washing!
—*Lezli Braswell, MD, a mom of a six-year-old daughter and four- and one-year-old sons and a family physician, in Columbus, GA*

My daughter had a few colds during her first year. It was really hard to see her uncomfortable and hurting. It was also difficult to stand by and let her body heal itself. The only thing we could do to help her was to suction her nose out, and that was torture for her and for us!
—*Melody Derrick, MD, a mom of a 17-month-old daughter and a family physician in private practice with Central DuPage Physician Group, in Winfield, IL*

No randomized controlled clinical trial shows that over-the-counter cold medications have any efficacy in children under six years old, according to the American Academy of Pediatrics. The side effects of these medications outweigh any benefits of using them.

My sons got nothing for colds except suctioning of their noses. Suctioning the mucus out of the nose helps the ears drain properly. I used bulb suction to prevent accumulation of fluid in the inner ear, thus averting ear infections as much as I could.
—*Sonia Ng, MD, a mom of seven- and two-year-old sons, a pediatrician, and a sedation attending physician at the Children's Hospital of Philadelphia Pediatric Care and the University Medical Center at Princeton in Princeton, NJ, and the Pediatric Imaging Center in King of Prussia, PA*

One of my daughters is often very congested and sniffly, with a lot of mucus. I run a humidifier in our home, especially when the air is dry. It makes it a lot easier for her to blow the mucus out of her nose.

When my baby has a cold, I put a little saline in her nose, and often suction isn't needed. The saline devices with the quick squirt action are best because it's over and done with before your baby has time to get upset about it.

—*Gabriella Cardone, MD, a mom of five-, three-, and one-year-old daughters and a pediatric emergency physician at Texas Children's Hospital, in Houston*

My husband and I were blessed not to encounter any significant health issues during my baby's first year, but she definitely caught colds. Our home treatment was nasal bulb suction. This is easy to tell other parents to do, but it's much harder to do to your own baby!

I did give my daughter acetaminophen (Tylenol) or ibuprofen (Motrin) for fever or if she seemed uncomfortable. (Talk with your doctor before giving your baby this or any medication.)

—*Kathleen Moline, DO*

For babies with colds, there's not much you can do. I would elevate the head of their cribs, run a vaporizer, and put saline drops in their noses.

I'd also keep an eye out for a fever or crankiness. Those can be signs of an ear infection, and they warrant a call to the doctor.

—*Heather Orman-Lubell, MD, a mom of 10- and six-year-old sons and a pediatrician in private practice at Yardley Pediatrics of St. Christopher's Hospital for Children, in Pennsylvania*

When my younger son was 2½ months old, he had bronchiolitis. It's a super-common viral respiratory infection that usually occurs in the winter. It's a little scary when babies are very young, but he was fine. It was pretty much just a bad chest cold, and he has had no ongoing problem since.

Suctioning his nose and using saline drops were the most helpful things, so he could breathe through his nose.

—*Rebecca Reamy, MD*

My older son started day care when he was three months old when I began my pediatric residency. We were all sick for the next 13 months! We probably had two colds each month! My husband and I just worked through it any way we could. We checked to make sure the baby's nose was clean before naptime, feedings, and bedtime. We gave him acetaminophen (Tylenol) only if absolutely necessary for a fever. (Talk with your doctor before giving your baby this or any medication.)

My husband was pretty quick to want to take the baby to the doctor, as most new dads are when something about the baby is not right. But I'd say, "*I'm* a doctor, and the pediatrician isn't going to do anything about a minor cold!"

I think it helped a lot that none of these medical conditions freaked me out. My husband was a lot more worried about things than I was, but that is probably because I saw all kinds of sickness in the hospital, the emergency department, and the pediatric clinic I was training in.

—*Leena Shrivastava Dev, MD*

During my daughter's first year, she was actually very healthy, and she didn't get serious respiratory infections. I would always get bad colds, while hers were very mild—presumably due to the antibodies she got from my breast milk. That's the strongest argument for continuing to nurse for as long as possible. Respiratory infections can be extremely scary in young infants.

However, be prepared for the shock of your kids suffering one respiratory infection after another once they start day care. Unless you or your partner is in a position to take off work to stay home with them, having a day care that can accommodate sick children is an absolute necessity.

—*Stuart Jeanne Bramhall, MD, a mom of a 30-year-old daughter and a child and adolescent psychiatrist, in New Plymouth, New Zealand*

In my babies' first years, I didn't give them any drugs for a cold. To help to ease their nasal congestion, I'd mix up a saltwater solution in a glass. Then I'd gently and slowly insert 10 to 20 drops of the salty water into the baby's nostrils, let it sit for a few minutes, and then suck the mucus out really well with a nasal aspirator. After that, my babies would nurse better, sleep better, and feel better. For more information on washing the nose, visit Nasopure.com/nasopure-for-kids/babies.

> —Hana R. Solomon, MD, *a mom of four, ages 35 to 19, a board-certified pediatrician, and the author of* Clearing the Air One Nose at a Time: Caring for Your Personal Filter, *in Columbia, MO*

For the few times that my daughters were sick with common colds their first year, I found A/B Otic invaluable for earaches. It's available by prescription from your doctor.

> —Darlene Gaynor-Krupnick, DO

Every illness lasts longer with twins because they pass it back and forth. A cold that should last five days lasts us about two weeks. We use a lot of hand sanitizer, and we avoid sharing cups. But you can't prevent kids from sneezing and coughing on each other, so once someone gets a cold, we all get ready. We all get more rest, and my husband and I increase our vitamin C intake. We try to avoid being around kids with runny noses like the plague, but catching colds is part of the day care experience. Interestingly, when I was a pediatric resident, I don't remember a week when I wasn't sick. When I started my dermatology residency, it was refreshing not to be sick for a year! Kids = germs

> —Brooke Jackson, MD

My babies got lots of colds, of course. Because I had such a menagerie at my house, when someone got something, the "quarantined" signs went up, and away we went, trying to prevent everyone else from getting sick.

I don't get sick too often. I'm not sure if it's because my immune system is so strong from being exposed to so many germs at work. Or if it's because I'm so stubborn and I ignore my illnesses and work right through them.

My husband and I have the philosophy that kids get sick, but as long as they're still playing happily and eating and sleeping normally, we don't treat them with any medications. Despite runny noses and coughs, we never really gave our kids any cold medicine. If they weren't complaining, we just let them go. Babies are much more resilient than most people give them credit for.

—*Susan Besser, MD*

Dealing with Separation Anxiety

You and your baby spent nine months inseparable. Now separation can be painful, for both of you.

⌇

At first, managing work and family was very trying. My husband was very supportive. Throughout the years, balancing these issues has been more or less trying.

—*Cathie Lippman, MD, a mom of 30- and 28-year-old sons and a physician who specializes in environmental and preventive medicine at the Lippman Center for Optimal Health, in Beverly Hills, CA*

⌇

One thing that helped me was to have really good help when I went back to work. I made sure to find people I really trusted.

—*Heather Orman-Lubell, MD*

⌇

I went back to work when my son was 12 weeks old. It was very difficult. I cried and cried and cried. But my son was at home with a very good nanny, and he was fine. It's very hard for a new mom because you're not always emotionally or physically ready to be apart from your baby. The only thing that made it tolerable for me was that I like my job so much.

I believe that being a working parent makes me a *better* parent.

I think that my time with my kids is quality time, and I feel that I'm setting a good example for my children. Also, the fact that I have something for myself allows me to feel better about myself.

—*Alanna Kramer, MD, a mom of an eight-year-old son and a six-year-old daughter and a pediatrician with St. Christopher's Hospital for Children, in Philadelphia, PA*

Probably the most difficult part of my sons' first years was leaving them at home when I went back to work. I was very fortunate to have very good caregivers, and I never worried about my sons' safety. But I really wanted to be with them. It wasn't that I felt they'd be better off with me, but I had waited so long to have them that it was really hard to leave them.

In retrospect, having to leave my sons each day to go to work also made me value the experience of having them. There wasn't any

MomMy TIME

Have a Spot of Tea

It can be hard to be separated from your baby, but it's inevitable. One thing that can help offer comfort on a number of levels is enjoying a cup of tea.

Taking the time to boil the water and steep the leaves can help to calm you. Filling a favorite mug, one that feels good in your hands, and then sitting and sipping the soothing warm tea comforts from the inside out.

More scientifically, tea can help you relax and concentrate more fully on tasks. Studies have shown that an amino acid in tea called L-theanine alters the attention networks in the brain and can have demonstrable effects on the brain waves. Tea has antibiotic and antiviral properties, lowers blood sugar, reduces blood pressure, and fights cancer. It also boosts the metabolic rate and promotes weight loss.

All that for a few cents and a cup of water!

drudgery at all for me because their caregivers cleaned their diapers and washed their clothes. I got to enjoy all of the fun parts of being a mom, playing with my sons and watching them develop.

I loved my profession too, and after two full days of being at home full-time with the boys on weekends, I must admit, I was ready to go back to work on Monday morning.

—*Sandra Carson, MD*

I went back to work when my son was five weeks old. When I left him with the babysitter for the first time, my knees were shaking. It was very tough.

One thing that helped a lot was the fact that the babysitter and I had a one-week overlap. The babysitter started working during my last week of maternity leave. That helped me to get to know her better. It's very scary to leave your baby in the hands of a stranger. You wouldn't give your most valuable diamond to a perfect stranger. Yet, we turn over our precious babies to babysitters we barely know. Our babysitter proved to be very nice and caring, but you never really know until you get to know a person.

My ex-husband is a musician, so he was able to spend a lot of time at home, and that really helped. It was comforting to have some kind of family presence there. I asked him to keep an eye on things.

I also tried to come home early from work whenever possible, and I called home a lot. I gave our babysitter very detailed instructions on what to do, and what not to do. That made me feel better. It's like when you tell someone, "Be sure to look both ways before you cross the street." People know to do that, but saying it makes you feel better.

—*Judith Hellman, MD*

Introducing Juice

Experts agree that breast milk or formula should be your baby's primary beverage for her first year. You could introduce a little water after your baby is four months old. Experts urge parents to wait to give babies juice until six months. Here's why: Babies who drink too much juice can develop diarrhea, gas, bloating, and

tooth decay. Worse, juice tastes very sweet and promotes a preference for other sweet-tasting foods and beverages, which can
increase babies' risk for becoming overweight or obese.

If you do give your baby juice, limit it to four to six ounces
of pasteurized fruit juice a day, and dilute it with water. Your
baby will never know the difference!

❦

During my daughter's first year, she drank mostly formula, and a little
watered-down apple juice. As she got closer to her first birthday, we
transitioned to the structure of meal and snack times. Juice is frowned
upon now because of the worry about childhood obesity, but 100 percent
fruit juice, maybe watered down and given with meals and snacks, is
fine. I tried to give my daughter around four ounces a day, but I didn't
worry if she got a little more on some days and a little less on others.
—*Katja Rowell, MD*

RALLIE'S TIP

*I started my babies on juice when they were about seven months old, and
like most babies, they loved it! Because juice is sweet and tasty, it's easy
for babies to drink too much, and this can lead to problems, including a
preference for sweet-tasting foods and beverages and a higher risk for tooth
decay. Drinking too much juice can also cause babies to have stomachaches and diarrhea because the high carbohydrate content can overwhelm
the ability of a baby's digestive tract to absorb all those sugars.*

*Juice can also impact a baby's weight. In babies who eat well and
drink lots of juice, the extra calories can promote excess weight gain. In
babies who would rather drink juice than eat nutritious foods, excessive
juice consumption can actually lead to poor weight gain or weight loss.*

*The American Academy of Pediatrics recommends adding juice to a
baby's diet only after six months of age. It's especially important to
choose 100 percent fruit juice that has been fully pasteurized.*

*I offered my children water when they were thirsty, and I made
juice a part of meals and snacks. When I did give my sons juice, I
diluted it with an equal amount of water to prevent some of the problems
that drinking too much juice can cause. They never knew the difference!*

I think juice is evil, and we rarely have it in our house. My kids can buy it themselves when they're old enough to want cocktail mixers.

> —*Amy Baxter, MD, a mom of 13- and 10-year-old sons and an 8-year-old daughter, the CEO of MMJ Labs, and the director of emergency research of Children's Healthcare of Atlanta at Scottish Rite, in Atlanta, GA*

I never really gave my daughters very much juice. They simply drank breast milk or water.

> —*Robyn Liu, MD, a mom of seven- and four-year-old daughters and a family physician with Greeley County Health Services, in Tribune, KS*

I never gave my daughter juice. It wrecks kids' teeth, and it's highly caloric. Instead, I only gave my daughter whole fruit.

I gave my daughter water to drink. I also gave her milk, but when she gave up her bottle, she refused to drink milk ever again. So I gave her a calcium supplement.

> —*Debra Jaliman, MD, a mom of a 19-year-old daughter, a dermatologist in private practice, and an assistant professor of dermatology at Mt. Sinai School of Medicine, in New York City*

I was not a juice mom. Juice comes with many risks—from promoting tooth decay to cultivating a love of sweet beverages, which can be a disaster. Plus, the more calories a baby drinks, the less food she's likely to eat. Drinking sugary beverages is not a good way to go.

I never put juice in my babies' bottles. They drank breast milk, formula, and water.

—*Ann Kulze, MD*

Getting Back into Shape

After nine months of pregnancy and six months of nursing if you're breastfeeding, you're probably ready to have your body back—now. One of the best ways to feel more like yourself is to exercise your body. You'll look better and feel better—and will have an easier time fitting back into all of your old clothes to boot.

In my son's first year, I exercised almost every day, taking my son and dog on long walks throughout the countryside where I lived. I would either put my son in the BabyBjörn, or push him in his jogging stroller, and he loved both of these! I also ran on my treadmill while my son napped.

—*Leigh Andrea DeLair, MD, a mom of a two-year-old son and a family physician, in Danville, KY*

When my twins were born, I went back to the gym as quickly as I could. I found a local gym with a kids' club. My kids have enjoyed going there since they were around three months old. People from all over Seattle go to that gym because it has such great child care.

—*Katherine Dee, MD*

I don't have to really work out because I work in the hospital, and I wear a pedometer. I walk 10,000 steps at work each day. That doesn't include walking around the house, or walking from the parking lot to the hospital. I think I take more steps than people who are trying to lose weight.

To lose the pregnancy weight, my motto was: Nine months on,

and nine months off—or more. I'm back to my pre-pregnancy weight now only after 25 months.

—*Sonia Ng, MD*

I found that jogging with a jogging stroller was a great way to get exercise. I started jogging with my twins in a jogging stroller when they were around six weeks old. One of the many benefits to jogging with your babies is that as the babies grow, you have a gradual buildup of the weight you're pushing.

If you are going to run or jog, it's important to use a jogging stroller. They roll much more easily than regular strollers, and they are designed for your hands to be at the proper height.

My twins were nine months old by the time summer arrived, and I loved to play with them in the pool. Once when I was in the swim club locker room, a high school girl looked at me and asked how I had gotten such awesome back muscles. I laughed and explained I carried around my twins, one on each hip.

—*Lillian Schapiro, MD*

RALLIE'S TIP

For moms who are anxious to return to their pre-baby weight, mimicking their babies' eating style is a great strategy. Babies tend to eat small, frequent meals. They eat whenever they feel hungry, and they stop eating as soon as they start to feel full. If adults ate only when we felt hungry and stopped eating as soon as we started to feel full, most of us would find it far easier to lose weight. Eating small, frequent meals helps stabilize blood sugar levels, resulting in less hunger, fewer carb cravings, and more energy with fewer energy crashes.

As babies grow older and adjust to schedules at day care and school, they tend to eat on cue (10:00 snack time, 12:00 lunchtime, etc.) rather than in response to hunger. Like adults, children learn to eat when they're told to eat, or according to societal "cues," rather than when they're actually experiencing hunger.

I'm a grazer, and I tend to eat small snacks and meals throughout the day. When my sons were babies, I'd usually sit down and eat a little snack when I fed them. I think it made feeding time feel more like a meal than a chore, and that was more fun for both of us. My babies always ate better if I was eating with them. The challenge, of course, was to make sure that I was eating food that was just as wholesome and nutritious as the food I offered my babies.

❧

Weight is a big issue. (Literally!) For some reason, I was under the impression that I'd be back in my size six clothes as soon as the baby popped out. Unfortunately, for most of us, this isn't exactly what happens. Much to my dismay, I was still wearing a lot of my *maternity clothes* in the weeks following delivery!

But, not to worry. I have had three children, gained about 50 pounds each time, and been able to lose all of my pregnancy weight every single time. I think that the golden rule of "nine months on, nine months off" is a great way to take the pressure off. I nursed all of my children—nine months for my daughter, and 12 months for my boys. Because I was breastfeeding, I knew that my nutrition was still majorly important, and I didn't want to go on a serious crash diet plan.

What I did was the following: I looked at my eating habits— eating a big breakfast, a mid-morning "cereal break," a big lunch, another snack, a big dinner, and then another snack before bed. (How do you think I gained 50 pounds!) Then I started to eliminate snacks, one by one—first the midnight snack, then the before dinner snack, and then the cereal break. Eventually, I started cutting out the unnecessary, "empty" calories in my main meals, and I returned to my usual eating habits.

—*Stacey Weiland, MD*

❧

Too many moms feel pressured to get right back to their pre-pregnancy weight because celebrities do it in six weeks. I have four children, and it took me years to get my body back. Today I weigh less than I did in high school! You must be patient with yourself.

—*Melanie Bone, MD, a mom of four, ages 16, 15, 14, and 13, a grandmom of one grandson, a gynecologist, the founder of the Cancer Sensibility Foundation, and the author of the syndicated column* Surviving Life *and the book* Cancer, What's Next?, *in West Palm Beach, FL*

Keeping Your Baby's High Chair and Dishes Clean

Who knew dried baby cereal could double as paste and that orange baby food is the most durable color on the planet? Babies aren't the neatest eaters, but it is possible to keep the mess (mostly) at bay.

I'm not so worried about germs. I do the best I can, and I keep a clean house. One thing that I think is very helpful is having a dishwasher. Besides washing the dishes, it also sterilizes them.

—*Sharon Giese, MD, a mom of a two-year-old son and a cosmetic plastic surgeon in private practice, in New York City*

I simply washed all of my babies' bottles and dishes in the dishwasher. Ten years ago, no one was concerned about heating plastics in the dishwasher. Now that the plastics used in baby bottles are bisphenol A (BPA) free, I still wouldn't worry about it.

I am careful not to use plastics labeled with the numbers 3, 6, or 7, which are the potentially dangerous ones. My husband laughs about this, but I feel that there are so many things out there that we have no control over, you have to control as much as you can.

—*Heather Orman-Lubell, MD*

My husband and I never had a full-size high chair. Instead, we had a portable high chair with a big tray that we strapped to a kitchen chair. That saved us a lot of money because high chairs are so expensive. Also it saved us a lot of space because high chairs are huge!

—*Robyn Liu, MD*

I never had a high chair for my children. Instead, I had a Sassy seat, which hooks onto the table. All of my babies used it—and my nieces and nephews too. It was one of my favorite baby items. It was easier to clean than a high chair, and it was quite portable.

—*Charlene Brock, MD*

I always hand-washed my baby's bottles and nipples. I didn't like the idea of the plastic going through the heat of the dishwasher, even if it was BPA free.

I also never microwave food in plastic dishes—only glass or ceramic. And I don't store food in the fridge in plastic either, only glass containers with lids.

My baby's high chair tray was such a pain to clean. As soon as she was physically mature enough, we got rid of the tray and pulled her right up to the table. Kids need to make a mess to learn to eat. I just had to accept it!

—*Katja Rowell, MD*

Nurturing Your Partnership

So much to do, so little time. Don't let your partner get lost in the shuffle.

My babies' first years, I made sure to have plenty of time for my husband. When you're taking care of a baby, it's very easy to forget about your spouse. But that other person needs some attention too. Every so often, we'd put the kids to bed early so we had some quiet time to ourselves.

—*Heather Orman-Lubell, MD*

One thing that was very helpful for my husband and me was that we weren't afraid to take our daughters places that we enjoyed going. We took them to church, to our friends' houses, and even hiking. We felt it was important to continue to live our lives, and now we had these two new people to include.

Even if we were going out late at night to meet friends at a restaurant, we took our baby along. We'd put her in a car seat, and she slept there. One time, we were kicked out of a bar because my daughter "wasn't of age." Of course she wasn't of age; she was four weeks old!

—*Robyn Liu, MD*

My husband and I had a very unique situation when our oldest kids were babies. My husband was an Army physician, stationed in

Germany, and we had three kids under age three. We lived "on the economy," in a tiny German village. Our neighbors spoke little English, and we spoke even less German. We could say "hello" and "good-bye" and order in restaurants, but that was about it.

In a way, it was a wonderful time for our family. We were in survival mode! We were so far from family and friends that my husband and I had to work together. That time together really strengthened our bond, and we learned to support each other. We spent a lot of time together just as a family, and we traveled all over Europe. We made so many wonderful memories.

—*Ann Kulze, MD*

Having your first baby changes your life. I was determined to continue my romantic life with my husband after we had our baby. Less than a week after our baby was born, we went out for dinner at a restaurant, leaving our baby in the very capable hands of my parents.

With our second and third babies, my husband and I were much braver and more creative in taking our kids along on our dates—when they would be asleep anyway! We'd take the babies along to the movies, and they'd sleep through the whole thing. My husband and I delighted in going out and feeling like the young couple that we had been before we had babies. Because, of course, we still *were* a young couple!

I think that our commitment to our marriage has also been a great lesson to our kids. We've modeled a healthy marriage, and we've shown them that working on your marriage is something that you need to do.

—*Ayala Laufer-Cahana, MD, a mom of 15- and 13-year-old sons and a 12-year-old daughter, a pediatrician, and the founder of Herbal Water Inc., in Wynnewood, PA*

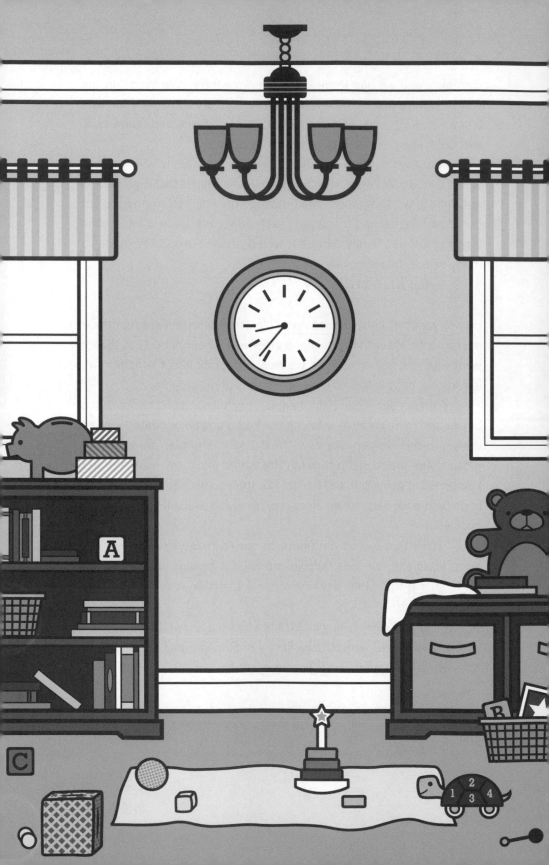

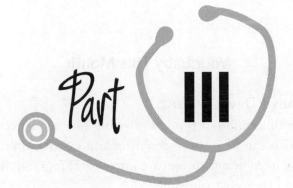

Part III

THE THIRD QUARTER

Chapter 7
7th Month

Your Baby This Month

YOUR BABY'S DEVELOPMENT

The seventh month is a time of growing independence for your baby, which can be both frightening and exhilarating for him. Your baby likely wants to venture into new things, but he's afraid to stray too far away from you!

Around this time, your baby's vision is almost as good as an adult's—an adult with 20/20 vision anyway! Your baby's eye color is just about fully set now as his body finishes depositing pigment into his irises. Don't be too surprised, though, if his eyes do still change a bit in color. A baby's eye color can still subtly change through his toddler years. They might even change again at puberty, when hormones kick in.

By seven months, your baby can probably sit without any support at all. Your baby can probably get up onto his hands and knees, maybe even crawl. Amazingly, around seven months, a baby can go from sitting, to lunging, to crawling! Your baby might even be able to stand while holding tightly on to something.

If you place a toy out of reach, your baby will likely work to try to get it. He can probably pass a small toy from hand to hand, delighting in this new trick. Babies this age love toys that they can shake, twist, drop, rattle, open, close, empty, and fill. Your baby is starting to understand that smaller objects fit into a larger one, and he probably loves filling up containers and dumping them back out.

Your baby now has a slight understanding of cause and effect. You can see this at work, for example, because if he drops an object, he'll look for it. He might join you in a game of peek-a-boo, now as more of a participant than just an observer.

Your baby now likely responds to his name. When you say, "No," he probably looks at you—though he's not likely to stop what he's doing in response! At this age, your baby understands the word "no" more by inflection and tone than by the actual word itself.

More than anything, though, your seven-month-old baby craves your attention. He's learning which behaviors, both good and bad, engage you and keep your attention.

At seven months, your baby's understanding of words far outpaces his ability to use them. Around seven months, many babies are babbling pros, combining consonants and vowels to say ga-ga-ga-ga, ba-ba-ba-ba.

Taking Care of You

Have someone watch your baby while you get your hair done. This could be your partner, a parent, or even a trusted friend. It's great to line up a few trusted babysitters to call upon when you need a break.

Justification for a Celebration

Once your baby starts crawling, he can come to *you*! What a wonderful reason to celebrate!

Eating Out with Your Baby

It can be challenging to eat out with a baby. But with proper planning and packing, it is possible. You don't have to limit yourself to restaurants with play places and cartoon characters. Buffets can be good options because you'll get your food quicker and spend less time waiting. Plus, there are more opportunities to get up and move around.

◦◦◦

I found that the best place to eat out was a buffet. That way, if my son got cranky, and I needed to walk him, I would just get up and go back to the buffet for more food. I would take turns with my husband.

We always took Purell with us because we didn't want our son to get sick. The number of people who touch their faces right before reaching for a food ladle is pretty amazing.

—*Sonia Ng, MD, a mom of seven- and two-year-old sons, a pediatrician, and a sedation attending physician at the Children's Hospital of Philadelphia Pediatric Care and the University Medical Center at Princeton in Princeton, NJ, and the Pediatric Imaging Center in King of Prussia, PA*

◦◦◦

My husband and I took our baby everywhere, even to restaurants. We always took along some of his favorite toys or books. Often we went out to eat with friends, and we all took turns holding him. I also brought along food that he liked to eat, and we made sure we didn't stay out too long. I think he enjoyed the change of scenery! Restaurants are generally very visually stimulating.

Taking our son out to eat with us was actually easier early on, before he started walking. After that, he didn't want to sit still, and someone had to chase after him.

—*Sharon Giese, MD, a mom of a two-year-old son and a cosmetic plastic surgeon in private practice, in New York City*

◦◦◦

When my oldest child was two days old, we went straight from the hospital to our country club to have lunch, even before going home. That might have been a little ridiculous.

It really is easier to take a baby out during his first year of life—compared with the toddler years. That first year, babies sleep so much that as long as they are fed and changed before going to the restaurant, they are usually quite content during the meal. I'd put my baby in the infant car seat and cover him with a blanket if necessary. During the first year, my husband and I even took our baby with us to see some movies.

Mommy MD Guides-Recommended Product
Table Toppers

If you spend too much time thinking about how clean a restaurant is—or isn't—you probably would never eat there. To make matters worse, babies touch everything and then put their fingers into their mouths, and they generally eat their food right off of the table. Ick. Who knows how many germs or cleaning chemicals are on that table?

Motherhood necessitates invention, and a clever mom came up with a handy solution: Table Toppers disposable placemats. You simply peel the backing off the adhesive and stick these plastic mats right to the table. (Don't worry, they come off cleanly and easily.) Instantly, you have a clean surface on which to feed your baby. After your baby is done eating, simply remove the Table Topper and throw it away.

Table Toppers come in lots of fun patterns, including Sesame Street, Dora the Explorer, and Disney Cars and Princesses. As a bonus, the fun, colorful designs help to keep babies entertained while they wait for their food.

Each Table Topper measures 18 inches x 12 inches. New eco-friendly Table Toppers are also available.

You can buy 50 Table Toppers in a reusable, pop-up plastic carrying case for around $19 online.

It gets much harder to eat out when kids are two and three years old. I always believed that you should expose children to lots of different experiences, and so my husband and I took our kids many places with us. In retrospect, I might have pushed that a little too hard. There were times that my children were highly disruptive! If you're a high-stress person, don't even try this! Get a sitter and go out for supper with your husband.

—*Melanie Bone, MD, a mom of four, ages 16, 15, 14, and 13, a grandmom of one grandson, a gynecologist, the founder of the Cancer Sensibility Foundation, and the author of the syndicated column* Surviving Life *and the book* Cancer, What's Next?, *in West Palm Beach, FL*

∽

My husband and I are both foodies, and we love eating out and trying new cuisines. When our three oldest kids were babies, we lived in Germany. We were constantly exploring new foods.

My husband and I took our babies with us to restaurants, but we were very strict. We never let them get out of control—or even anywhere close to out of control. I took along all sorts of things to keep my kids entertained, and my husband and I would take turns taking care of the kids and eating. I'd entertain the babies while he ate, and then we swapped.

One thing that we didn't do was use the restaurant's high chairs. They are nasty! Instead, we took along a portable baby seat that attached to the table.

—*Ann Kulze, MD, a mom of 22- and 15-year-old daughters and 20- and 19-year-old sons; a nationally recognized nutrition expert, motivational speaker, and family physician; and the author of the best-selling book* Eat Right for Life, *in Charleston, SC*

∽

I think that meals are social experiences. My husband and I would bring our infants with us into restaurants from the very beginning— even when they were so small that they would lie in those little plastic infant buckets right on the table.

This only works well if your infants have the right sort of temperament. If your babies aren't fairly easily pleased, or if they have protracted periods of fussing or crying, the other diners are going to be inconvenienced and this won't work at all. But many small infants are happy to go along.

When the baby is old enough to sit without being propped up, those special seats that attach to the table with supporting arms are wonderful. The youngster can take part in the meal, watching the grown-ups while munching on a cracker or a bit of age-appropriate food. Again, this is suitable only for a rested baby who has the right personality, and not necessarily every child at every stage of development. The curious crawler who needs a lot of big-muscle activity and tends to hurl objects to the floor is perhaps not the best restaurant guest until he passes this phase.

—*Elizabeth Berger, MD, a mom of a 28-year-old son and a 26-year-old daughter, a child psychiatrist, and the author of* Raising Kids with Character, *in New York City*

Babyproofing More

The key to babyproofing: Stay one step ahead!

A major challenge to babyproofing your home is that some of your safety measures can be undone by older kids. My husband and I put a safety gate at the top of our stairs. We were careful to buy one that only an adult can open. We didn't want our older sons unlatching it and leaving it open for the baby to topple down the stairs. We keep the gate at the top of the stairs closed at all times.

—*Amy Thompson, MD, a mom of four- and two-year-old and nine-month-old sons and an ob-gyn at the University of Cincinnati College of Medicine, in Ohio*

I remember that when my sons were around eight months old and more mobile, we had to step up our babyproofing. My husband and I put latches on our kitchen cabinets and covers in the outlets.

But if you have smart kids, they figure out how to get around those babyproofing efforts in a few months. It's the first IQ test.

—*Sandra Carson, MD, a mom of two grown sons and the director of the Center for Reproduction and Infertility of Women and Infants Hospital, in Providence, RI*

A great product for us was the type of baby gate that you can clip together, such as the Secure Surround Play Safe Play Yard. We could bend it into various shapes and move it around where we needed it. It was very helpful for us in our living room to keep our daughter away from the glass-door bookcases and fireplace. In a pinch, we also made it into a playpen. It was big enough for my daughter to crawl around in while I took a shower. I've seen friends put it up around a Christmas tree so the babies wouldn't bring the tree down on themselves.

You can buy the Summer Infant Secure Surround Play Safe Play Yard online and in stores for around $55.

—*Katja Rowell, MD, a mom of a five-year-old daughter, a family physician, and a childhood feeding specialist with FamilyFeedingDynamics.com, in St. Paul, MN*

My baby figured out how to undo all of our safety measures by the time he was 18 months old. I moved all chemicals and medications to higher shelves and got a lockbox for the medications.

When we took a family trip to the Grand Canyon, I put a baby leash on my son, but he just held the leash and cried, refusing to walk. Once I took it off, he would dash away. I nearly had a heart attack. Meanwhile, my older son and my husband were shoving each other while they were atop some of the natural arches. (Men!)

—*Sonia Ng, MD*

When my oldest kids were babies, we lived in Germany. On the weekends, we loved to walk through the historic, charming streets. Sometimes we pushed our kids in strollers, but they didn't have double or triple strollers back then, and we had three kids under age three, so that was a challenge.

To keep our kids safe, we did something the Germans thought was appalling: We put our son (who was wildly rambunctious) on a baby leash. To us, it was safe and practical, and our son didn't mind a bit. We sure got looks from other people, though! Their jaws would drop. It was like they were thinking, *What are you doing to that child?*

—*Ann Kulze, MD*

∽◌

I didn't buy a toilet lock, but in hindsight perhaps it would have been a good idea. When my third child was about a year old, I was in the shower, and my husband was getting dressed. Someone had used the toilet and flushed, but neither of us realized that it wasn't flushed completely.

We had put our daughter near the bathroom with some toys, but she came into the bathroom and pulled herself up to stand next to the toilet. Then she put her hand in the toilet, grabbed some poop, and ate it.

The good news is, our daughter is 22 now, and she was just invited to an interview as part of her application to complete her doctorate of nursing degree. The toilet experience didn't hurt her brain at all. My point is that you never know when a baby is going to take a developmental leap and pull herself up, for example. You have to stay a step ahead with the babyproofing.

—*Hana R. Solomon, MD, a mom of four, ages 35 to 19, a board-certified pediatrician, and the author of* Clearing the Air One Nose at a Time: Caring for Your Personal Filter, *in Columbia, MO*

∽◌

I think that the best advice I received regarding babyproofing was getting down on all fours and crawling around the house so that I would be at the same level as my baby. It's amazing what you can find when you are down at a baby's level.

All electric sockets need to be covered with outlet protectors. All electric cords, telephone cords (does anyone have phones like this anymore?), and drape cords need to be out of reach. Anything that is top-heavy and that can be pulled down needs to be moved. Doors to steps need to be closed, and safety gates should be put up. Any poisonous substances should be removed.

Babyproofing some things can be a little difficult. We always had an issue with the dog food. The dogs had to eat, and their food had to be on the floor. My kids always had a lot of fun putting the dry dog pieces in the dog's water bowl and making nice little floaters. One of my kids actually seemed to like the taste, and several times I had to remove the kibble piece by piece from his little chipmunk cheeks!

—*Stacey Weiland, MD, a mom of a 12-year-old daughter and 7- and 5-year-old sons and an internist/gastroenterologist, in Denver, CO*

Feeding Your Baby Fruits and Vegetables

What a wonderful time, introducing your baby to all sorts of delicious, nutritious foods. It's best to talk with your baby's doctor to find out if your baby is ready to start eating fruits and vegetables.

Even though you probably don't eat green peas for breakfast, morning is a good time to offer your baby new foods. That way, you have all day to watch him for signs of an allergic reaction. Plus, babies are usually hungriest in the morning, and conventional wisdom says they're usually in the best mood then for social interaction, including feeding. Above all, enjoy this special time with your baby, and get your camera ready.

⁓

After oatmeal, we added a single new type of baby food each week to make sure that our baby didn't have allergies. We started with vegetables. Squash was our son's favorite. He never liked the fruits.

—*Sonia Ng, MD*

⁓

When my sons were six months old, I introduced baby foods. I started with orange and yellow vegetables first, and then I went through green vegetables, then fruits. I gave them one new food every five days to watch for allergic reactions. It went very well. My sons might not have been good sleepers, but they were good eaters!

—Jill Wireman, MD, a mom of 14- and 11-year-old sons and a pediatrician in private practice at Johnson City Pediatrics, in Tennessee

∽◦∽

My babies were both incredibly great eaters. They loved everything. My husband is the main cook in our home, and he pureed a lot of vegetables for them. We didn't buy a lot of baby food. Our babies especially loved pureed white and sweet potatoes, squash, and carrots. Once the vegetables are cooked, you can use a small food processor or hand mash them with a fork.

—Ann V. Arthur, MD, a mom of a nine-year-old daughter and a seven-year-old son, a pediatric ophthalmologist in private practice at Park Slope Eye Care Associates, and a blogger at WaterWineTravel.com, in New York City

∽◦∽

I started to feed my daughter vegetables and meat when she was five months old. I used a food grinder because I was concerned about MSG and preservatives that are added to prepared baby foods. So my daughter always had the same foods the adults ate for dinner. I had to grind her vegetables up with soft cheese, though, or she wouldn't touch them.

—Stuart Jeanne Bramhall, MD, a mom of a 30-year-old daughter and a child and adolescent psychiatrist, in New Plymouth, New Zealand

∽◦∽

When I started to give my babies vegetables and fruits, I wanted to limit commercially prepared baby foods as much as possible. I used a BabySteps Hand Crank Food Mill to grind up food. To save time, I would grind up a larger batch of food and then freeze it in single-serving ice cube trays. Then I could just defrost a cube of peas in the microwave, for instance, and presto, instant baby food.

You can buy a BabySteps Hand Crank Food Mill online for around $12.

—Robyn Liu, MD, a mom of seven- and four-year-old daughters and a family physician with Greeley County Health Services, in Tribune, KS

With both of my kids, I practiced exclusive breastfeeding for the first four months, and then I introduced them to rice cereal and fruits like peaches, mashed banana, and applesauce. I know conventional wisdom says to start with vegetables. But I chickened out. I watched a lot of green peas go to waste. Fruits are sweet,

Mommy MD Guides–Recommended Product
Sprout Organic Baby Food

Why shouldn't your baby eat food that's as delicious and nutritious as your food? That's probably what the folks at Sprout Foods, Inc., were thinking when they launched their new line of baby foods.

Sprout was cofounded by Executive Chef Tyler Florence, 15-year Food Network veteran, father of three, and author of seven cookbooks, including one based on his baby food expertise (*Start Fresh: Your Child's Jump Start to Lifelong Healthy Eating*). Sprout is unique in that its food features gourmet recipes and 100 percent USDA-certified organic ingredients, and it is the only pouch to have separate fruit and vegetables. Then Sprout uses homemade cooking methods like roasting and baking to bring out the natural flavors of the food. Because of Sprout's innovative, BPA-free packaging, their cooking process is substantially shorter than what would be required for food stored in glass containers. This process helps Sprout to preserve more flavor, color, and nutrients, as well as energy.

For babies, Sprout offers a selection of "starter" foods, including roasted pears, roasted bananas, baked sweet potatoes, sweet peas, and roasted butternut squash. Sprout foods contain no artificial flavors, colors, or preservatives, and they're 100 percent USDA-certified organic.

You can buy Sprout foods in grocery and baby stores across the United States as well as at major online retailers. Visit their site, **SPROUTBABYFOOD.COM**, for more information.

and I found that my babies developed their sweet teeth early and responded well to the fruits.

—*Bola Oyeyipo, MD, a mom of three-year-old and six-month-old sons, a family physician in private practice, and the owner of SlimyBookWorm.com, in Highland, CA*

During my daughter's first year, she was such a good eater. Now she's a candy monster, but that first year, she really *liked* food. I could get her to eat lots of foods then that she won't touch anymore, like kale and spinach.

I'm a vegetarian, and my daughter was a vegetarian too until last year. To feed her a balanced vegetarian diet, I made sure to give her plenty of egg yolks, yogurt, and tofu. She also ate rice and beans.

—*Dina Strachan, MD, a mom of a five-year-old daughter, a dermatologist and director of Aglow Dermatology, and an assistant clinical professor in the department of dermatology at Columbia University College of Physicians and Surgeons, in New York City*

I was very by-the-book when introducing foods, especially with my oldest baby. She was a very good eater with a welcoming palate.

My second baby was critically ill when he was born, and he was a *very* finicky eater from the start. Feeding him was awful. I couldn't get him to eat vegetables, so I skipped ahead to fruits. I didn't like that idea, but I wanted to get *something* into him. He'd usually eat fruit mixed into rice cereal.

If I could go back and do it over, I would have done some things differently, including strictly avoiding any foods not certified organic and only feeding them plain (not fruit-flavored) yogurts. Fruit yogurts are loaded with sugar that can exploit an infant's highly developed taste buds for sweet flavors.

—*Ann Kulze, MD*

My daughter has never had a problem with eating. One thing that was interesting is she didn't like stage 3 baby foods. So I simply kept her on the stage 2 baby foods a little longer. Sometimes you have to use trial and error to find out what works with each kid.

—Jeannette Gonzalez Simon, MD, a mom of a two-year-
old daughter who's expecting another baby and a pediatric
gastroenterologist in private practice, in Staten Island, NY

With my older son, I carefully followed the standard recommendations about introducing table food. With my younger son, though, we did things a bit differently. If we were eating any single-food items, my husband would mash them up for the baby. Our son is none the worse for wear. People have been feeding babies that way for generations.

My mom lives close to my sister, and she was very helpful to my sister when my nephew was born. She would prepare a food, like peas, and mash them up and freeze them in ice cube trays. Then she'd give Ziploc bags full of the baby food cubes to my sister, who would thaw them out a cube at a time. It was a wonderful way for my sister to feed her baby healthy foods easily and inexpensively.

—Carrie Brown, MD, a mom of seven- and five-year-old sons and
a general pediatrician who treats medically complex children
and specializes in palliative care at Arkansas Children's Hospital,
in Little Rock

I never gave my daughter processed, store-bought baby food. Instead, I softened foods, like sweet potatoes or squash, by baking them. I also microwaved foods, such as avocados or bananas, and then added a little water and mashed them. I steamed a lot of foods, including vegetables, because steaming helps preserve the nutrients in the food. I also used a mini Cuisinart food processor for fruits like plums.

Early on, I introduced my daughter to all kinds of exotic fruits and vegetables. Even as a baby, she ate artichokes and asparagus. I know lots of people who feed their kids a steady, bland diet of pizza and pasta. But we never did.

—Debra Jaliman, MD, a mom of a 19-year-old daughter, a
dermatologist in private practice, and an assistant professor of
dermatology at Mt. Sinai School of Medicine, in New York City

I had thought that I'd be one of those moms who grind up organic food, but I couldn't get my act together. I felt disappointed in myself at first, but a huge lesson in parenting for me was to let go of guilt. Guilt is such a joy-killer. Making my own baby food felt overwhelming with everything I had going on, so I just bought mostly organic baby food instead.

Sometimes I did blend or mash up food for my daughter, such as squash or sweet potatoes. By the time she was nine months old, she was eating most of our table food. I just mashed or cut up food so that it was safe for her to chew and swallow. If you want your child to grow up liking vegetables, then find ways that you like to eat them and make them part of regular, enjoyable family meals. Kids *want* to grow up to eat the foods the family enjoys.

When my daughter was starting to eat table food, I introduced new foods by putting a blob on her lip to taste. I gave her a minute to taste the food before popping a spoonful into her mouth. Most important, I remained calm, pleasant, and reassuring throughout the meal, and I always waited for her to open her mouth for the spoon. Forcing, tricking, or stuffing it in when they are distracted will backfire. I've found sneaking and using tricks aren't the way to go. If you're being sneaky about it, I think you need to step back and look at the big picture. We enjoy a variety of wonderful foods, including vegetables. I think that eating meals together and modeling the enjoyment—without pressure—is the key.

—*Katja Rowell, MD*

? When to Call Your Doctor

As you introduce each new food to your baby, keep an eye out for allergies. Signs and symptoms include a rash, diarrhea, or vomiting. If any of these occur, call your baby's doctor the next business day.

If your baby has trouble breathing, it could signal a severe allergy. If that happens, call 9-1-1.

My husband and I were very vigilant with our first baby about following our pediatrician's recommendations about when to start cereal, vegetables, and fruits, and only adding one food at a time for a week or so.

I definitely became more mellow with the boys. After giving them cereal, we were pretty quick to add the other foods. (I always used Gerber.) None of my kids developed any food allergies, and they are all exceptionally adventurous eaters.

I attribute this to two things. I ate a lot of variety while I was pregnant, and I think even more importantly, we always ate *with* our children. Even when they were babies, they would see what we were eating, and we would give them a taste. We took them out to a lot of restaurants—Italian, Chinese, Indian—and we would always encourage our children to experiment with new things. Even now, I always ask them to at least *try* something they have not had before. If they don't like it, I'll give them a break and let them have something else.

Another thing that I found, especially with my daughter, who is now 12, is that their tastes will change. I distinctly remember her trying and *hating* certain things at one point, but then loving them several months later.

—*Stacey Weiland, MD*

After we got our babies used to eating cereal, we went on to introduce fruits and vegetables, in the standard way that pediatricians recommend. Of course, our children preferred the fruits and the sweeter vegetables! They liked sweet potatoes better than green beans, for instance.

My husband and I are Orthodox Jews, and we keep kosher. Back when our kids were little, there was very little out there in the way of kosher baby foods. Today you can buy more kosher baby foods. I think Beechnut has some kosher items, as does Gerber.

—*Susan Besser, MD, a mom of six grown children, ages 26, 24, 22, 21, 19, and 17, a grandmom of one, a family physician, and the medical director of Doctors Express-Memphis, in Tennessee*

Any food on a baby's face can irritate and redden the skin. This is especially true for partially chewed food that smears on your baby's face. The best remedy is to apply a thin coating of Vaseline to your baby's cheeks and chin prior to feeding.

—Amy J. Derick, MD, a mom of two-year-old and nine-month-old sons and a dermatologist in private practice at Derick Dermatology, in Barrington, IL

Napping

During the first six weeks after her baby's birth, the average new mom spends 20 percent more of her day awake than she did before her baby was born. If you're so tired that the only thing keeping you awake is lots of strong coffee, take a cue from your baby and catch a nap. Naps are a great way to catch up on lost sleep. Here are some of the many benefits of naps.

- Moms who nap along with their babies might be less likely to suffer postpartum depression.
- Moms who nap are more likely to have babies who nap, because newborns tend to adopt their mothers' circadian sleep rhythms.
- Napping can make being a mom a little easier. Sleep deprivation can hinder a mother's ability to care for her infant because her judgment and concentration decline.
- Naps might help new moms lose their pregnancy weight. Lack of sleep produces changes in appetite-regulating hormones, which tend to make you feel hungrier in general and less satisfied after you do eat. Studies show that with less sleep, we tend to increase our caloric intake.
- Babies who nap during the day are more likely to exhibit an advanced level of learning, and the same is true for new moms.
- Napping improves memory and performance on new tasks, and there are plenty of those for new moms to learn. As it turns out, taking a short siesta helps "engrave" new information into the long-term memory.

- Taking a midday snooze along with your baby can boost mood, memory, reaction time, and alertness, especially when you're sleep deprived.
- Naps are good for your heart. Studies show that napping might lower the risk of death due to heart disease by more than a third.

∽

My husband loves to play video games, which was not my favorite thing, but it has suddenly come in very handy. He puts our baby on his chest, with her arms and legs splayed out. He calls it the "tree frog." He'll sit for hours with her like that with him playing video games and her napping. That's great for all of us! But I admit, I still do give him a hard time for playing video games so much.

—*Jennifer Bacani McKenney, MD, a mom of a two-month-old daughter and a family physician, in Fredonia, KS*

∽

Nothing was harder on me during my baby's first year than the sleep deprivation. My first daughter was born when I was in my internship, which is already a sleep-deprived part of life. Adding a newborn who didn't sleep well on top of that was brutal.

The thing that saved me was that my daughter and I learned to take naps together. I'd come home from being on call at the hospital all night, and I'd take my daughter to bed with me to nurse, and we'd both fall asleep. That is a very special memory for me. I took the adage "Sleep when your baby sleeps" to heart because I really wanted to be awake when she was awake.

—*Robyn Liu, MD*

∽

I was really protective of my babies' naps. Sleep is really crucial. I find to this day that when my kids are well rested, they are happy. Rather than sticking to a rigid nap schedule, I watched my babies for signs that they were getting tired. If I caught them at the first yawn, before they got overtired, they didn't cry much at all when I put them down for a nap.

To make this work, I tried as much as possible not to be out of the house at naptime. It was a sacrifice in terms of the rest of life, though.

—*Michelle Paley, MD, PA, a mom of two and a psychiatrist and psychotherapist in private practice, in Miami Beach, FL*

༚

It's difficult to find time for self-care, but it's absolutely necessary for both your and your baby's well-being. As a breastfeeding mom, I found myself constantly tired. The disrupted sleep and late hours began to take a toll on my health and energy level. I began to follow the old adage, "Sleep when the baby sleeps."

This was very easy to do with my first child, but when my second son was born 21 months later, I found that it was much harder to do. I learned that keeping naptime flexible with the older child meant that I could put him down during one of the baby's naps, which allowed time for me to nap while both slept. I could have used that time to clean the house or do laundry or any number of household chores, but the reality is I needed the sleep more than I needed a clean house. Those family nap sessions became a standard at our house and helped to keep all of us well rested and happy.

—*Saundra Dalton-Smith, MD, a mom of six- and four-year-old sons, an internal medicine specialist, and the author of* Set Free to Live Free: Breaking Through the 7 Lies Women Tell Themselves, *in Anniston, AL.*

༚

When my twins were first born, they took 10- to 15-minute catnaps. It drove me crazy. One mistake I made was making my house too quiet for naptimes. I'd require it to be dead silent! I think that backfired a bit because as the twins got older, they had to have silence to sleep. I don't recommend complete silence.

To try to get my twins to nap longer, I'd put them down at the scheduled naptime for a couple of hours. It was a bit like sleep training; they cried some but then they fell asleep. It started to get better once I put them into their cribs for naps, rather than letting them fall asleep in the living room in their swings. The key was consistency, in terms of timing and place, which paid off as they got older.

—*Ann Contrucci, MD, a mom of 12-year-old boy-girl twins who works as a pediatric emergency physician, in Atlanta, GA*

RALLIE'S TIP

When my first two sons were babies, I always tried to catch up on work or exercise the minute I put them down for their naps. I didn't want to "waste" one minute of my precious free time sleeping! I found out the hard way that sleep is a necessity, not a luxury. I was exhausted most of the time. By the time my youngest son was born, I had learned my lesson. Whenever I put him down for a nap, I'd be right behind him. The funny thing is that when you get plenty of sleep, it seems as if you can do twice as much in half the time. Spending a little more time sleeping actually saved me time in the long run.

◯

My son was very fussy. He never napped a day in his life. It was very troublesome—and very tiring. It wasn't for lack of trying. I would put my baby down for naps, but he would just cry.

To this day, my son still won't nap, even though he's old enough to know that some days he could really use one. I've always believed that my son was afraid he'd miss something if he took a nap. But fortunately, since my son was about 10 weeks old, he's slept like a baby through the night.

—*Alanna Kramer, MD, a mom of an eight-year-old son and a six-year-old daughter and a pediatrician with St. Christopher's Hospital for Children, in Philadelphia, PA*

Dealing with Isolation

It's so ironic: Probably at no time in your life have you been closer to someone than now with your new baby, yet if you're spending lots of time alone at home with your new baby, you might never have felt more alone. If you're feeling lonely and isolated, don't just wallow. Reach out to a friend or family member.

◯

I was surprised by how isolated I felt in the first weeks of my baby's life. Getting up every couple of hours in the middle of the night while my husband is sleeping and the house is so quiet can feel very lonely. My husband wants to help as much as possible, but when you're breastfeeding, there's really no way for anyone to help you with feeding the baby early on.

Also, during the day, I'm used to being at work around lots of people. It's so weird to be home all by myself! One thing that has really helped is calling into my office and checking my messages remotely. That way I still feel like I'm being a doctor, and I still have connections with people.

—*Jennifer Bacani McKenney, MD*

Give Curves a Try

If you're feeling isolated, a simple fix is to find a reason to get out of the house and meet other folks, especially other moms. Chances are very good that you'll see other moms at a Curves near you. With nearly 10,000 locations in more than 85 countries, Curves has found a winning formula for helping women get—and stay—in shape. Created specifically for women, Curves works every major muscle group with strength training, cardio, and stretching in a 30-minute circuit, three times a week. Although you generally can't bring your baby to a Curves, getting together regularly with other new moms can be a welcome, and healthy, activity just for you in baby's first year.

Many moms feel guilty about spending time away from their babies. The great thing about a Curves workout is that it's very efficient. A single 30-minute session can burn up to 500 calories. The circuit is made up of resistance machines that work every major muscle group, two muscle groups at a time. A circuit coach to teach and motivate will help you to reach your fitness goals.

Here's another Curves plus: the company's interest in charitable causes. You can feel great—in both body and spirit—at Curves.

Monthly membership fees vary, and sign-up fees can be affected by promotions and coupons. The best way to get the actual cost at your local Curves is to call or stop in.

I am not the kind of person who likes to be stuck at home. Spending days alone at home with my new baby was not my thing.

To maintain my sanity, I found very good babysitters, and I trusted them to watch my babies for a few hours while I went out for a bit of alone time. This is actually easier to do when your baby is very young. I don't even think my babies noticed who was taking care of them! Some moms might not be comfortable doing this. I'd suggest packing their babies up and taking them out somewhere, such as to Starbucks. I believe that moms who don't do this, who allow themselves to become isolated, are more likely to experience postpartum depression.

—*Melanie Bone, MD*

As a new mom at home for long stretches of time, you start to feel very isolated. I remember whenever anyone would call for whatever reason, I would try to engage them in conversation. "What are you selling? Oh, how long have you been doing that? Where are you calling from?, etc." Not good. Possibly even pathetic.

When my daughters were small, we often went to story time at the local library. One day I met another mom who had two little boys. We discovered we were both physicians working part-time, and we exchanged phone numbers. I was beside myself with joy, thinking we might be friends. I waited a day to call her so I wouldn't look desperate. Later, she confessed that she had done the same. To this day, we remain friends.

Another thing that helped me with isolation was learning that we had an elderly neighbor who had no family. She was easy to "adopt." We often seemed to have an extra serving of everything at dinner, so we would fix a plate and I would take it over to her. Then we would visit and talk, and occasionally she watched the girls so my husband and I could go out. When I went into labor at 11:30 at night, we called her and she walked across the street, up the stairs, and into our bed while we dashed off for the delivery.

We loved having her as part of our family, and we know she

enjoyed it as well. I think my advice would be to reach out to someone else. "If you want to make a friend, be a friend."

—*Lesley Burton-Iwinski, MD, a mom of 20- and 18-year-old daughters and a 14-year-old son, a retired family physician, and a parent and teacher educator with Growing Peaceful Families, in Lexington, KY*

I wanted to be at home to raise my own children, and I was fortunate enough to have a partner and a financial situation that allowed me to do so. But even so, I found that being at home in the house with babies all day very quickly became solitary confinement with infant cell-mates.

I hired a sitter for two, three, or four hours every day so that I could run to the office to work on a very limited basis. Being able to take a brief breather every day from that "indoors full-time mother" role was lifesaving. It is unnatural to be isolated with newborns in four walls, waiting for your husband to come home for dinner day after day with nothing but the perplexing variety of laundry detergents to occupy your thoughts. The easy accessibility of an extended family, neighbors, and other moms who will watch your brood for a while is closer to the universal human experience.

The monotony and loneliness of staying indoors with babies as a steady diet can be soul-crushing. So I think that mothers who are not currently involved in professional or working capacities should still make arrangements to escape each day, if only for a brief period of time, to air out their spirits for a fresh start.

—*Elizabeth Berger, MD*

Preventing and Treating Diarrhea

You are the world's foremost authority on your baby. Because you also are probably his chief diaper changer, you are also the world's foremost authority on his poop. (Isn't motherhood fun?)

Because a baby's stool is often runny and soft, what you're looking for is a *change*. Look for a sudden increase in the frequency of bowel movements. If it changes noticeably within only a few days, your baby might have diarrhea. Also watch for a sudden increase in the water content of your baby's stool.

Babies can get diarrhea from a change in diet, or from a change in *your* diet if you're breastfeeding. Diarrhea can also be a side effect of antibiotics, and it can be caused by infections. Generally, diarrhea will resolve within the week, but watch your baby carefully because it can become serious.

As with vomiting, diarrhea can be dangerous for babies because it can cause a baby to lose too much body fluid and become dehydrated. To prevent dehydration, continue to breastfeed your baby. If you feed your baby formula, your doctor might advise switching to a lactose-free one, which is easier for your baby to digest. Also talk with your doctor about giving your baby an oral rehydrating solution, such as Pedialyte.

One more crummy side effect of diarrhea can be diaper rashes. Normal stool contains some of the enzymes that help us to digest our food. But when a baby has diarrhea, the stool is zipping through the body faster than usual, and so the poop contains more of those enzymes than usual. They can actually start to digest the sensitive skin on your baby's bottom. So be especially vigilant about changing your baby's diaper.

❧

My mother came to spend a month with me when my daughter was born. I remember two of my sons developed diarrhea when my newborn was just a few days old. My mom was a gem, and she took care of them so that the baby's risk of getting sick was minimized. One night, that involved removing my older son's extremely messy pajamas and giving him a shower in the middle of the night.

—*Charlene Brock, MD, a mom of 28-, 25-, and 23-year-old sons and an 18-year-old daughter and a pediatrician with St. Chris Care at Falls Center, in Philadelphia, PA*

When my daughter was 10 months old and had stopped breastfeeding, she developed persistent diarrhea, and also eczema. The pediatrician was stumped by this. I happened to find a book in a health food store about eczema being linked to milk intolerance. When I weaned my daughter, it became apparent that she was allergic to milk.

—*Stuart Jeanne Bramhall, MD*

Mommy MD Guides-Recommended Product
Pedialyte

When your baby has diarrhea or is vomiting, the last thing that you want to do is to have to haul her to the store. That's why Pedialyte is a good thing to have on hand at all times.

Pedialyte is the number one pediatrician-recommended oral rehydration fluid. Pedialyte is therapeutic hydration because it is specially formulated to replenish vital minerals and nutrients lost during diarrhea and vomiting to help prevent dehydration.

You might be surprised to learn that sports drinks, sweetened sodas, and juices don't meet medical guidelines for helping prevent dehydration due to diarrhea and vomiting in children. In general, these drinks are too high in carbohydrates (sugar) and too low in the mineral sodium, which is an important electrolyte that is lost when a child has diarrhea and vomiting. Plus, drinks containing too much sugar can actually make diarrhea worse. (Talk with your doctor before giving your baby this or any medication.)

You can buy Pedialyte in various package forms, and it comes in several flavors, including fruit, grape, strawberry, and apple. You can buy Pedialyte in stores and online for around $5.50.

For more information, visit **PEDIALYTE.COM**.

When to Call Your Doctor

If your baby develops diarrhea that is accompanied by any of the following other signs and symptoms, call your doctor or take your baby to the emergency department.

- Fever (any fever in a baby younger than three months old or a fever of 101°F or higher in a baby three months old or older)
- Signs of dehydration, including dry mouth, crying with few or no tears, fewer than four wet diapers per day, going four to six hours without urinating, or if the soft spot on your baby's head looks sunken or flatter than usual
- Vomiting
- Blood, mucus, or pus in the stool

If your baby has more than eight stools in eight hours or if the diarrhea lasts longer than a week, call your doctor.

When my daughter was four months old, she developed severe diarrhea. I knew that something was wrong because her stool really didn't look right. I took her to the pediatrician. It turns out she had a bacterial infection in her digestive tract. She was prescribed antibiotics, and after that she was fine. This is very uncommon, but the lesson is, if something doesn't look or feel right to you, have it checked out.

—*Alanna Kramer, MD*

My older son got rotavirus just before his first birthday. My husband and I worked diligently to make sure he was well hydrated. We made sure he got 5 cc (one teaspoon) of fluids every few minutes, using a syringe. But it would all come out anyway. We watched him carefully for signs of dehydration. For example, we watched to make sure he was peeing at least three times in 24 hours and that his mouth wasn't too dry, and that he was making tears.

My husband and I hoped so much that our son would be better

by his birthday. He was, but meanwhile my parents had caught his rotavirus, and so they missed his party.

—*Leena Shrivastava Dev, MD, a mom of 14- and 10-year-old sons, an assistant professor of medicine at Drexel University College of Medicine, and a general pediatrician, in Philadelphia, PA*

Changing a Wriggly Baby's Diaper

No doubt about it, a determined baby is a *strong* baby. A baby has far more interesting things to do than have his diaper changed, so around this age, diaper changes can become quite the power struggle.

I never used the changing table. I did everything low to the ground because I was afraid my son would fall. If your baby rolls at floor level, he can't hurt himself.

—*Sonia Ng, MD*

My middle baby was so strong that he'd fight me whenever I was changing his diaper, so much that he'd roll right off the changing table! If this is a concern for you, don't be afraid to hold your baby very firmly by the leg. I've never seen anyone dislocate a baby's hip by holding the baby's leg firmly. If you're still concerned, change your baby's diaper on the floor.

I found it helpful to keep a toy on the changing table. Something like Buzzy (See "Mommy MD Guides–Recommended Product: Buzzy for Shots" on page 72) is helpful because it vibrates and tickles the baby and distracts him.

—*Amy Baxter, MD, a mom of 13- and 10-year-old sons and an 8-year-old daughter, the CEO of MMJ Labs, and the director of emergency research of Children's Healthcare of Atlanta at Scottish Rite, in Atlanta, GA*

RALLIE'S TIP

My youngest son was very active from the minute he was born. When he was older, he didn't like sitting still for anything, especially a diaper change. Fortunately for me, he was mesmerized by my car keys. I only

let him hold them while he was having his diaper changed, and he was
so happy to have them in his little hands that he would forget about
everything else and concentrate on those keys.

Even if we were away from home having a diaper change in a restroom
at a restaurant or a store, I always had my car keys with me, and they never
failed to keep my son's attention long enough for me to change his diaper.

Keeping Your Baby Cool in Summer and Warm in Winter

A comfortable baby is a happy baby, and a happy baby makes for
a happy mom. When dressing your baby, let your own outfit be
your guide. Dress your baby in the same weight of clothing and
number of layers as you're wearing, plus one extra layer.

I live in Florida, so my challenge was keeping my babies cool in
summer and coping with the often extreme temperature changes
going from hot outside to air-conditioned inside. I dressed my babies

in loose clothing so that the air could circulate around them. Also, I took a lot of clothes with me so I could layer my babies up or layer down as necessary.

—*Melanie Bone, MD*

We live in Louisiana, and it's hot. When my daughter was a baby, we played a lot of water games outside. We'd hook a sprinkler to the hose so she could play in the water and stay cool. I'd also give her cool things to eat, like popsicles and juice frozen in cups.

—*Christy Valentine, MD, a mom of a five-year-old daughter, a specialist in pediatrics and internal medicine, and the founder of the Valentine Medical Center, in Gretna, LA*

When it was cold outside, I dressed my son in one additional layer of clothing than I wore to keep his temperature normal. Babies lose body heat faster than adults because of their smaller body surface area.

—*Sonia Ng, MD*

During my baby's first year, I found baby cardigan sweaters to be wonderful. They're soft and warm, they're great for layering, and they're easy to take on and off.

—*Leigh Andrea DeLair, MD, a mom of a two-year-old son and a family physician, in Danville, KY*

We lived in Michigan, and it's really hard to keep warm in the winter. During my son's first year, it was often too cold to go out. My husband and I didn't want to expose him to anything, so we just kept him inside as much as possible.

When we did have to go outside, I put my son into a front carrier or sling, and then I wrapped a big coat around both him and me. My body heat kept my son warm and cozy.

—*Lennox McNeary, MD, a mom of a two-year-old son, a specialist in physical medicine and rehabilitation at Carilion Clinic, and a cofounder of the Mommy Doctors Bakery (makers of Milkin' Cookies), in Roanoke, VA*

It's been very cold here in Kansas! I love baby sleep sacks, and I put one on my daughter each night for bed. We also run a humidifier in her room at night because moist air feels warmer than dry air.

I never knew how many baby blankets there are! When you're having a baby, you get a gazillion blankets. You'll never be short on blankets. I received so many beautiful handmade blankets, and I'll never part with them.

—*Jennifer Bacani McKenney, MD*

Dressing babies can be tricky, especially babies younger than four to six months. The general rule is as long as the baby wasn't born prematurely and he doesn't have any underlying medical issues, you should dress him just like you are dressed, plus one layer, plus a hat.

At one time, I might have questioned the hat part, but about two years ago I lost all of my hair because of chemotherapy. I know what it's like to be bald. It's amazing how much colder you feel. I could have been wearing the same amount of clothing as seven other people, and they'd all be fine, but I'd be frozen. Put a hat on that baby!

—*Hana R. Solomon, MD*

When my son was five months old, I had the opportunity to lecture in Romania. I was still breastfeeding, and my son had two sets of immunizations, so I took him with me. It was a little chilly in Romania while we were there.

While I was out walking my son in his stroller, a Romanian doctor leaned over and said, "He needs to wear a hat." Everyone there seems to smoke, and at the same time, this doctor exhaled a cloud of cigarette smoke right into my baby's face! I looked at the doctor and said, "I think there are worse health risks than not wearing a hat!"

—*Amy Baxter, MD*

Crawling

Babies don't meet milestones on the clock, but in general, most babies crawl between seven and 10 months. If your baby isn't crawling, though, don't panic. Crawling isn't technically a milestone because some babies skip it altogether, going straight to standing and cruising or making up their own little scooting maneuver. If that's the case, give your baby extra points for creativity!

෦෴

It was fascinating that my twins reached just about every developmental milestone, such as smiling for the first time and crawling, within days of each other!

 —*Ann Contrucci, MD*

෦෴

I tried to encourage my babies to reach their milestones. For example, I remember getting down on the floor with my oldest baby and asking her, "Do you want to come to me? Well, baby, you've got to make it over here." That helped to motivate her to crawl or scoot over to me.

 —*Ann Kulze, MD*

෦෴

Crawling can irritate your baby's hands and knees. Not only can physical abrasion irritate the skin, but dust mites in carpeting can irritate too. I have no special advice other than to dress your crawling baby in pants, and make sure your carpeting is frequently vacuumed.

 —*Amy J. Derick, MD*

෦෴

Parents today are often urged to take on a technical role in their child's development. The parent is advised to be a teacher, coach, administrator, and manager of various functions. I heartily disapprove of this mentality because it often makes parents feel anxious and inadequate and because it puts the emphasis on the wrong things.

 Babies need parents to be enthusiastic, to be empathic, to be loving, to be tuned in, to be joyful, and to be sensitive—whatever the baby is up to. Your baby needs your watchful eye, with the gleam that only mothers can have. Your own heart will tell you to reach out your hand to support your baby, if your baby needs it, or if your baby needs to be jiggled or to be soothed. Mothers are experts at this kind of love. Crawling isn't an athletic event or a physical therapy session or a school lesson. Babies will crawl in due time.

 —*Elizabeth Berger, MD*

Chapter 8

8th Month

Your Baby This Month

YOUR BABY'S DEVELOPMENT

Your baby's vision is now almost adult-like in clarity and depth perception. By eight months, most babies' vision is 20/40, so she's only slightly nearsighted.

Also, around this time, your baby starts to produce real tears. Not that there has been any shortage of crying before this, but your baby was previously producing a thicker kind of tear, called mucin, that stuck to her eyes and kept them moisturized.

By around eight months, your baby's arms and hands have loosened up, and she can probably hold a bottle. You're probably working your way through baby foods at this point, but your baby still gets a lot of her nourishment from formula or breast milk. Around this age, some babies also start to eat finger foods. Cheerios, anyone?

At this age, your baby can probably stand with some help. An eight-month-old baby might be able to lean up against something, such as a sofa, for five to 10 minutes. Interestingly, at this age, babies lean up against things for balance, not for support. Once your baby discovers how fun it is to be standing, she'll start to figure out how to pull herself up to a standing position all by herself. Also, your baby can get into a sitting position from her stomach.

Your baby probably continues to practice raking small objects toward her and picking them up in her fist. Some babies can pick things up between their thumbs and forefingers at this point. Then if the object falls on the floor, your baby will look to see where it went.

At this age, babies' babbling changes from sounds made with the lips (like ba-ba) to sounds made with the tongue (like da-da). Even though some eight-month-old babies can say "DaDa" or "MaMa," it's more by accident than on purpose. They likely get the words mixed up, calling MaMa "DaDa" and vice versa.

One word that some babies are starting to understand is "No." At this age, babies understand the word "no" to mean "stop"—though that doesn't mean babies will actually stop doing what they're doing! A favorite game of babies this age is patty-cake.

TAKING CARE OF YOU

Meet a friend for coffee or lunch. Because babies are not always great restaurant-goers, consider leaving your little one with your partner, a parent, or a trusted babysitter.

JUSTIFICATION FOR A CELEBRATION

The first time you hear "DaDa" is sure to be a reason to celebrate; just wait until you hear "MaMa"!

Enjoying Holidays and Special Events

A baby's first year is such a wonderful series of firsts. Some of the most memorable firsts are the first time you celebrate holidays and special events, things that are meaningful to you and your family, with your baby. Even silly holidays can become big events if you get a little creative. How will you celebrate your baby's first Groundhog Day (February 2), Incredible Kid Day (March 15), Mother Goose Day (May 1), Sneak Some Zucchini onto Your Neighbor's Porch Day (August 8, and no, we did not make this up), and National Dessert Day (October 14—now that's something to celebrate!)?

When our twins were babies, my husband and I started a tradition of having an annual summer party, inviting all of our friends with kids. The party has grown to be quite enormous now that all three of our kids are in school with friends of their own. This year we had about 60 people over!

—*Katherine Dee, MD, a mom of six-year-old twin daughters and a four-year-old son and a radiologist at the Seattle Breast Center, in Washington*

My twins were born in September. The year they were born, I sent a message to my parents and my in-laws to say that whoever called the caterer first could come visit us at Thanksgiving!

—*Lillian Schapiro, MD, a mom of 14-year-old twin girls and an eight-year-old daughter and an ob-gyn with Peachtree Women's Specialists, in Atlanta, GA*

Even when my son was very small, my husband and I dressed him up for Halloween. It might not have been his very first year, but I remember one year he was Spiderman, and we dressed our dog as a frog!

—*Judith Hellman, MD, a mom of a 13-year-old son, an associate clinical professor of dermatology at Mt. Sinai Hospital, and a dermatologist in private practice, in New York City*

My daughter was born on Halloween, and her first Halloween was a lot of fun. I bought a costume on Etsy.com. That website has tons of vendors who make one-of-a-kind things. I ordered an Abby Cadabby costume with a tutu and wings, hair puff, and wand for my daughter. It was adorable! We had a costume party for all of her friends, and even the adults dressed up.

Especially during my baby's first year, I took every chance I could to dress her up in a special outfit, such as a green one for St. Patrick's Day. Every outfit was an excuse to take tons of pictures.

—Jeannette Gonzalez Simon, MD, a mom of a two-year old daughter who's expecting another baby and a pediatric gastroenterologist in private practice, in Staten Island, NY

My kids have no idea what religion they are. I celebrated whatever holidays I wanted to, regardless of what religion they represented. We celebrated both Passover and Christmas. We lighted a candle on Christmas Eve, and we left cookies for Santa.

—Nancy Rappaport, MD, a mom of 21- and 16-year-old daughters and an 18-year-old son, an assistant professor of psychiatry at Harvard Medical School, an attending child and adolescent psychiatrist in the Cambridge, MA, public schools, and the author of In Her Wake: A Child Psychiatrist Explores the Mystery of Her Mother's Suicide

At Christmas time, my family passed a tradition to us that we have continued. Together we set the Nativity when Christmas season starts, and everyone eagerly waits for the baby Jesus's birthday. We have special dresses and even have our hair bows picked out. On December 25th, the youngest child present (if family is visiting) puts baby Jesus on the manger. We sing a traditional Italian song, "Tu scendi dalle stelle." The youngest child carries baby Jesus and places him on the Nativity. We love building those family bonds and celebrating special traditions.

—Gabriella Cardone, MD, a mom of five-, three-, and one-year-old daughters and a pediatric emergency physician at Texas Children's Hospital, in Houston

One tradition we started during our twins' first year was taking an annual family Christmas picture. We send it as a card if I plan well enough in advance to get the picture taken in November. Usually we have the photograph taken in December, and our friends get their cards in February. It's the thought that counts, right?

Also each year we have a mother-daughter Christmas dinner for our friends and their children. We have the dinner at the American Girl Store, and the girls all dress up. It's really cute!

—*Brooke Jackson, MD, a mom of 3½-year-old twin girls and a 14-month-old son and a dermatologist and medical director of the Skin Wellness Center of Chicago, in Illinois*

∽

My son came home from the NICU just before Christmas, so that first holiday season is a blur to me. The second Christmas wasn't much better. For his third Christmas, he'd just turned two and he loved to sit by the tree and watch the lights. He also loved to play I Spy and search for different ornaments on the tree.

—*Lennox McNeary, MD, a mom of a two-year-old son, a specialist in physical medicine and rehabilitation at Carilion Clinic, and a cofounder of the Mommy Doctors Bakery (makers of Milkin' Cookies), in Roanoke, VA*

Tracking Your Baby's Growth

At every well baby visit, your baby's doctor will check her growth, including her weight, length, and head circumference. The doctor will then plot these measurements on a standardized growth chart to see how your baby measures up. Experts agree that the most important thing is not where your baby falls on the charts, but that her growth pattern remains consistent over time. In other words, whether she's a small, medium, or large baby, chances are excellent that she is growing just fine as long as her growth pattern stays consistent over time.

∽

My twins were born in September. During their first few months, I took pictures of them sitting next to pumpkins. As they got older, I found bigger pumpkins. I did that as long as I could find pumpkins that were bigger than the girls.

—*Lillian Schapiro, MD*

⤬

My husband and I love watching our daughter grow and develop ever-changing interests. We have enjoyed taking pictures of her every month with a sign that tells how old she is. Then we line up the pictures and see how fast she's already grown.

—*Kathleen Moline, DO, a mom of a 20-month-old daughter and a family physician in private practice with Central DuPage Physician Group, in Winfield, IL*

⤬

My twins were small when they were born, but they remained on their growth curve. Some breastfed babies are big ol' chunky, Buddha babies. Other breastfed babies are lean. Mine were lean. The key to using the growth curve is making sure the baby is staying on track on his own growth curve, and not "falling off," which can lead to concerns. Small babies may just be small due to their genetics, for instance. As long as they are proceeding on their particular growth curve, no worries!

—*Ann Contrucci, MD, a mom of 12-year-old boy-girl twins who works as a pediatric emergency physician, in Atlanta, GA*

⤬

My second baby was critically ill when he was born. When he left the hospital, he was two pounds lighter than when he was born. He was a very picky eater; he flat-out didn't seem to have any appetite.

I agonized over this baby's eating habits and his growth. He did gain weight and grow appropriately, but he was always a very skinny baby. I think it was likely related to his very rocky start in life. The developmental pediatrician warned me that his body had taken a huge hit, and he might be delayed in his growth and development. Today he's a very healthy and bright young man—6-foot-4 and on track to enter medicine in the next year and a half.

—*Ann Kulze, MD, a mom of 22- and 15-year-old daughters and 20- and 19-year-old sons; a nationally recognized nutrition expert, motivational speaker, and family physician; and the author of the best-selling book* Eat Right for Life, *in Charleston, SC*

◦◦◦

My younger son is small for his age. He was 5 pounds, 15 ounces when he was born. He was born at 37 weeks, so technically he was full-term and perfectly healthy. He was able to go home from the hospital with me.

Early on, my son was only at the 3rd percentile for weight on the growth curve. When he was six months old, his pediatrician told me to supplement my breast milk with formula to see if he gained more weight. We went back to see the doctor when my son was seven months old, and he had gained a bit of weight, but he was still at the bottom of the growth chart. Developmentally, he's always done great; he's just small.

At my son's nine-month visit, he had moved up to the 10th percentile in weight, and his head went from the 10th percentile to the 50th percentile. Because that represented a crossover of two percentiles on the growth chart, my pediatrician now had a new worry. The pediatrician sent my baby for an ultrasound to make sure he didn't have hydrocephalus. My son screamed the whole time he was getting the ultrasound, like we were pulling his arms and legs off, but it turned out just fine.

My son is still very small. He weighs 19 pounds at 13 months, but he's dancing and waving and doing all of the things he's supposed to be doing. He might just be a small kid, and that's okay. We joke that he'll be a jockey instead of a football player.

—*Rebecca Reamy, MD, a mom of six- and one-year-old sons and a pediatrician in emergency medicine at Children's Healthcare of Atlanta, in Georgia*

Monitoring TV Time

Must-see TV? Not for babies! The American Academy of Pediatrics urges parents to limit children's television watching to less than two hours of "quality programming" per day. Yet the average child watches three hours a day.

The problem is that the more time a baby or child spends watching TV, the *less* time she spends playing. Babies need active play time to develop their mental, physical, and social skills. The results of a study published in the journal *Child Development* revealed that if you have the TV on for background noise, it's harder for babies to hear and learn individual words.

Interestingly, young children don't know the difference between programs and commercials. Ronald McDonald is every bit as trustworthy to them as an educational program.

~

I managed to hide TV from my kids for quite a while. But the gig was up when my older daughter turned forward-facing in the car and we let her watch DVDs on trips. Then it was all over.

—*Cheri Wiggins, MD, a mom of four- and two-year-old daughters, a specialist in physical medicine and rehabilitation at St. Luke's Magic Valley, and a cofounder of the Mommy Doctors Bakery (makers of Milkin' Cookies), in Twin Falls, ID*

~

I did let my babies watch some TV. But do I think babies should watch Baby Einstein DVDs every day to stimulate their brains? Absolutely not!

—*Melanie Bone, MD, a mom of four, ages 16, 15, 14, and 13, a grandmom of one grandson, a gynecologist, the founder of the Cancer Sensibility Foundation, and the author of the syndicated column Surviving Life and the book* Cancer, What's Next?, *in West Palm Beach, FL*

~

I love *Sesame Street.* I think it's wonderful, and I swear watching it is why my older son was able to read so early. I watched it with him. It's safe, it's educational, and it's timeless. And when it was on, I could go to the bathroom by myself.

—*Heather Orman-Lubell, MD, a mom of 10- and six-year-old sons and a pediatrician in private practice at Yardley Pediatrics of St. Christopher's Hospital for Children, in Pennsylvania*

I did let my babies watch TV for short periods of time, such as while I took a quick shower. I let them watch programs that are educational, such as *Sesame Street*. They also loved *Yo Gabba Gabba* and *Super Why*.

TV watching is a point of contention with my mother-in-law, though, because she was a second grade teacher. She watches the kids for us, and if she comes over and the kids are watching TV, she shuts it off and says, "You've watched enough TV for now." She never says anything directly to me, but she gets her point across. She is wonderful with our kids, and we are so lucky to have her, so I don't mind.

—*Jennifer Gilbert, DO, a mom of 18-month-old twins and an ob-gyn at Paoli Hospital, in Pennsylvania*

Be a Knifty Knitter

Even though experts might say TV time isn't the *best* stress-reliever, it's certainly one of the most *common* ones. If you're looking for a way to make TV time more relaxing, make it productive, and prevent yourself from snacking to boot, here's a simple solution: the Knifty Knitter. Even if you're not crafty and you haven't been able to knit in the past, the Knifty Knitter is so simple that practically anyone can do it. It comes in kits, either round looms to knit hats, socks, slippers, and mittens, or what they call long looms that are really skinny ovals to knit baby blankets, shawls, and scarves.

With a Knifty Knitter, you don't need long, pointy knitting needles. Instead, the kits come with loom hook tools and plastic needles. The kits come with simple instructions, and their website, **PROVOCRAFT.COM**, offers easy-to-follow videos. If you search for "Knifty Knitter patterns" online, you'll find plenty of project ideas.

You can buy Knifty Knitter kits and replacement parts online and in stores. A round loom kit costs around $16. Looms sold separately cost around $4.

Recently, we brought a TV upstairs into our family room. Before that, we only had a TV in the basement! I try to minimize TV time, but I realize it's a cultural experience that my children will want to eventually share with their friends. The key is to balance that with family time.

At this point, we let our two older sons have a bit of a voice in what they watch. They like Pixar movies and Thomas the Tank Engine. Nemo is big in our house. But our boys aren't ready for shows like *Star Wars*, even though they might think they are. We also try to avoid shows with guns and violence. We try to watch any new movies or shows with the boys for the first time to screen them.

> —*Amy Thompson, MD, a mom of four- and two-year-old and nine-month-old sons and an ob-gyn at the University of Cincinnati College of Medicine, in Ohio*

Since 1995, we haven't had cable, and my husband and I limited our children's TV time. If I had it to do over, I'd have limited it even more.

When we did allow our children to watch TV, my husband or I sat and watched with them. We only watched family movies or videos that contained appropriate material for children.

> —*Michelle Storms, MD, a mom of 24- and 20-year-old sons and a 21-year-old daughter, the assistant director of the Marquette Family Medicine Residency Program, in Marquette, MI, and a member of the health professionals board for Intact America*

Organizing Your Baby's Clothing

Babies outgrow clothing quicker than you can say, "Osh Kosh B'Gosh." Keeping clothing neat and orderly and accessible is practically a full-time job.

My twins share a room. I hang up most of their clothing because that makes it easier for me to see at a glance what I have. I hang my son's clothing on the left side of the closet and my daughter's clothing on the right. I stash their pajamas in drawers, though, and I put all of their socks in baskets—blue for my son and pink for my daughter.

> —*Jennifer Gilbert, DO*

We were fortunate to inherit a lot of beautiful clothes from my brother and his wife, who have two young daughters. I actually used the boxes from our wedding china to separate clothes by sizes—newborn, three, six, and nine months. I stored the boxes in my daughter's closet and packed and unpacked the clothes into and out of her dresser drawers as she grew. When my daughter was born, she was already too big for many of the clothes that she received as gifts, so we exchanged new outfits that were too small.

—*Rachel S. Rohde, MD, a mom of a five-month-old daughter, an assistant professor of orthopaedic surgery at the Oakland University William Beaumont School of Medicine, and an orthopaedic upper-extremity surgeon with Michigan Orthopaedic Institute, P.C., in Southfield, MI*

My husband and I didn't find out that we were having a girl until our baby was born. Once we announced that to our friends and family,

Mommy MD Guides–Recommended Product
Lil' Dressers Drawer Labels

If it feels like your baby's socks, onesies, and shirts are multiplying like rabbits and taking over your house, you're not alone. Organizing, and reorganizing, all of those tiny pieces of clothing can be a joy to some moms, but a royal pain to others.

One way to help keep things straight is Lil' Dressers Drawer Labels. You place the adorable labels on the outside of drawers to indicate what's stashed inside. They come in boys' packages and girls' packages, and each pack includes 18 labels, with illustrations of items such as shirts, pants, and socks.

Who knows, they might make it easy for your partner, and someday your child, to help put away the laundry.

You can buy Lil' Dressers Drawer Labels for less than $10 a pack at **MOMMYMDGUIDES.COM**.

they started to bring us all of these baby clothes. People love buying baby clothes, so they keep on coming!

About a week after our daughter was born, my husband and I bought a bunch of plastic storage containers at Walmart. We put all of our daughter's three- to six-month clothes into one bin, the six- to nine-month clothes into another bin, and so on. We put all of the bins into our daughter's closet.

As our daughter outgrows a size of clothes, we put it back into a bin. Then we put that bin in the basement. It's amazing how quickly babies outgrow the small sizes! My baby is two months old now, and she has outgrown some zero- to three-month clothes already!

—*Jennifer Bacani McKenney, MD, a mom of a two-month-old daughter and a family physician, in Fredonia, KS*

RALLIE'S TIPS

Organization is definitely not my strong suit, and I've always struggled to keep closets, drawers, and shelves neat and tidy. My two youngest sons were born just 13 months apart, so I had lots of little outfits to wash, fold, and organize when they were babies and toddlers. I started out using a chest of drawers to hold all of their clothes, but I found that when I put everything in drawers, my boys ended up wearing the same three or four outfits over and over. My husband and I would just grab the outfit on top of the stack (or crumpled pile) of clothes, and the outfits at the bottom of the drawers never saw the light of day. With this "system," my boys were outgrowing a lot of their clothes before they ever wore them!

I finally figured out that it worked better for us to hang most of their clothes in their closet. That way, when I opened the closet door, I could see most of their outfits at a glance. I used the dresser drawers for smaller items, such as socks, shorts, T-shirts, hats, and mittens. I also found that it was easiest for me to organize my sons' clothes if I washed them in a separate load of laundry. It was just too easy for those teeny tiny baby socks to get lost in the sleeves of my husband's flannel shirts or in the legs of my fuzzy pajama pants.

Unfortunately, my two youngest sons appear to have inherited their mother's organization skills, and as teenagers, they haven't yet mastered the art of maintaining neat and tidy drawers. To this day, I still put most of their clothes on hangers after I've washed them. The good news is that now they're old enough to put their own clothes in their closets!

Watching Out for Bumps and Bruises

When you're a baby and you're learning to do *everything*, bumps and bruises are bound to happen. Just about every parent has an I-couldn't-believe-this-happened-to-my-baby story of a little one rolling off of a couch or crashing into a piece of furniture. Fortunately, babies are close to the ground, and they really are quite durable little creatures. For minor bumps, the best thing you can do for your little one is avoid showing your own fear, because your baby will take her cue from you. If you can see that your baby is unharmed, a cheerful, "Oops!" along with a reassuring smile and a kiss will go a long way to setting your baby's world right again.

⁓

When my baby gets a scrape, I clean it with soap and water to wash away the dirt. Ice helps reduce any pain and swelling, and I use acetaminophen (Tylenol) or ibuprofen (Motrin) if needed. (Talk with your doctor before giving your baby this or any medication.)

I didn't use Band-Aids on scrapes when my children were babies, because they would pull them off and put them in their mouths.

We've been lucky that we haven't needed to go to the emergency room for any injuries. My son did fall the day before his first birthday and got a big scrape under his nose. That looked great for his birthday photos.

—*Rebecca Reamy, MD*

⁓

When my babies got bumps and bruises, I treated them with a homeopathic remedy called arnica, which you can find in cream or tablets. It's a wonderful over-the-counter, natural, anti-inflammatory remedy. You can buy it online and in stores. To use it, just follow the instructions on the package. Don't put arnica cream on broken skin.

—*Lauren Feder, MD, a mom of 17- and 13-year-old sons, a nationally recognized physician who specializes in homeopathic medicine, and the author of* Natural Baby and Childcare *and* The Parents' Concise Guide to Childhood Vaccinations, *in Los Angeles, CA*

∾

All children fall down at some point, and you just have to do the best you can to babyproof your home to prevent major injuries.

When to Call Your Doctor

Accidents happen, but it's important to know when to get medical help. If your baby gets a cut, head to the emergency room or call 9-1-1 if the cut bleeds profusely or doesn't stop bleeding after you've applied direct pressure to the area for five minutes.

If your baby bumps her head, don't panic. The skull is designed to withstand the hard bumps of childhood. However, trust your inner voice to decide whether or not to call the doctor. If your child is experiencing any of the following signs and symptoms, call your doctor right away or go to the nearest emergency department.

- Lost consciousness or blacked out, for even a few seconds
- Vomits
- Just doesn't seem right, for example, isn't focusing on you or is responding oddly
- Sense of balance is off
- Prolonged crying
- Worrisome eye signs, such as crossed eyes or rolling eyes or if your baby seems to have trouble with vision
- Weakness on one side of the body or any impaired motor function, such as inability to nurse, sit up, or crawl
- Seizure

I had big children. Our worst fall happened when my older son was toddling across the floor upstairs. He fell and hit the baby gate with such force that the gate detached from the wall! As I watched helplessly from a few feet away, my son rode that baby gate down the entire flight of stairs! I winced, thinking, *Is this going to be an ER visit*? Thankfully, my son laughed the whole ride down the stairs, and he was still laughing when he reached the bottom, unharmed.

I wondered, *Was there something else I could have done*? No, I can't wrap him in Bubble Wrap and lock him in his room. You think you've babyproofed, but accidents still happen.

—Carrie Brown, MD, a mom of seven- and five-year-old sons and a general pediatrician who treats medically complex children and specializes in palliative care at Arkansas Children's Hospital, in Little Rock

One Friday afternoon, we were getting ready to go to lunch, and my daughter tripped and fell on the carpet, hit her head on the door hinge, and cut open her forehead. I called every single plastic surgeon I knew in New York City, and they were all in the Hamptons for the weekend. The only doctors in the hospitals were interns!

So I sewed up my daughter's cut myself. Then I treated the wound very carefully to prevent scarring. I cleaned the wound every day with rubbing alcohol. Instead of using a topical antibiotic, I put Aquaphor on it daily to keep it moist. Unlike with antibiotics, no one in the history of mankind has been allergic to Aquaphor.

I then covered the wound with DuoDERM Extra Thin, which you can buy online and in drugstores. You cut the bandage into the shape and size you need, and it speeds wound healing by 80 percent. My daughter's cut healed perfectly, without a scar.

—Debra Jaliman, MD, a mom of a 19-year-old daughter, a dermatologist in private practice, and an assistant professor of dermatology at Mt. Sinai School of Medicine, in New York City

One day when my kids were very small, my husband was in the backyard shooting some video of the kids. I took our son inside to change his diaper, and our daughter fell off of the porch and hit her head on a rock. My husband brought her inside for me to see, and even though she had stopped crying, she had a thumb-sized dent in her skull, so it was clear she needed to go to the ER. At first my husband wanted me to go along, but it made more sense for me to stay home with our other two children.

That was the right decision because they waited a while in the ER to be seen. Our daughter toddled around the waiting room as happy as could be. She had to have a CAT scan, but even that went well. They told us little kids do okay during CAT scans because there are lots of colored lights for them to look at. The techs popped a bottle in her mouth, slid her in the scanner, and she was fine. She had a depressed skull fracture all right, called a Ping-Pong ball fracture, but they told us it would take care of itself as she grew, and it did.

Last year, when our daughter was a senior in college, she was trying to get a soccer ball that had landed on a porch roof, and she fell 12 feet onto a pile of rocks. She went to the ER, and all turned out to be fine. I jokingly asked her, "Did you tell the ER folks that you have a habit of falling off porches?"

—*Penny Noyce, MD, a mom of 23- and 21-year-old daughters, two 21-year-old sons, and a 13-year-old son, the author of the preteen novel* Lost in Lexicon, *and an internal medicine specialist, in Weston, MA*

Keeping Your Baby and Your Pets Safe and Happy

If you have pets, there's a good chance your pet was your baby before your baby was born. Pets truly are part of the family. Introducing your baby to your pet was likely a big deal, and now as your baby is becoming more mobile, keeping everyone safe and happy can be a challenge. The most important thing to keep in mind is that babies and pets shouldn't be alone together at any time.

Here are some tips to consider to keep your baby and your pet both safe and happy.

• Never leave your baby and a pet together unattended.

- Install a sturdy gate to keep your pet out of the nursery when unsupervised.
- Keep your pet up to date on vaccinations and have your pet checked regularly for parasites.
- Provide a comfortable, special area for your pet inside your home, such as a dog crate or a cat bed.
- Move your pet's food and water bowls to a location out of your baby's reach. The food is a choking hazard, the water is a drowning hazard, and both are unsanitary for your baby to be playing in.
- Be sure to keep any pet medications, brushes, and leashes away from your baby.
- Keep your baby and pet toys separate. Don't give your pet plush toys or rattles, or she might be more likely to mistake your baby's toys for her own.
- If you haven't done so already, consider having your pet spayed or neutered, which might decrease aggression.
- If your dog or cat will tolerate it, teach your baby from a very early age how to gently pet your dog or cat by stroking the pet's back and sides but not reaching toward or over her head. Don't allow your baby to pull at your pet's fur or poke her eyes, or disturb your pet when she is eating, drinking, or sleeping.
- If your baby's crying upsets your pet, encourage your pet to go to her safe retreat place, such as her crate or bed.
- Because your baby will be touching your pet, keep your dog or cat as clean as possible.
- Keep your cat indoors to minimize exposure to fleas and ticks.
- Don't let your dog or cat run loose in the woods during poison ivy season. It's possible to get a poison ivy rash from touching a pet that has brushed up against the leaves.
- Certainly, keep your baby far away from the cat's litter box or the dog's poop!
- If there will be times you need to take both your baby

and your pet in the car, come up with a way to keep them separate, such as by confining your pet to a crate or carrier.

• Reward your pet's good behavior around your baby with treats.

❧

Our two cats are very special to us, and my husband and I were concerned about introducing them to the baby. We started furnishing our baby's room a few months before our baby was born. We also cut "windows" in the door to the nursery and placed mesh over the holes. That way, we could see and hear through the door, but the cats could not get into the room if the door was closed. We had heard scary stories about pets jumping into cribs, and we had read bad reviews of the tents that supposedly fit over cribs and playpens.

Before our daughter was born, I started using some baby lotion to get the cats used to the smell, and my husband brought a receiving blanket home from the hospital before we brought our daughter home. The cats actually slept on the blanket!

The cats have been so great with our daughter that she recently has started petting their fur a little, and we don't routinely keep her door closed anymore.

—*Rachel S. Rohde, MD*

❧

When my daughter was born, we had dogs at home. My husband and I wondered, *How do we bring our baby home to our dogs, who were our babies before our baby was born?*

My husband asked his brother to bring a baby blanket home from the hospital so that our dogs could smell it before we brought our baby home. We hoped that way they could get a sniff and realize, "Okay, this kinda smells like Mommy and Daddy."

When we brought our baby home, my husband went in first to talk the dogs down. Then we brought the baby in. We let them interact a bit, letting the dogs sniff her. We tried to give them a little bit of bonding time, but by then it was time to breastfeed her again!

We were careful to never put the baby on the floor because we were never quite sure where the dogs would be. Upstairs, she was pretty much in her crib, and downstairs, if I wasn't holding her, she was in her Pack 'n Play.

—*Jeannette Gonzalez Simon, MD*

❧

When we were thinking about getting a dog, our son was very small. I sought a lot of advice on what type of dog to get. Lots of dogs are great for grown-ups but not safe for kids. My son was a small baby, so we got a Maltese, which is a small breed of dog.

More than the dog, though, I worried about my baby and the cat. Cats are not great with babies. They are more likely to lash out at them in anger. I watched my cat very carefully anytime she was near my son.

Also, cats carry more diseases because of their litter boxes, and I always taught my son to wash his hands after he petted the cat. I taught him to be very kind and sweet to the cat, and he usually kept a respectful distance from her.

When my son got a little older, I was able to relax. I have a great photo of my son at a year and a half, dangling a shoelace in front of the cat. I call that photo "The Taming of the Wild."

—*Judith Hellman, MD*

Rallie's Tip

My dogs were very tolerant of my babies, even when my sons started crawling around and pulling on their ears and tails. For the most part, I didn't worry that my dogs would bite my children, but I did take extra precautions to prevent this from happening by never feeding my dogs meals or treats when my children were nearby. I had seen too many children in the emergency department who had been bitten by dogs when the dogs were trying to eat. When it was time for me to feed my dogs, I'd scoop up my babies and take them in the other room so that the dogs could enjoy their food without feeling threatened.

Working with Your Nanny, Babysitter, or Day Care

Probably the most important person you will ever hire is your child's caregiver. Working with that person is a bit of an art, requiring the utmost care.

Returning to work was difficult for me. It took quite a while for my family to settle into a routine. My husband and I both worked full-time, so we had to figure out who would be taking the baby to day care and who would be picking her up. Eventually we found that it worked best if I dropped my daughter off every day, and my husband picked her up because his schedule allowed him to leave work at a predictable time. I think having the routine is important for our daughter, because she knows what to expect. She went through a period where she would get upset when I dropped her off, but this comes and goes. Most of the time she's excited to see the other children at day care and she runs into the playroom without looking back, which reassures me that she has a good time while she's there.

—*Kathleen Moline, DO*

When I had to go back to work, thank goodness I was able to find a good babysitter who helped me for years. She came to my house for an hour each morning to help me get the babies up and ready for day care.

The day care is right across the street from the hospital where I work, which is very convenient. After work, I'd pick the babies up on my way home, and my babysitter would come back to my house in the evenings from 5 to 8 p.m. to help me with dinner, baths, and getting the babies to bed.

—*Sadaf T. Bhutta, MD, a mom of a five-year-old daughter and three-year-old triplets and an assistant professor and the fellowship director of pediatric radiology at the University of Arkansas for Medical Sciences and Arkansas Children's Hospital, both in Little Rock*

We had a nanny who came to our house. When my older daughter was a baby, I couldn't get her to go to bed at night. I asked our nanny what their day was like, and I found out the baby was napping five hours each day! No wonder she wasn't tired at night.

After that, I asked our nanny to keep a daily log for me of my daughter's activities during the day: when she ate, napped, and even when she went to the bathroom. Having that information was so helpful, and things went much better after that.

I also did surprise visits, where I'd just pop in unexpectedly to see how everything was going. I ended up firing two nannies because of those visits. One time I caught our nanny sleeping. When I went to wake her, my daughter said, "Oh no, Mommy, don't wake her up. She gets really mad when you do that!"

Another time, my daughter had colored all over our dining room walls with red marker. I thought, *It takes a long time for a two-year-old to draw that much! She must have been unattended for a long time.*

—*Lisa Dado, MD, a mom of three children, ages 21 to 16, a pediatric anesthesiologist with Valley Anesthesiology Consultants, and a cofounder and CEO of the Center for Human Living, which teaches life skills and martial arts training, in Phoenix, AZ*

When my sons were born, I was already working in private practice. I was actually able to take three whole months off to be with them. (For my daughter, I could only take six weeks off.) My husband and I also had enough money to afford to hire a nanny for our sons. My daughter had to be in day care. She was always the first one to be dropped off and the last one to be picked up. Whenever I had any free time at work, particularly during my "lunch hour" (you don't really get a "lunch hour" when you are a doctor), I would drive over to my baby's day care just to hang out with her and nurse her. It definitely made the time away from her easier.

Child care sure hasn't been cheap. When our boys were babies, my husband was a radiology resident and then a radiology fellow, and we used to joke that our nanny made more money than he did!

—*Stacey Weiland, MD, a mom of a 12-year-old daughter and 7- and 5-year-old sons and an internist/gastroenterologist, in Denver, CO*

Coping with Sibling Rivalry

Whoever coined the phrase "love/hate relationship" was probably talking about siblings. We all want our children to get along, but the best-laid plans do sometimes go awry. Sibling rivalry often starts before a second child is even born, and it continues as kids compete for everything, from toys, to attention, to *you*. It can be hard to promote harmony. But the solution begins with you.

❧

The first two weeks after my daughter came home from the hospital, my son had a rough time. He had just turned two, we had moved into a new home, and I was home during the day for the first time that he could remember. After about two weeks, though, my son adjusted to his new routine, and he was his happy self again.

> *—Michelle Hephner, DO, a mom of a two-year-old son and eight-month-old daughter and a family physician in private practice with Central DuPage Physician Group, in Winfield, IL*

❧

The biggest challenge with my second son was to try to make his older brother not feel left out. My second son was a very easygoing baby, so caring for him was pretty simple. But every time the baby needed me, my eight-year-old son would come over and say that *he* needed me. I'm sure it was sibling rivalry.

I tried to avert the sibling rivalry by taking my older son to a community class that introduces children to the care of babies and shows them how they can participate in the care of a little brother or sister. The instructors pointed out opportunities that older siblings might have to be the helper. In the end, the kids received a T-shirt and certificate for being an outstanding older sibling.

I try to equalize everything. I offer my sons equal shares of everything, and if the little one doesn't want it, his brother can have it. I also tell my sons very often that I love them.

> *—Sonia Ng, MD, a mom of seven- and two-year-old sons, a pediatrician, and a sedation attending physician at the Children's Hospital of Philadelphia Pediatric Care and the University Medical Center at Princeton in Princeton, NJ, and the Pediatric Imaging Center in King of Prussia, PA*

❧

When my second baby was born, my oldest was 21 months old. I was very successful in helping my first child welcome the baby. She tells me today that she never remembers feeling left out or jealous.

Before my second baby was born, I read a book called *Welcoming Your Second Baby* by Vicki Lansky. I implemented a few pieces of her advice. The most important thing was that when my baby cried, if I was occupied with her sister, I never rushed away from my older child to tend to the baby. When the baby cried, I'd tell my older daughter, "Listen to that! Can you hear the baby? Let's finish this up, and we'll go see what she needs." Then we had closure on what we were doing, and together we went to see the baby.

Also I included my older daughter as often as possible when I was tending to her sister. For example, my older daughter loved to get the diapers out of the changing table. She'd put a diaper on the floor, smooth it out with her hands, and say, "Mommy, I'm making this nice and flat for you." I welcomed any help that my daughter could give me.

When my son was born, it was a challenge to keep him safe from his very loving, very involved "other mothers." I think my younger daughter would have hugged the very life out of him with her loving exuberance if I hadn't been there to make sure she let go long enough for him to breathe. For his part, he took it like a champ.

—Lesley Burton-Iwinski, MD, a mom of 20- and 18-year-old daughters and a 14-year-old son, a retired family physician, and a parent and teacher educator with Growing Peaceful Families, in Lexington, KY

For many years, I used to keep in my wallet along with the photographs a little wad of blond hair that our daughter had pulled out of our son's head, and a little wad of light brown hair that our son had pulled out of our daughter's head. I am pretty sure that these represented two different occasions. I always found these little mementos hilarious and enjoyed pointing them out to people who looked at the photos. Our children are a year apart in age, and as children as well as adults, they have always been very close and deeply devoted to one another. But naturally, children are full of hate as well as love, and lively, robust children will be full of lively, robust hate at times.

I think it's important for parents not to get overly drawn in by everyday sibling conflicts. Parents can say, "Oh, quit it!" to the warring siblings or refuse to arbitrate petty squabbles, "Oh, work it out between yourselves!" Getting alarmed and aiming to get to the bottom of minor quarrels can deliver the message that these tiffs are terribly important and alarming, and thus just add fuel to the fire. In addition, it must be observed that it's usually impossible to get to the bottom of these quarrelsome matters and that the intense interest on the part of a concerned third party often just escalates the drama as well as the confusion. The goal is to just patch it up somehow and get on with the next thing.

Of course, it's important to make sure that one child isn't regularly bullying and exploiting another.

The answer is not for the parent to focus on fairness and dividing up the candy bar or the TV shows with exactitude. The answer might be for the parent to be more attentive and involved with each child individually. The core of the sibling rivalry is usually that the sib is perceived to stand in the way of the parents' availability. It is not "You stole my candy bar!" so much as "You stole my mother!" that has fundamentally enraged the jealous sibling. The child might not have the courage to level the reproach directly at the parent. The sibling is, in this sense, just a stand-in for the elusive parent, who is really the source of the frustration. The fact that an exact division of the candy bar into two molecularly equal pieces never satisfies the participants is a sign that the candy bar is only a symbol of the real loss—the parent's full attention and devotion. Of course, Dad too plays a role here—so you might say that the child's jealousy of the sibling is also a reflection of the universal magical wish of every child to have each parent all to himself or herself.

—*Elizabeth Berger, MD, a mom of a 28-year-old son and a 26-year-old daughter, a child psychiatrist, and the author of* Raising Kids with Character, *in New York City*

Playing with Your Baby

As your baby becomes more mobile—and more communicative—play becomes more and more fun.

My daughter loves to play with any toy that has a tag on it. (These are the cloth tags that are sewn onto toys such as small stuffed animals and are securely attached to the toy—not the store sales tags that are easily removed.) She turns the toy around until she finds the tag and then sucks on the tag. The tags must feel good in her mouth.

—*Michelle Hephner, DO*

One thing that wasn't a big hit with my kids was the automatic baby swing. Whenever I put them into it, they'd get impatient. They wanted to be out doing something. We had another swing hanging from the

Mommy MD Guides–Recommended Product
Discovery Toys

For more than 30 years, moms have turned to Discovery Toys for high-quality, educational toys, books, games, and music. With age-appropriate products for children ranging from infancy to school years, Discovery Toys are reliable, safe, learning-centered, and, best of all, fun. They really do live up to the company's mission to Teach, Play, and Inspire.

What else is great about Discovery Toys? The company's reputation for excellence makes selling their toys a great business opportunity for stay-at-home moms, or for moms looking for extra income. As you might expect from a company committed to children, Discovery Toys is committed to serving the needs of children with autism and special needs. It's where many moms go for products to make learning fun for their children.

Discovery Toys are sold online at **DISCOVERYTOYS.COM** and in the United States and Canada by thousands of independent education consultants, many of whom are teachers, parents, or both. A final perk: Discovery Toys' reasonable pricing. Most Discovery Toys products cost less than $20.

porch outdoors, and that one my kids loved, probably because it required a parent to push it!

—*Penny Noyce, MD*

RALLIE'S TIP

I loved playing with my babies, and it was so much fun discovering what they enjoyed most. My oldest son was an explorer, and as soon as he could crawl, he rarely stayed still. His idea of a good time was wriggling under the coffee table or worming his way behind the couch.

My middle son didn't mind sitting still. He really enjoyed stacking blocks and giant Legos.

My youngest son loved the water, and splashing around in the bathtub was one of his favorite things to do. The funny thing is that none of my children were drawn to expensive toys or games. The simplest activities were the ones they enjoyed most.

Chapter 9
9th Month

Your Baby This Month

YOUR BABY'S DEVELOPMENT

At nine months, babies start to be able to remember people and things that are out of sight. This is why separation anxiety often begins to get stronger around this age. Your baby knows you from others, and he feels abandoned when you leave. Most babies this age are active and need lots of stimulation, but they don't like to be away from Mommy and Daddy.

By nine months, most babies need just one morning and one afternoon nap. Most babies at this age sleep for around 2¾ hours during the day and for around 11¼ hours at night. Hopefully this means you are getting more beauty sleep too!

At this age, most babies have perfected whatever method of crawling or scooting is most efficient—and likely most fun—for them. For many babies, this means the standard cross-crawl, moving the opposite hand and foot in concert. Other babies come up with their own baby locomotion. Some babies creep, wriggle, drag with their arms (the baby commando crawl), or scoot on their bottoms. Give them extra points for creativity! Some babies never crawl at all; they go straight to walking!

Around this time, about half of babies can pull themselves up to stand. Some even begin cruising around the room, holding on to furniture. Most of the time, babies don't know how to get back down, and they simply fall back down on their behinds.

Plop! Some babies start to figure out how to lower themselves without falling.

Definitely keep an eye out for small things within your baby's reach. At this time, it's likely that your baby can pick up a tiny object with his thumb and finger, using a pincer grasp. Coins, beads, and crumbs are all very close to his level and totally irresistible. It's no secret where these tiny items will end up if your baby gets his hands on them!

Nine-month-old babies love predictable things that they can do over, and over, and over. Many babies this age love passing games, where they give you a toy only to take it right back. Peek-a-boo is still a favorite game of nine-month-olds. Your baby might put his own hands over his eyes to try to hide his face. He's trying to master imitation.

By nine months, most babies have developed their own language to communicate with you. This is probably a combination of sounds and gestures that no doubt you understand quite well, but strangers have no clue how to decipher it.

As you can probably tell, your baby knows his name now. He's also starting to learn the meaning of many words that are associated with familiar and loved people or objects, such as "dog" and "car." At this age, some babies can follow simple one- or two-word commands.

Your baby might start to say even more consonants now, such as p and f. Babies babble their way through the whole consonant alphabet, ba-ba, da-da, ga-ga, and then they start to make combinations. Someday soon, you'll hear "ah-ba-di-da-ga-ma."

Taking Care of You

Get a mani/pedi. You spend so much time taking care of your baby, it's important to take time to take care of yourself also.

Justification for a Celebration

"Ah-ba-di-da-ga-ma" means "I love you."

Going to an Amusement Park

To those people who say, "Why take a baby to Walt Disney World, he'll never remember it anyway?" we say, "What about us? *We'll* remember it." And we'll have the 2,131 photos to show him when he gets older.

‿◦‿

We live in Florida, and when my kids were small, we had yearly passes to Walt Disney World. We went there often, but we didn't take the babies on any rides. Going there was more for us! I don't think kids get much out of amusement parks until they're around six or seven years old.

> —*Melanie Bone, MD, a mom of four, ages 16, 15, 14, and 13, a grandmom of one grandson, a gynecologist, the founder of the Cancer Sensibility Foundation, and the author of the syndicated column* Surviving Life *and the book* Cancer, What's Next?, *in West Palm Beach, FL*

‿◦‿

When my kids were babies, we lived in Germany. Over there, small carnivals travel from town to town. They were so simple and so endearing—usually just a carousel, a live pony ride, and face painting.

We loved taking our babies to the small zoos in Germany. Many of them had petting areas where we had lots of "hands-on" fun and laughs together. Of course, washing hands afterward was a must.

> —*Ann Kulze, MD, a mom of 22- and 15-year-old daughters and 20- and 19-year-old sons; a nationally recognized nutrition expert, motivational speaker, and family physician; and the author of the best-selling book* Eat Right for Life, *in Charleston, SC*

‿◦‿

We have a great photo of our son at three months old wearing Mickey Mouse ears, drinking pumped breast milk in front of Cinderella Castle at Walt Disney World. My husband and I found it easy to take our children on vacation when they were infants. They were more like accessories at that age! They fell asleep in the car or on the plane that first year, and they weren't walking yet. It was a great time to travel. My husband and I took our babies everywhere we could, and we photographed their every move.

After our babies had gotten their first round of shots and I was still breastfeeding, I felt that their immune systems were boosted enough to protect them from most illnesses. At that point, I wasn't worried about exposing them to unfamiliar bugs.

—*Amy Baxter, MD, a mom of 13- and 10-year-old sons and an 8-year-old daughter, the CEO of MMJ Labs, and the director of emergency research of Children's Healthcare of Atlanta at Scottish Rite, in Atlanta, GA*

My number one recommendation for amusement parks is to go early in the day. Try to be there when the parks open, because the lines are much shorter, and you can whiz through the whole Magic Kingdom, for example, before noon, have a relaxed lunch, and go back to hang out at your hotel! Sometimes, in addition, because both parents can't go on the rides with the babies, the park staff will allow the parent who stayed behind the first time to skip the lines and take his or her turn. This also gives the older sibling a chance to ride twice without waiting the second time.

Many amusement parks have family areas and nurseries, which are great for nursing, napping, or just taking a quiet break in the middle of a hectic day. Remember to bring sunscreen and lots of water.

—*Michelle Paley, MD, PA, a mom of two and a psychiatrist and psychotherapist in private practice, in Miami Beach, FL*

Buying Baby Shoes

Most doctors recommend holding off on buying baby shoes until your baby is actually walking outside. In fact, some doctors say that walking barefoot helps a baby to learn to walk and minimizes falls. But that doesn't keep most parents from delighting in buying cute little baby shoes.

I remember buying my son's first sneakers: baby Nike tennis shoes that were about one inch long. I still have them!

—*Sandra Carson, MD, a mom of two grown sons and the director of the Center for Reproduction and Infertility of Women and Infants Hospital, in Providence, RI*

I remember buying a lot of shoes because my daughter grew so fast. I'd try to buy them a half size larger than she needed because otherwise I was lucky if she got a few good wearings out of them. I bought some of my daughter's shoes at Stride Rite because I think their shoes are sturdier and offer extra support. I also bought her everyday shoes at Target.

—*Christy Valentine, MD, a mom of a five-year-old daughter, a specialist in pediatrics and internal medicine, and the founder of the Valentine Medical Center, in Gretna, LA*

〜

I found that with baby shoes, investing a little more money paid off. My daughter had really wide feet as a toddler. We'd buy the cheaper shoes, but we found that buying one or two pairs that were made for wider feet from Stride Rite worked best and saved money over the long haul.

—*Katja Rowell, MD, a mom of a five-year-old daughter, a family physician, and a childhood feeding specialist with FamilyFeedingDynamics.com, in St. Paul, MN*

〜

My sister-in-law had given me a pair of hand-me-down white dress shoes for my son, and I had put them on him simply because they matched his outfit on that particular day. He wasn't walking yet. When a shoe salesman saw them, he chastised me, "We aren't using those shoes anymore. The soles are too stiff." Who knew? I still laugh about the fact that I dressed my son in the "wrong" shoes. Thankfully, it was the first and only time he wore them, and he was not walking yet.

—*Amy Thompson, MD, a mom of four- and two-year-old and nine-month-old sons and an ob-gyn at the University of Cincinnati College of Medicine, in Ohio*

RALLIE'S TIP

I didn't keep shoes on my boys' feet regularly until they were old enough to run and play outdoors. I really felt that my babies needed to use their toes to push themselves around or up to a standing position. I wanted them to develop and exercise the muscles in their feet and legs, and I wanted them to experience all the wonderful sensations of being barefoot.

Plus, I loved playing with their tiny little toes and feet.

When my two youngest boys were babies, I had them in a double stroller at my husband's softball game, and of course they were both barefoot. One of my friends said, "I guess it must be hard to buy shoes for those boys on two doctors' salaries!"

⌇

I remember taking my baby to Stride Rite early on. The salesperson told me, "Shoes in the first year are like jewelry; they're accessories." Babies love to kick their shoes off. You put shoes on them just to lose them.

It's not until a baby is actually putting weight on his feet and walking outdoors that he really needs shoes. But, if you want to spend money on losing baby shoes, by all means, go for it.

—*Melanie Bone, MD*

Preserving Memories

First smile, first food, first haircut, first tooth—you're capturing them all in your memory and in your heart, and probably also with your camera. This is a wonderful idea because in a few short years, your toddler will love to look at photos and videos of himself. Plus, you'll have plenty of fun things to tease your teen about someday.

⌇

During my son's first year, I enjoyed watching him grow and change over the months. I took many photographs of him, and I enjoy seeing the changes he made over time.

—*Leigh Andrea DeLair, MD, a mom of a two-year-old son and a family physician, in Danville, KY*

⌇

I tried to take a lot of pictures of my son. I didn't have any set schedule of when to take photos. I simply took pictures whenever, wherever we were.

Today I wish I had kept up better with his baby book, though. I have to go back and catch up!

—*Sharon Giese, MD, a mom of a two-year-old son and a cosmetic plastic surgeon in private practice, in New York City*

I've been scrapbooking since before my sons were born. I really enjoy it. I have a room with all my scrapbooking supplies and space to work. I have my sons' baby photos and other mementos, like the wrist bands from the hospital, in a baby book.

—Rebecca Reamy, MD, a mom of six- and one-year-old sons and a pediatrician in emergency medicine at Children's Healthcare of Atlanta, in Georgia

I really like to take pictures of my kids! I'm not a professional photographer by any stretch of the imagination, but one thing that made it easier to capture good photographs of my constantly moving children was the purchase of a digital single-lens reflex (SLR) camera. It has very little delay from the time you press the button to the time the picture is snapped, so you don't miss those precious moments.

—Lezli Braswell, MD, a mom of a six-year-old daughter and four- and one-year-old sons and a family physician, in Columbus, GA

During my babies' first years, I loved all the "firsts" and how much the girls changed that first year of life! I still can't believe that kids go from a big lump to a walking, talking little person in just 365 days. I took a lot of pictures. You think you will remember what they looked like at six months, but it is impossible!

My first daughter has a scrapbook for her first year. My second daughter has a scrapbook with photos inside of it just needing to be organized. My third daughter has a scrapbook that's still in the wrapper.

I figure one day I will have the time to organize everything. For now, I have photos, and photo discs, just waiting to be organized and displayed. Life happens!

—Marra S. Francis, MD, a mom of seven-, six-, and four-year-old daughters and an ob-gyn, in The Woodlands, TX

I loved watching my daughter develop and change and grow. It's so great to see her learn new things and develop into a little person!

One thing I did that was fun and memorable was take pictures of her in all the different outfits that people bought us. My daughter has two grandmas who *love* shopping, so she had a lot of clothes! I made sure to take a picture every month on her month "birthday," and then we put the photos in an album online and shared it with friends and family. It was really fun to see how she changed from month to month. Sometimes instead of a thank-you note, I would e-mail people a picture of her in the outfit they bought her with a message from us saying thanks!

—*Melody Derrick, MD, a mom of a 17-month-old daughter and a family physician in private practice with Central DuPage Physician Group, in Winfield, IL*

With my older son, I wrote down a lot of memories. I had put some loose-leaf paper in the back of his baby book, and I noted funny things he did or later said.

I also took tons of pictures. I think with my oldest I took a picture every time I changed him into a new outfit! I didn't have a digital camera then, and I took rolls and rolls of pictures. After I got them developed, I put them into three-ring photo albums. I put the really good ones into frames. Now that I have a digital camera, I don't print out so many bad pictures.

It's so much fun to record those memories so that you can look back and see the funny things your children said or did and the faces that they made. Kids love to look at photos of themselves, too, when they get older.

—*Heather Orman-Lubell, MD, a mom of 10- and six-year-old sons and a pediatrician in private practice at Yardley Pediatrics of St. Christopher's Hospital for Children, in Pennsylvania*

RALLIE'S TIP

My two youngest boys were born so close together that I didn't have time to even think about organizing a photo album or a scrapbook for the first several years of their lives. I did make sure that I took plenty of photos along the way, and I stored them in shoeboxes in a safe place. When our sons were both in school, my husband and I finally found the time to sit down and put the photos into scrapbooks and photo albums. By that time, the boys were old enough to help, and we had so much fun looking at all their baby pictures and reliving our memories of those moments. Before that, I had always felt a little guilty that I hadn't taken the time to make scrapbooks and photo albums, but as it turns out, I wouldn't have had it any other way.

Cleaning Up Messy Eating

Someday your child will sit nicely at the table, eat with a fork and spoon, and dab at his lips with a napkin. That day is *not* today.

In general, when my daughters started eating solid food, I learned to tolerate a little mess. One thing that helped to contain the mess of my babies' eating was never feeding them over carpets!

—*Robyn Liu, MD, a mom of seven- and four-year-old daughters and a family physician with Greeley County Health Services, in Tribune, KS*

My husband and I joke that our daughter is such a messy eater that we need five hands to feed her. Last night she started a new trick: She blows raspberries when she's eating. There were bananas everywhere! I just take the approach that there are going to be messes, so just clean them up.

—*Michelle Hephner, DO, a mom of a two-year-old son and eight-month-old daughter and a family physician in private practice with Central DuPage Physician Group, in Winfield, IL*

The mess simply goes with the territory! My husband and I made sure that our baby's high chair was on a washable surface, such as the linoleum floors in our kitchen. If we were having a "formal" meal in the dining room, we would put the high chair on a plastic sheet or shower curtain to contain the mess.

—*Susan Besser, MD, a mom of six grown children, ages 26, 24, 22, 21, 19, and 17, a grandmom of one, a family physician, and the medical director of Doctors Express-Memphis, in Tennessee*

I am a sloppy feeder, and it drives my husband nuts. I would always put bibs on my babies when they were eating. But better still, a friend gave me a bib shirt, which I thought was very neat. It's a long-sleeved shirt that covers the baby's entire outfit! It really keeps the mess down.

　　—*Jennifer Gilbert, DO, a mom of 18-month-old twins and an ob-gyn at Paoli Hospital, in Pennsylvania*

I got my sons used to eating with utensils very early on. How? I simply gave them spoons and forks! My mother was a bit horrified, but they were hard plastic utensils with dull tips for goodness' sake! To this day, my middle son prefers to eat just about everything with a fork.

　　We also eat as a family. We try to sit down to dinner together on the nights I am not on call, so our children see my husband and me using our utensils properly.

　　—*Amy Thompson, MD*

When we started giving our twins cereal, we got them those baby seats that clip on the side of the table, and they sat side by side. It was a huge mess. My husband wanted to install a sloping floor that led to a drain. But that wasn't too practical, so he put a big plastic bin under their chairs to catch the mess.

　　—*Penny Noyce, MD, a mom of 23- and 21-year-old daughters, two 21-year-old sons, and a 13-year-old son, the author of the preteen novel* Lost in Lexicon, *and an internal medicine specialist, in Weston, MA*

I invested in a great high chair. The tray was very large and easy to clean. I also bought big plastic bibs with open pockets on the bottom to catch the food. If I was feeding a baby a food that was really messy, I'd simply take his shirt off!

When I fed my children, I moved the high chair into the middle of the kitchen floor, as far from the walls, rugs, and furniture as I could get it. It was messy, but I got good at cleaning up quickly and efficiently.

—*Ann Kulze, MD*

Preventing and Treating Ear Infections

The most common reason for hauling one's baby to the pediatrician is an ear infection. Almost two-thirds of babies will get at least one ear infection before their first birthdays.

There's good reason why babies are more likely to get ear infections than adults. The Eustachian tubes, which connect the inner ear to the back of the throat, are small. Plus, a baby's immune system is still developing, so it has a harder time battling off the viruses and bacteria that cause ear infections.

Often, babies get ear infections after they've had colds. Ear infections aren't contagious, but colds that cause them sure are.

My kids rarely got ear infections. I kept their noses clean by dropping in 10 to 20 drops of a saltwater solution and then sucking it out with a nasal aspirator. By the time my two younger kids were born, I knew about nasal irrigation, which is basically washing the nose. I washed their noses quite frequently, and I think that's why they rarely got ear infections. For more information on washing a baby's nose, visit Nasopure.com/nasopure-for-kids/babies.

—*Hana R. Solomon, MD, a mom of four, ages 35 to 19, a board-certified pediatrician, and the author of* Clearing the Air One Nose at a Time: Caring for Your Personal Filter, *in Columbia, MO*

My younger son had two ear infections in his first year of life. He seems to have a high threshold for pain. He had an ear infection that perforated his eardrum, and he never cried or had a fever.

—*Sonia Ng, MD, a mom of seven- and two-year-old sons, a pediatrician, and a sedation attending physician at the Children's Hospital of Philadelphia Pediatric Care and the University Medical Center at Princeton in Princeton, NJ, and the Pediatric Imaging Center in King of Prussia, PA*

My boys were both pretty healthy, especially in their first years. My second son had a few more ear infections than his older brother, but luckily they weren't too severe. He gave me the classic signals: After having cold symptoms for a few days, he became fussy, especially when we laid him down, and he had a fever. That let me know what was going on.

—*Jill Wireman, MD, a mom of 14- and 11-year-old sons and a pediatrician in private practice at Johnson City Pediatrics, in Tennessee*

RALLIE'S TIP

My oldest son had a couple of ear infections before his first birthday. He was so miserable, and I felt helpless to make him feel better. We both cried! That was before I was a doctor, and I didn't know the first thing about preventing ear infections.

By the time my youngest two sons were born, I had graduated from medical school, and I understood the benefits of nasal saline rinses. Whenever my youngest boys got stuffy noses, I'd mix up a saline solution, dissolving ¹/₂ teaspoon of iodine-free salt in ¹/₂ cup of warm water. Using one of the bulb suction devices that the hospital gave me when my sons were born, I'd gently squirt ¹/₂ teaspoon or so of the saline solution into each nostril and then gently suction it out. Because the rinse helps remove bacteria and allergens from the nasal passages, it reduces the risk of ear infections. The salt water reduces inflammation and removes excess mucus, which makes it easier for babies to breathe comfortably and also reduces the risk of ear infections. My two youngest sons rarely had ear infections when they were babies, and I'm sure that the saline rinses were a big factor in preventing them.

∽⌒∾

My daughter had a bunch of ear infections her first year. She had four ear infections in both ears in four months. That was tough. I didn't want to take her temperature for every little thing, and she also has a very high pain threshold, so it was tricky to even know when she had an ear infection.

One thing that I found helpful was to have her receive antibiotics by an injection, rather than having to take medication by mouth for days. I think the antibiotic shots work more quickly. My daughter would need to have one antibiotic injection the day of her doctor visit, and then we'd go back the next day for her follow-up shot. But still I think that's easier than giving a baby antibiotics by mouth two or three times a day for 10 days.

? When to Call Your Doctor

Some ear infections clear up on their own; others require antibiotics. It can be hard enough for a *doctor* to tell the difference, let alone a parent. If your child has the following signs and symptoms of an ear infection, call your doctor for advice.

- Pulling on ears (although one study found that only 15 percent of babies pulling on their ears had ear infections)
- Does not seem to hear normally
- Crying, especially during feeding, when lying down, and at night
- Fever (any fever in a baby younger than three months old or a fever of 101°F or higher in a baby three months old or older)

Ear infections can also be accompanied by diarrhea and vomiting.

—*Jeannette Gonzalez Simon, MD, a mom of a two-year-old daughter who's expecting another baby and a pediatric gastroenterologist in private practice, in Staten Island, NY*

⟳

When my boys started day care at about a year of age, they started to get ear infections. They all had their share of antibiotics.

Most children get ear infections in their first two years of life—more frequently if they are in day care, if they are formula-fed instead of breastfed, or if they are exposed to cigarette smoke. A baby should never be given a bottle while he is lying down, because that can predispose him to ear infections.

It can't be stressed enough that frequent handwashing helps to minimize colds, which usually precede ear infections. Sick children should not attend day care.

—*Charlene Brock, MD, a mom of 28-, 25-, and 23-year-old sons and an 18-year-old daughter and a pediatrician with St. Chris Care at Falls Center, in Philadelphia, PA*

⟳

I love ear tubes, and the need for tubes tends to run in families because it has to do with the shape of the head and how well the Eustachian tubes drain.

My sons had multiple ear infections early on, and I was very proactive about getting them ear tubes. The tubes made a tremendous difference. One day we noticed my older son couldn't hear out of one ear when he was talking on the phone. We discovered that one of his tubes had fallen out, and his ear was full of fluid. He simply had a new tube put in, and all was well.

—*Amy Baxter, MD*

⟳

My youngest daughter had a severe ear infection her first year, but her symptoms weren't pointing to that. I didn't know what was wrong with her. I took her to the ER and practically walked out when the nurses tried to restrain her on a stretcher so they could draw her blood and perform tests.

My gut said "No," and luckily the Motrin kicked in and my

daughter stopped crying. A mother's gut saying "No" loudly is usually correct.

—*Darlene Gaynor-Krupnick, DO, a mom of five- and two-year-old daughters, a female urologist fellow trained in pelvic reconstruction and neurology, and the inventor of Valera, a USDA-certified organic vaginal lubricant, in northern Virginia*

⌒

My youngest two babies had repeated ear infections and ended up having ear tubes put in. Back then, our pediatrician treated the ear infections with antibiotics.

But the recommendations for treating ear infections have changed over the years. Now the research suggests that even if an ear is very red and horrible-looking, it might be caused by a viral infection, and so antibiotics won't help. More and more pediatricians recommend waiting a bit to see if the ear infections resolve on their own, without using antibiotics.

When my babies had ear infections, I usually watched them closely for a few days to see if they improved. If they didn't get better on their own, I went the antibiotic route.

—*Susan Besser, MD*

⌒

My older son had a lot of ear infections his first year. I'm not a huge fan of ear tubes. I believe that they are put into babies more often than they should be. A lot of research suggests that ear tubes don't make a baby hear or speak any better or change his outcome later in life.

I frequently got calls from my son's day care that his eardrum had ruptured, goop was all over his shirt, and the staff wanted to know what to do.

"Nothing," I'd reply. "The pressure on the eardrum is gone now, and he's probably happy as can be." My son's ear infections progressed very rapidly. I could have him at the doctor and his ears would look fine, but six hours later his eardrum would rupture. In some kids, the pressure behind the eardrum builds up faster than in others. Just because their ears look fine today doesn't mean they won't be infected tomorrow. (Ruptured eardrums normally heal just fine.)

After a few eardrum ruptures, we did have tubes put in my son's ears. He's fine today. The tubes fell out when he was around a year and a half old, and he hasn't had an ear infection in a really long time. As babies get older, their head shape changes, and they spend more time sitting up, so they have fewer ear infections.

—*Carrie Brown, MD, a mom of seven- and five-year-old sons and a general pediatrician who treats medically complex children and specializes in palliative care at Arkansas Children's Hospital, in Little Rock*

Watching for Signs of Allergies

If allergies run in your family, you have plenty of company. Up to 50 million Americans, millions of them kids, are allergic to something.

When a person has an allergy, his body reacts to a substance that's harmless to most people. His body releases chemicals to defend against the allergen "invader." These chemicals cause allergy symptoms, such as sneezing, itchy nose, throat irritation, nasal congestion, and coughing. Some common allergens are dust mites, insect venom, medicines, molds, pollen, and pets.

In babies, the type of allergies you hear about most commonly are food allergies. About four out of every 100 children have a food allergy. When a person is allergic to a food, the body overreacts as if the food was harmful. A person can be allergic to any food, but interestingly almost all food allergies in children are caused by the following worst offenders.

- Cow's milk (Between 1 and 7 percent of infants are allergic to the proteins found in cow's milk.)
- Eggs (Most kids outgrow egg allergies by the time they start kindergarten.)
- Fish
- Peanuts (Along with tree nuts, peanuts cause some of the most severe food–related allergies.)

- Shellfish
- Soy (About 30 to 40 percent of babies who are allergic to cow's milk are also allergic to soy milk.)
- Tree nuts (These include almonds, pecans, and walnuts.)
- Wheat

Children who are allergic to cow's milk, eggs, soy, or wheat usually outgrow the condition. But children who are allergic to peanuts, tree nuts, fish, or shellfish usually remain so for life.

&

Food allergies run in my family, and when my son was a baby, I was very concerned he might develop them. I took the recommendations about when to introduce which foods very seriously. For example, I waited to give my son shellfish and nuts until he was three years old.

As an extra precaution, I asked my son's pediatrician for a prescription for an EpiPen. I took it with us, especially when we traveled away from home. This might not be practical for all parents, but all parents should learn the signs and symptoms of an allergic reaction.

—*Sharon Giese, MD*

? When to Call Your Doctor

If your baby has a food allergy, introduce new foods very carefully. It's best to try new foods in the morning so you can watch your baby all day for signs of an allergic reaction. Be on the lookout for the following signs and symptoms, and call your doctor if you see any of them.

- Hives (itchy, red welts on the skin)
- Swelling of the tongue, lips, face, or any other area of the body
- Coughing
- Trouble breathing or wheezing

If your baby has trouble breathing, call 9-1-1 or go to the nearest emergency room immediately.

My older daughter has food allergies. Our first clue that she had them was when we were on vacation in Taiwan. We had gone to a restaurant, and I had ordered a stew with little cubes of tofu in it. I gave a cube to my daughter, and she loved it, so I gave her a bunch of them.

The next morning, my daughter started vomiting, and her face broke out in hives. She was miserable. We had no idea what had caused it—until later when we learned those tofu cubes had crabmeat mixed into them. We had unwittingly been feeding her tons of shellfish!

Over the next year and a half, my daughter had a few episodes like this, usually after eating in restaurants. When she was three years old, we took her to an allergist for testing and discovered that she was allergic to peanuts and fish.

—*Robyn Liu, MD*

❧

Every pregnant woman is told to drink lots of milk. I followed this advice, and I continued to drink milk as I breastfed my baby. I also ate a lot of frozen yogurt.

When my son was old enough to eat solids, I gave him some yogurt, and he immediately became hoarse. He had developed a sensitivity to dairy foods, having been exposed to them so much in utero. That's when I started to learn more about clinical ecology, which is now called environmental medicine, which suggests that any symptom might be a result of a sensitivity or intolerance to a food, chemical, or something else in the environment.

I took my son off all dairy foods for two years, and now he can eat them without any difficulty.

—*Cathie Lippman, MD, a mom of 30- and 28-year-old sons and a physician who specializes in environmental and preventive medicine at the Lippman Center for Optimal Health, in Beverly Hills, CA*

❧

The biggest challenge I had during my son's first year was his nonstop crying spells. He had gotten multiple diagnoses, from colic to gastroesophageal reflux to possible food allergies.

I was breastfeeding, so changing my son's "formula" was not an option. After trying multiple medications for colic and reflux, I finally decided to take a more drastic approach. I put myself on an elimination diet, avoiding all of the common allergens—dairy, nuts, corn, wheat, soy, and shellfish.

Once these foods were eliminated from my diet, all of my son's crying stopped. Over the course of a few weeks, I slowly added back each of the eliminated foods. My son's crying returned when I added wheat and dairy products. I completely removed these two items from my diet for the remainder of my time nursing. Breastfeeding was much easier with a calm baby whose tummy was not gassy. I definitely missed eating wheat and dairy foods, but I found some great alternative products at the supermarket. My son outgrew his wheat allergy within a year, but the dairy allergy lasted until he was five. During the time of my son's allergies, he would get a rash within 30 minutes of eating anything with dairy in it. I would treat his symptoms with liquid diphenhydramine (Children's Benadryl), at an age- and weight-appropriate dosage.

—*Saundra Dalton-Smith, MD, a mom of six- and four-year-old sons, an internal medicine specialist, and the author of* Set Free to Live Free: Breaking Through the 7 Lies Women Tell Themselves, *in Anniston, AL*

Stressing Less

We must confess, stress makes us a mess. That's why we deal with it as best we can!

∽

I find that taking deep breaths and spending a few minutes alone can do wonders for stress.

—*Rachel S. Rohde, MD, a mom of a five-month-old daughter, an assistant professor of orthopaedic surgery at the Oakland University William Beaumont School of Medicine, and an orthopaedic upper-extremity surgeon with Michigan Orthopaedic Institute, P.C., in Southfield, MI*

To reduce my stress about my kids, I tried very hard not to compare them to other peoples' kids—or even to their own siblings. Every child is beautiful in his or her own way. Each child is a unique flower, and like all flowers, they bloom at various times and have different attributes.

—*Hana R. Solomon, MD*

? When to Call Your Doctor

If you feel intensely anxious, or if anxiety or stress is interfering with your day-to-day life, contact your doctor or midwife.

When I feel myself getting anxious or angry, I try to remember my girls' smiles. This calms me down and helps me to be more patient. When you're feeling anxious or guilty, you transmit that to your kids. But if you are able to keep calm, it's amazing how your kids' attitudes will change, and how much better they'll cooperate.

—*Gabriella Cardone, MD, a mom of five-, three-, and one-year-old daughters and a pediatric emergency physician at Texas Children's Hospital, in Houston*

My husband and I faced *a lot* of challenges during the first year of our three children's lives. Our oldest child had to be our guinea pig, because she was the first. I was so much more relaxed when our boys came, and especially with our youngest. By the time he came along, I could nurse him, prepare dinner, and help the older children with their homework all at the same time! It does get easier!

—*Stacey Weiland, MD, a mom of a 12-year-old daughter and 7- and 5-year-old sons and an internist/gastroenterologist, in Denver, CO*

When my first child was born, I expected myself to do everything "just right"—as if there is such a thing. But with my little one, I cut myself a lot more slack. I think that it's actually better for the kids to see us being more flexible.

A lot of rigidity that new parents have comes from anxiety.

When people are anxious, they cling to books, rules, and schedules. Kids really pick up on our anxiety. While consistency is important for kids, rigidity is not helpful. I believe there needs to be some flexibility.

—*Michelle Paley, MD, PA*

I'm a very organized person, and keeping things in order makes life feel less stressful for me. Other people might find that taking the time to organize things is *more* stressful. You have to find what works for you.

Also keep in mind that the parenting tip that worked wonders for your friend might not work for you. Don't stress out just because you need to do something differently than someone else does.

—*Heather Orman-Lubell, MD*

Looking back now, I see how important it is that first year to give yourself a break. We moms want to do everything perfectly, and we can pile on the guilt if we don't feel like we measure up. Did I wear her in a sling enough? Did I make organic homemade baby food? Did I let her cry too long? We spend so much time beating ourselves up, and usually that guilt and worry make us less effective as parents.

I'm glad I let certain things go, such as not making my own baby food and cooking from scratch every night. My husband and I got takeout a couple times a week that year; now it might be a few times a month. It gets easier as they get older. The kinder we are with ourselves, I think the better we are as parents.

—*Katja Rowell, MD*

Relaxing is tough for me. I'm a type A person, and I'm not happy unless I'm burning the candle on five different ends.

Even though my husband worked as hard in his career as I did when our kids were babies, he pitched in around the house all of the time. He's an attorney, and he worked a lot from home. I couldn't see patients at our house, after all! He shuttled the babies around and stayed home with them when they were sick.

—*Susan Besser, MD*

Try Yoga

Yoga is a perfect MomMy Time activity. (Okay, an extra hour of sleep on Saturday still is the absolute best!) Yoga originated in India more than 5,000 years ago, and it is now one of the fastest-growing health practices. More than 30 million people practice yoga on a daily basis.

Many of our Mommy MD Guides say that yoga is a great way to tone your body, build strength, and gain flexibility after having a baby. Certainly, the basis of modern yoga—proper relaxation, proper exercise, proper breathing, proper diet, positive thinking, and meditation—is ideal for new moms during baby's first year.

Pregnancy is a major nine-month transformation, and the postpartum period also is accompanied by a number of physical changes. Getting your body back into shape after pregnancy takes time. If you didn't work out regularly during your pregnancy, you'll want to ease into an exercise routine. And even if you were exercising regularly, the initial demands of feeding and caring for your baby around the clock don't leave much time for trips to the gym.

As long as your doctor or midwife says it's okay for you to exercise, your baby's first year is a wonderful time to start yoga as you adjust to the physical and emotional changes going on in your life. In fact, many yoga stretches can even be done while holding or nursing your baby. Some stretches help ease the back and shoulder strain that results from carrying your little one.

One much-practiced pose for new moms is the downward-facing dog pose. Start on the floor on your hands and knees. With your hands shoulder-width apart, spread out your fingers, distributing your weight evenly through your hands. Spread your feet hip-width apart, tuck your toes under and forward, and arch your hips towards the ceiling. Keep your back, shoulders, and head aligned while extending your hips back. This energizing position stretches the spine, the legs, and the entire body.

For all moms, yoga can be just what your body—and soul—need.

RALLIE'S TIP

Here's some good advice for new moms who feel anxious or overwhelmed from time to time: When your mind drifts, it's hard to remember what was going on or what you were thinking about before you stopped paying attention. If there's something you don't feel like thinking or worrying about, it might be helpful to recall a pleasant memory, such as your honeymoon trip or your wedding day.

Scientists demonstrated that the content of your daydreams affects your ability to access a recently acquired memory. They found that if you want to put something stressful or unpleasant out of your mind, you're better off remembering a more distant event than a close event, because it can help you feel like you're in a different situation. So if you're feeling stressed, you might want to let your mind drift to a happy memory.

Saving for College

Brace yourself: College costs increase about *twice* as fast as the inflation rate. To better plan for your baby's college tuition, Google "college cost calculators." For example, the website SavingForCollege.com has the "world's simplest college calculator." All you enter is your baby's age. For a newborn, the site predicts that total college costs will be $312,166. It calculates that a parent would need to make monthly contributions of $602 to meet this cost.

~

I regret not starting college savings plans for my children. In Florida, we have a great pre-paid tuition program. My husband said, "I can make more in the stock market!" so he didn't want to sign up. But in hindsight, I wish we had participated in the tuition program. If your state doesn't have one of these, consider investing in a 529 plan. It's a good idea to start saving for college right from the beginning so you're not faced with an enormous bill when your "babies" go to college.

—*Melanie Bone, MD*

~

My husband is definitely the money expert in our family. We met with our financial planner before our daughter was born to set up her 529 fund for college and to figure out how much we need to contribute each year. Plus, we've got her little piggy bank for collecting spare change too!

—*Jennifer Bacani McKenney, MD, a mom of a two-month-old daughter and a family physician, in Fredonia, KS*

We have a piggy bank for our daughter, and when she receives money as a gift, we tell her that it's for college, and we put it in the bank. Once the piggy bank is full, we put the money into her account at the bank. I think it's important to start this process at a very young age so kids get into the habit of saving money.

—*Christy Valentine, MD*

RALLIE'S TIP

My husband's parents have a wonderful tradition of buying all of their grandchildren U.S. savings bonds for their birthdays and Christmas gifts. We've kept all of those savings bonds in a safe place over the years, and by the time my boys are ready for college, they'll have enough to pay for their first year of tuition. My husband and I also started a college savings account for each of our children when they were born, and we make regular deposits into those accounts. We might not have enough saved to fund an entire college education for each child by the time he graduates from high school, but we'll be able to get our sons off to a good start. And we won't be the least disappointed if our children earn scholarships or get involved in work-study programs to help finance their college educations.

Making Time for Yourself

You! Remember you? The you before you were Mom? Be kind to yourself—make time for yourself.

My babies' first years, I did a lot of walking. I also enjoyed catching up on reading while I was breastfeeding.

—*Bola Oyeyipo, MD, a mom of three-year-old and six-month-old sons, a family physician in private practice, and the owner of SlimyBookWorm.com, in Highland, CA*

When my kids were babies, it was really important for me to get a run in as often as possible. As soon as my kids were old enough, at six months, I'd get up early in the morning, put them into the baby jogger, and go for a run.

—*Nancy Rappaport, MD, a mom of 21- and 16-year-old daughters and an 18-year-old son, an assistant professor of psychiatry at Harvard Medical School, an attending child and adolescent psychiatrist in the Cambridge, MA, public schools, and the author of* In Her Wake: A Child Psychiatrist Explores the Mystery of Her Mother's Suicide

∽

I don't feel bad about leaving my sons with a babysitter once a week while I'm not at work. That way I have time to read a book or do something for myself.

—*Carrie Brown, MD*

∽

I know women who never leave their babies with other family members or sitters. I try to reassure them that having a little time to yourself is not a bad thing. It makes you a more relaxed mother.

—*Marra S. Francis, MD*

∽

I think many new moms feel the need to give their whole lives to their babies. This seems to be especially true for older moms who put off childbearing for a career. They can lose all sense of themselves and make their children their next career. I think you need to block out time for you.

I wasn't very good at this when my kids were babies, but when I was diagnosed with breast cancer, I sure learned it in a hurry. While I was undergoing treatments, I was too tired to spend long hours with my children, but they don't remember it now. You are not helping your children by holding on to them and not letting them have their own alone time.

—*Melanie Bone, MD*

∽

I never understood why people said that they were so busy with a newborn that they couldn't take a shower—until I had a newborn.

However, I always made time to eat and to take a shower, even if it meant putting my daughter in her bouncy seat and taking her into the kitchen or bathroom with me.

I also make sure to have my "alone time" to decompress after our daughter goes to bed.

—*Rachel S. Rohde, MD*

My husband and I are very good at reading each other and knowing when we need a break. He'll say, "Why don't you go to the gym? I'll watch the baby." Or he'll encourage me to meet a friend for lunch, and I do the same for him. We try to do as many things together as a family as we can, but we know that we need time away too. It's important to give your partner that time to recharge.

—*Jeannette Gonzalez Simon, MD*

My mom offered me some great advice when I had my first baby: Get out of the house every day, even if it's just to walk down the street. Getting "out" forced me to get out of my pajamas, brush my teeth, take a shower, and put some clothes on. It helped me to feel like myself!

I have also been fortunate enough to have great nannies and babysitters, so I was able to schedule time for myself to do errands alone. Going to the grocery store without kids can really be a treat!

—*Lezli Braswell, MD*

One way that I make time for myself is by scrapbooking. It's something that I really enjoy, and because I have something to show for it at the end, I don't feel too guilty about spending time doing it.

It can be hard to find the time to scrapbook. When my babies were young, the only way I could find time was to actually go somewhere, such as to a friend's house. (One of my friends happens to have a Creative Memories business!) I'd spend a few hours there and get a whole bunch of scrapbooking done at once. Some people are good at working with a few minutes here and there, but I really need to set aside a big chunk of time to focus on one project.

—*Rebecca Reamy, MD*

RALLIE'S TIP

Playtime shouldn't just be for babies. New moms still need to have fun to reduce stress levels and to maintain their physical and emotional health. The first step is for moms to define what counts as "play," because it's different for everyone. It might be enjoying a game of tennis or losing yourself in a brand-new video game.

When my babies were little, my personal playtime involved reading a few chapters of a good book or going for a run—sans jogging stroller. Once the baby is born, playing becomes less spontaneous, so moms need to plan for it.

෧෧

Make sure to make time for yourself. You can't live 24/7 for your kids. That's not good for anyone. You have to get past the guilt of taking time away. If mom's happy, everyone's happy.

I'm a runner, and I tell my husband that running is a lot cheaper than therapy. My family knows that I need to run to stay sane. They've been known to say, "Mom's cranky; she needs to go run."

—*Heather Orman-Lubell, MD*

෧෧

I wish that I could say I did a good job taking care of myself when my babies were small, but I didn't learn how to do that well until I was almost 50. The advice I have given to all young mothers since then is to never use baby's naptime as a chance to fold laundry, pay bills, exercise, bake dinner, volunteer somewhere, or run errands. Sit still or lie down and drink a cup of tea or read or take a bath or nap. Doing nothing is difficult for a lot of high-powered "do-ers," but it's important because it might prevent a physical or emotional disaster down the road. Self-care is not self-ish. It is essential for all women if they are to be the mothers, wives, friends, and citizens that they want to be.

—*Lesley Burton-Iwinski, MD, a mom of 20- and 18-year-old daughters and a 14-year-old son, a retired family physician, and a parent and teacher educator with Growing Peaceful Families, in Lexington, KY*

I used to feel bad taking time for myself, but now I realize it's an important part of maintaining a healthy family environment. As they say, "If mama's not happy, no one's happy."

To recharge my batteries, I spend time each day doing something I love to do. I enjoy writing, so in the evenings after I put my sons to bed, I make time to write. Writing is an outlet for me to express myself; it helps me work through thoughts and emotions. I've actually written so much that I submitted some of my writing to a literary agent and got a book contract for *Set Free to Live Free: Breaking Through the 7 Lies Women Tell Themselves*.

I think it's great for mothers to preserve a creative outlet during the early parenting years. It's very easy to forget your own needs as you spend so much time focusing on the needs of your child. Whether it's music, painting, poetry, writing, reading, or any number of creative options, having a way to express your individuality helps to remind you of your own needs and the importance of self-care.

—*Saundra Dalton-Smith, MD*

Prepare for parenthood by ensuring that you have a strong network of female friends and extended family members to help with the stress of child care and general emotional support. Couples who embark on parenthood with inadequate external support are at high risk for emotional difficulties.

My labor coach (another woman) continued to be closely involved with helping me with child care. She and one other friend made sure that I got out to play tennis regularly. I was also involved in a feminist book group and a folk dance club, and I traded child care with a friend who delivered her baby three days after I did.

—*Stuart Jeanne Bramhall, MD, a mom of a 30-year-old daughter and a child and adolescent psychiatrist, in New Plymouth, New Zealand*

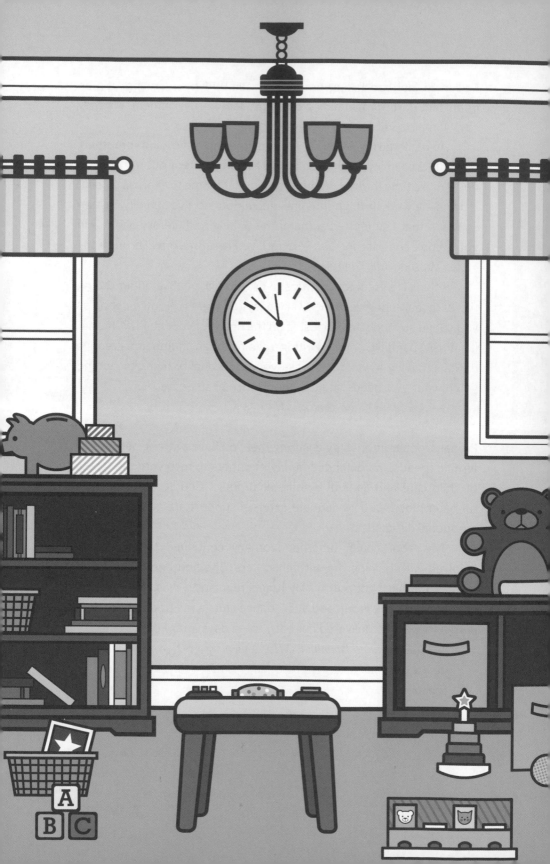

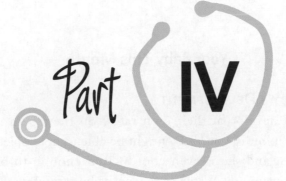

Part IV

THE FOURTH QUARTER

Chapter 10
10th Month

Your Baby This Month

YOUR BABY'S DEVELOPMENT

All babies develop at their own rates, on their own time. By around 10 months, your baby might be able to hold objects in her tiny hands, and she is even coordinated enough to bring her hands to her mouth. Watch as she learns how to blow you a kiss! Besides being a sign of physical development, this shows a healthy emotional development because she's showing she likes to give affection.

Around this age, many babies become attached to a comfort item, such as a stuffed animal or soft blanket. If you can, buy two, or three, of them! That will prevent you from an exhaustive eBay search if the cherished item is ever lost. The cuddliness of the lovey reminds your baby of the comfort she gets from you. Plus the familiar smell and feel are reassuring.

At 10 months old, creeping and crawling might give way to cruising around the furniture. Your baby might be able to stand alone for a few moments, holding onto something.

Who's that? A really fun development around this time is that your baby probably recognizes herself in a mirror now and smiles. Babies love to look at themselves in mirrors.

It's around this age that babies start to be able to indicate what they want in other ways than by crying. What a tremendous relief! A wonderful stage begins around now where babies speak gibberish that sounds like babies are talking in their own made-up language.

Your baby might be able to say "DaDa" and "MaMa." She might be able to say "DaDa" discriminately, on purpose. She might be able to wave bye-bye.

TAKING CARE OF YOU

Think of something that someone can help you with—and ask for it. Take a cue from your baby! When a baby needs something, she cries. Moms don't have to turn on the tears, but they shouldn't be shy about asking for help when they need it. Some moms wear their independence like a badge, but there are no prizes for maternal martyrdom!

If you need help, ask someone—your partner, your mother, your sister, your friend, or your neighbor. Most people are willing, happy even, to pitch in, especially when you're very specific about the type of help you need.

JUSTIFICATION FOR A CELEBRATION

Your baby is starting to learn to play more interactively! Why not celebrate with a game of patty-cake?

Corralling Your Baby's Toys

If the toy invasion hasn't begun, brace yourself. It starts inno-cently enough, probably with some cute, furry, soft stuffed ani-mals. Then come the large wooden toys. Then the noisy toys. Just when you think you might be able to contain the madness to one small playroom, your baby will be a toddler and past the choking danger. Just blink, and your house will be overrun by millions of teeny tiny Lego-sized toys. Don't say we didn't warn you.

∽

It's very hard to keep toys neat. It's a constant battle, and it makes us want a magic wand! When faced with a choice between toys with mul-tiple small pieces and toys with larger, fewer pieces, we get the latter.

—*Amy Thompson, MD, a mom of four- and two-year-old and nine-month-old sons and an ob-gyn at the University of Cincinnati College of Medicine, in Ohio*

Mommy MD Guides-Recommended Product
Tot Tutors Toy Organizer

One of the many challenges of organizing kids' toys is creating a system that's effective enough for Mom, and easy enough for Baby. For bonus points, you probably want to find something that looks nice in your home.

The Tot Tutors Toy Organizer is a wonderful compromise. It's a four-tier wooden frame with a natural finish with dowels that sup-port the toy bins. The bins themselves are plastic, so they are both durable and easy to clean. The bins come in two color palettes: pri-mary colors and pastels. The units measure 34 inches wide, by 11 inches deep, by 31 inches high. *Note:* The manufacturer says it's for kids ages three and up, so don't let your baby play with it unattended.

The toy organizers cost around $60 online and require some assembly.

I have baskets in our living room to keep all of our kids' toys in. But every morning, my son dumps all of his toys into a heap. We have a rule that before nap and before going to bed, we sing a song and pick up all the toys. Even from a young age, my son has been very compliant—though sometimes he gets distracted and starts playing with the toys instead of picking them up.

> —*Michelle Hephner, DO, a mom of a two-year-old son and*
> *eight-month-old daughter and a family physician in private practice*
> *with Central DuPage Physician Group, in Winfield, IL*

One reason I put my younger son in day care is because he emulates others. I thought he would learn to put away his toys and sit in circles. He doesn't rip books at school, and he doesn't throw food there either. He saves all that for home.

We use an octagonal baby gate to corral all his toys. We have one in our living room. We also have a coffee table with huge hidden drawers. In the guest room, my son has a bunch of plastic boxes from Bed, Bath, and Beyond that we use to store his Thomas trains and tracks.

> —*Sonia Ng, MD, a mom of seven- and two-year-old sons, a*
> *pediatrician, and a sedation attending physician at the Children's*
> *Hospital of Philadelphia Pediatric Care and the University*
> *Medical Center at Princeton in Princeton, NJ, and the Pediatric*
> *Imaging Center in King of Prussia, PA*

RALLIE'S TIP

I wanted my babies to have access to their toys, and that meant keeping them on the living room floor where my boys could see them and reach them. I didn't mind having toys scattered around the living room floor during the day while the boys were awake, but I did like putting them up after their bedtime so it wouldn't seem like my house was always a total disaster. I kept a few wicker laundry baskets in the living room, and after putting the babies to bed, I'd just scoop up all the toys and toss them in the baskets.

When the floor was free and clear of toys, it gave me the feeling that my house had some semblance of order, and I could sit down on the couch and relax with my husband.

My husband and I keep most of our babies' toys in our family room. I bought interlocking foam floor mats online. I put them on one side of the room, and I designated that area the "toy area." I put our Pack 'n Play over there, and we store most of the toys inside of that. It works well because it keeps the toys contained, yet our kids can get their own toys out. In theory, they could put their toys away too, but at the end of the day, I just throw all of the toys back into the Pack 'n Play.

—*Jennifer Gilbert, DO, a mom of 18-month-old twins and an ob-gyn at Paoli Hospital, in Pennsylvania*

Changing Doctors

Before your baby was born, you probably took a lot of time and care in choosing your baby's doctor. With a little bit of luck, this very important relationship has been going well. Both you and your baby enjoy going to the doctor, and you feel that your questions are answered and your needs are met.

Unfortunately, this isn't always the case. You might find yourself resuming your doctor search long before you imagined—or hoped. This can happen even if you love your baby's physician. Doctors retire, and sometimes they move away.

On the other hand, sometimes things don't turn out the way you thought they would. Maybe it's not worth a 40-minute drive in the snow to see one particular pediatrician. Or maybe you discover a family practice is too small, or too large. It's time to find another doctor. One who's just right.

&

I jokingly say that pediatricians are really practicing veterinary medicine in the first year of a baby's life. The baby can't talk or say what's wrong, so the pediatrician has to be a detective, much like a vet.

I put a lot of thought and care into picking my baby's pediatrician, choosing a physician in a small, boutique practice because I wanted to know the doctor well. I didn't think of the need for after-hours care and weekend help. In a small group, you're stuck because the pediatrician is unavailable, so you have to take your baby to the emergency room. After that happened to me, I changed to a big group practice that had office hours seven days a week and in the evenings.

—Melanie Bone, MD, a mom of four, ages 16, 15, 14, and 13, a grandmom of one grandson, a gynecologist, the founder of the Cancer Sensibility Foundation, and the author of the syndicated column Surviving Life *and the book* Cancer, What's Next?, *in West Palm Beach, FL*

We had one scary time during my son's first year, which was a lesson in how to interact with your baby's doctor. My son had a cold and a fever. We took him to the doctor, who diagnosed an upper respiratory infection and prescribed "Tylenol and lots of steam."

Despite running our humidifier near constantly, my son's cough got worse and worse. We took him back to the doctor and asked for an antibiotic. The doctor lectured us on antibiotics resistance and refused to prescribe an antibiotic. I didn't want to "play doctor," and I let the pediatrician manage my son's care. For the next two months, my son continued to cough.

One night, my baby turned blue in front of my eyes. "That's it!" I said, and I took matters into my own hands. I gave him a dose of antibiotic, and within just two hours, he was able to breathe better and started improving. The next day, I insisted the doctor give my son a chest X-ray, and it turns out he had pneumonia. And the doctor had been treating him with Tylenol and steam!

As soon as my son started to take the now-finally-prescribed antibiotic, he started to get better. I changed pediatricians right away after that. Also I realized that as a doctor mom, you can't be polite when you don't agree with your child's pediatrician. You've got to stand up for your opinion and speak up to protect your child.

—Judith Hellman, MD, a mom of a 13-year-old son, an associate clinical professor of dermatology at Mt. Sinai Hospital, and a dermatologist in private practice, in New York City

Making New Family Traditions

With our 140-character Twitter attention spans, it can be hard to find the time to make—let alone to savor—family traditions. But traditions are what hold families together. They're often what we remember from our own childhoods. Traditions don't have to be complicated or take a long time. Children enjoy and remember the simple things in life: a prayer before a meal, a secret gesture that means "I love you," a lullaby before bed, a gentle kiss good night.

∽◌∾

During our twins' first year, my husband and I started a holiday tradition of getting everyone a new pair of pajamas on Christmas Eve. Everyone has those new pj's on when they open up their stockings on Christmas Day.

> —Penny Noyce, MD, a mom of 23- and 21-year-old daughters,
> two 21-year-old sons, and a 13-year-old son, the author of
> the preteen novel Lost in Lexicon, and an internal medicine
> specialist, in Weston, MA

∽◌∾

Each night before bedtime, my two older daughters give a blessing to their baby sister before she goes to sleep. They all look forward to that special time each night.

First we pray for our family and our loved ones, then for people who don't have anything, then for people who don't know God, and then for everyone, and last my youngest says, "Amen." As I take the youngest to bed, my three- and five-year-olds pray a Hail Mary and the prayer to the Guardian Angel.

> —*Gabriella Cardone, MD, a mom of five-, three-, and one-year-old daughters and a pediatric emergency physician at Texas Children's Hospital, in Houston*

∽

One wonderful ritual my family enjoyed during my babies' first years was going to the local farmers' market each Saturday morning. We were living in Germany, and as in most European countries, the farmers' markets there are stunning and filled with yummy fresh foods. Those farmers' market visits were the highlight of our weekends. I can remember to this day that they had the best pommes frites ever.

> —*Ann Kulze, MD, a mom of 22- and 15-year-old daughters and 20- and 19-year-old sons; a nationally recognized nutrition expert, motivational speaker, and family physician; and the author of the best-selling book* Eat Right for Life, *in Charleston, SC*

RALLIE'S TIP

The older I get, the more I cherish our family traditions. Some of my favorites are camping out in the living room with tents and sleeping bags and watching movies on Friday nights, hiding and finding eggs on Easter, and making waffles on Saturday mornings.

The great thing about family traditions is that they don't have to be expensive or elaborate. It's usually the simple things that mean the most, and the memories they create will bring a lifetime of joy to parents and children.

⤨

Even more than big holidays and celebrations, I find that quiet rituals are important for our family. Each year, we took a camping trip to a really special place called Pine Valley in Los Padres National Park. We'd stay there for three or four days and visit a Zen monastery with hot tubs and a waterfall. It has a lot of special meaning for us.

Even less grand than that, rituals like reading together each night before bed or singing my baby a song I grew up singing were special as well. I used to sing "Seven Golden Daffodils" to my baby. I'm not that good of a singer, and I made up most of the words, but it wasn't until my kids were five or six that they realized I wasn't the next Barbra Streisand.

Doing simple things like taking your child to a café for tea or for a stroll around the block might not be momentous, but moments like that imbue strength in the relationship. Small intimacies like that are very important.

—Nancy Rappaport, MD, a mom of 21- and 16-year-old daughters and an 18-year-old son, an assistant professor of psychiatry at Harvard Medical School, an attending child and adolescent psychiatrist in the Cambridge, MA, public schools, and the author of In Her Wake: A Child Psychiatrist Explores the Mystery of Her Mother's Suicide

Teaching Your Baby Sign Language

Back in the 19th century, a linguist named William Dwight Whitney made an interesting observation: Babies of deaf parents were able to communicate earlier than children of hearing parents. In fact, Whitney observed that children of deaf parents were surprisingly on a similar speaking development path as children of hearing parents.

This curiosity was largely ignored until the 1970s, when an ASL (American Sign Language) interpreter named Joseph Garcia noticed that the children of his deaf friends were using sign language as early as six months to communicate with their parents. Dr. Garcia also found that these children had substantial vocabularies at nine months old, which is several months sooner than most children. In 1987, Dr. Garcia began to research using sign language to teach the children of hearing parents to communicate.

Several interesting studies have been published on teaching babies to sign. One small study published in the *Journal of Nonverbal Behavior* found that baby signers had an advantage on learning to talk over babies who did not sign. Another small study showed that babies who had been encouraged to use sign language when they were two years old scored 12 points higher on IQ tests during their summers after second grade than second graders who hadn't used sign language as babies.

Today you'll find a plethora of websites, books, and DVDs on teaching your baby to sign. Or you could simply come up with simple signs of your own—your own secret language to share with your baby. How will you sign, *I love you*?

❧

My kids were born before teaching kids to sign was in vogue. However, I always have been careful to listen to my kids' nonverbal signals. It's important to begin doing this when they are newborn babies and to continue it all the way through adulthood. Parents can often read the nonverbal cues way before their children verbalize their emotions or needs.

—*Hana R. Solomon, MD, a mom of four, ages 35 to 19, a board-certified pediatrician, and the author of* Clearing the Air One Nose at a Time: Caring for Your Personal Filter, *in Columbia, MO*

❧

I did try to teach sign language to my son because he was having difficulty talking. I taught him how to sign simple words, such as grapes, bread, and cheese. Ironically, when I took him to a speech therapist, she recommended *not* teaching him to sign, because it would hinder his efforts to overcome his condition of verbal apraxia and make it more difficult for him to learn to talk. She believed he needed to focus on communicating verbally.

—*Lesley Burton-Iwinski, MD, a mom of 20- and 18-year-old daughters and a 14-year-old son, a retired family physician, and a parent and teacher educator with Growing Peaceful Families, in Lexington, KY*

Teaching your baby sign language was beginning to be popular when my kids were babies, but I didn't teach mine. Could we be rushing our kids to learn too much, too soon for their own good? Studies show that American children are not smarter even with all the intervention. I support playing and regular interaction with both children and adults. They will learn without any specialized teaching.

—*Melanie Bone, MD*

Preventing and Treating Croup and Whooping Cough

Both croup and whooping cough seem like conditions of a bygone time, something that your grandmother might have treated with a little honey and a lot of love—and worried about till her hair turned gray. Sadly, both of these conditions are still with us, although croup is generally much less serious than whooping cough.

Croup is usually caused by a virus. It causes an inflammation in the voice box (larynx) and windpipe (trachea). This inflammation causes a barking cough or hoarseness, especially when a baby cries.

Because children have small airways, croup is most common—and most severe—in children who are six months to five years old. But croup can affect younger babies and older children too. Croup is most common between Halloween and St. Patrick's Day, but it can occur anytime.

Croup usually starts with cold symptoms, such as a runny nose, nasal congestion, and a fever. Then the voice becomes hoarse, and the child develops a harsh, barking cough that sounds like a seal. Like so many scary things in life, symptoms of croup are often worse at night and when a child is upset. Croup usually lasts from three days to a week.

Some children are prone to croup, and they get it again and again. Most of the time, croup can be treated at home and is mild, with no lasting effects. Occasionally, however, croup can cause constriction of a child's airways, making breathing difficult. When this happens, getting immediate medical attention is critical.

Whooping cough is a respiratory infection that's also called pertussis. In China, it's called the 100-day cough—for good reason, because it lasts a *long* time.

Before a vaccine was available, whooping cough killed 5,000 to 10,000 people in the United States each year. The vaccine reduced that to fewer than 30 deaths a year in the 1970s. But in recent years, those numbers have climbed.

By 2004, the number of whooping cough cases in the United States topped 25,000. It mainly affects infants younger than six months old because they aren't fully protected from whooping cough until they've received at least three vaccines, typically at two, four, and six months old. Whooping cough also often affects teens and adults, whose immunity to the bacteria has faded.

Whooping cough is aptly named: It causes severe, hacking coughing spells that end in a high-pitched whooping sound when the person inhales. A child with whooping cough might cough so hard that she throws up. Initially, whooping cough starts like a cold with a runny nose, nasal congestion, sneezing, watery eyes, dry cough, and a mild fever. After a week or two, the nasal symptoms go away, and the nature of the cough changes to severe, hacking spells. A baby might not develop the classic whoop sound, but instead have a persistent hacking cough and a red face, and look like she's gasping for air. She might even stop breathing for a few seconds.

Generally, a person with whooping cough will have this

severe type of cough for two to four weeks, or even longer. Some children take months to get well. Babies are at high risk for complications of whooping cough, which include ear infections,

? When to Call Your Doctor

If you think that your baby might have been exposed to whooping cough, call your doctor right away or take your baby to the closest emergency department, even if your baby has been vaccinated. Antibiotics don't cure whooping cough, but they can help to prevent the spread of the disease if given in time.

Immediately call your doctor if your baby has any of the following signs or symptoms.

- Croup that has lasted for more than a week or that recurs frequently
- Difficulty breathing, including rapid or labored breathing
- Stridor: a high-pitched squeaking noise when inhaling
- Retractions: the skin between the ribs pulls in when she breathes
- A pale or bluish color around the mouth
- Signs of dehydration, including dry mouth, crying with few or no tears, fewer than four wet diapers per day, going four to six hours without urinating, or if the soft spot on your baby's head looks sunken or flatter than usual
- Drooling
- Difficulty swallowing
- Coughing spells that cause her to vomit, make her turn red or purple, or are accompanied by a whooping sound
- Fever (any fever in a baby younger than three months old or a fever of 101°F or higher in a baby three months old or older)
- Seems agitated or especially irritable
- A very fatigued or sick appearance

pneumonia, slowed or stopped breathing, dehydration, and even brain damage.

Whooping cough is *extremely* contagious. Experts think that up to 80 percent of nonimmunized family members will develop whooping cough if they live in the same home as someone who has it.

If you hear someone with a dry, hacking, violent cough, get your baby far, far away.

❧

We didn't have to worry about whooping cough because my kids got the vaccine for that disease.

But when my oldest was a baby, I was living on a commune called the Farm. One night, my son developed a horrible, croupy cough. It was scary. We were living in a trailer in the woods, and my son was barking and coughing and couldn't catch his breath.

I bundled my son all up to take him to the emergency room, but when we got out into the night air, his cough got better. Now I know that two common treatments for croup are turning on hot water in the shower to steam up the bathroom and then bringing the baby into the steamy room, and taking the baby out into cold night air. These two remedies seem so opposite, but the cold air shrinks the swelling, and the warm air moisturizes the membranes. Maybe it's all BS, and only a change in scenery is the key!

—*Hana R. Solomon, MD*

RALLIE'S TIP

My youngest son had croup several times when he was a baby. Running a humidifier with a few drops of eucalyptus oil in the water helped. If the coughing woke him up at night, I'd turn on the hot water in the shower and let it steam up the bathroom. We'd sit in the bathroom and read books and breathe steam. In the winter, we'd bundle up and go outside and breathe the cold air for a few minutes, and sometimes that seemed to help more than breathing the steamy air. Fortunately, my son's croup never got so bad that it interfered with his breathing, but I was fully prepared to rush him to the hospital if it did.

My second child developed croup when he was around three months old. It was New Year's night, and I knew what to do to help him breathe: Get him out in the night air or into a steamy shower.

But my son started to turn a dusky blue color. I don't want to be my kids' doctor, so I phoned the pediatrician on call. He didn't want to get out of his warm bed, and he told me to put my son in a steamy bathroom and "He'll be fine." Wanting to be a "good" patient, I stayed up with my baby all night, making sure he was breathing. It was a very scary night. At 10 the next morning, I was standing with my croupy, hazy blue baby on the clinic's doorstep waiting for it to open. The doctor took one look at my son from across the waiting room desk, and they sent us by ambulance to the emergency room, and my son spent several days in the hospital. It was a really bad case of croup, but thank goodness he recovered just fine.

—*Susan Besser, MD, a mom of six grown children, ages 26, 24, 22, 21, 19, and 17, a grandmom of one, a family physician, and the medical director of Doctors Express-Memphis, in Tennessee*

Solving New Sleep Challenges

Ah, remember sleep? Some babies really *do* sleep well early on. We're sure they will trouble their parents later on with plenty of other things. But for most babies, sleep doesn't come easy, and the sleep challenges evolve over time. Just when you have one sleep scenario licked, your baby comes up with a new trick. Babies don't have hobbies, after all!

❧

From birth, my sons weren't good sleepers. We had a lot of nights that we simply didn't sleep. As my sons got older, they napped less during the day, and they did start to sleep better at night. By the time they were toddlers, they were sleeping well. Now as a teen and pre-teen, they're great sleepers. That's probably not too comforting for new moms though.

—*Jill Wireman, MD, a mom of 14- and 11-year-old sons and a pediatrician in private practice at Johnson City Pediatrics, in Tennessee*

My daughter had started sleeping through the night when she was 10 weeks old. But when she was three months old, I took her on a 2,000-mile plane trip to my father's funeral. After that, she began waking up two or three times each night, demanding to be fed.

I had a very supportive pediatrician who reassured me this was the oldest con in the world. He had me start some rice cereal in addition to breast milk, and he told me to just let her cry if she woke up. This happened only one time, and after that she began sleeping through the night again.

—*Stuart Jeanne Bramhall, MD, a mom of a 30-year-old daughter and a child and adolescent psychiatrist, in New Plymouth, New Zealand*

Mommy MD Guides–Recommended Product
Comfort Silkie

"We had sleep trained each of our babies when they were between three and five months old," says Katherine Dee, MD, a mom of six-year-old twin daughters and a four-year-old son and a radiologist at the Seattle Breast Center, in Washington. "When the twins were around seven months, we took them on their first trip. I was concerned that the big change of sleeping somewhere other than their cribs would throw their sleep off. So before we left, I got them each a Silkie for their crib, and we took it along. I thought it would help them to sleep if they had something with them that they identified from their cribs.

"Interestingly, my one daughter glommed on to that Silkie as her lovey. But her sister didn't. While we were on that trip, a friend gave them each small stuffed kitties. My other daughter totally took to that kitty and made it her lovey. Actually, she took both hers and her sister's!"

You can buy Comfort Silkies at **COMFORTSILKIE.COM** for around $17.

When my daughter was around nine months old, she discovered the neat trick of throwing her "lovey" out of her crib, or pushing it between the bars. Then she would cry until someone retrieved it for her—several times a night! As soon as she got her lovey back, she would fall asleep again.

We put a stop to that quickly! I put a crib net over her crib, which a mom at the park recommended because she had cats. My baby didn't mind it, and she could throw her lovey all she wanted, and it bounced back at her. She could comfort herself and fall back to sleep.

—*Katja Rowell, MD, a mom of a five-year-old daughter, a family physician, and a childhood feeding specialist with FamilyFeedingDynamics.com, in St. Paul, MN*

Talking!

Your baby might have more in common with a cowbird than you think. Researchers have discovered that babies learn to talk much in the same way that cowbirds learn to sing.

Once upon a time, researchers thought that babies learned to talk by imitating. Mom says, "Mama," baby says, "Mama." Not so, says new research. It seems that as babies make certain sounds and they receive positive feedback from their parents—a gentle hug from Mom, a pat on the back from Dad—babies learn that *those* sounds were well received, and that encouragement edges them further along in the development of language.

But what does this have to do with a cowbird? Only male cowbirds learn to sing, but they are taught to sing by females, who never sing at all. While the adult male cowbirds are off doing cowbird things, the females teach the baby male cowbirds how to sing by observing their singing and encouraging them when they do it right.

Encouragement: It's not just for the birds.

❧

It was very important to me that our sons be trilingual. I feel it's best to start this early. So my husband only spoke to our sons in French, our nanny only spoke Spanish, and I spoke English. Today, both of our sons speak all three languages very well.

—*Lauren Feder, MD, a mom of 17- and 13-year-old sons, a nationally recognized physician who specializes in homeopathic medicine, and the author of* Natural Baby and Childcare *and* The Parents' Concise Guide to Childhood Vaccinations, *in Los Angeles, CA*

⌒⌒

My son generally did things on his own schedule. When he was around a year old and he wasn't talking, my father urged me to have him evaluated for a speech delay. I knew that was not what I needed to do. My son was just waiting to talk until he could say a whole sentence.

—*Nancy Rappaport, MD*

⌒⌒

My younger son has a speech delay, but it turns out he had so much earwax that it took 20 minutes per ear to dig out. I hadn't looked at his ears before he had his ear infections, so I now dig it out every six weeks, and he is talking better. (Note: If you think that your baby might have wax in her ears, take her to the doctor.)

My son always waited until he was face-to-face before he would smile and then he would babble. He wanted your full attention, and he would babble like he had something really important to say.

As my baby got older, I got worried about his speech delay, and I purchased the *Your Baby Can Read* DVD set. He cried every time I put it on, so I stopped putting it on. My son does like the *Your Baby Can Read* books, and he likes animal flash cards, but he rips everything up. I ended up just bringing down his brother's plastic animals, and he would just make the animal noises. Now, though, he does say their names. He still won't watch the videos, though! He only watches *I Love Toy Trains*.

—*Sonia Ng, MD*

⌒⌒

Both of my daughters learned to talk early, and talking seemed to come very easily to them. My parents were British, and my mother used to come and stay with us for a few months at a time. My mom spoke the Queen's English, and she would recite oodles of poetry to

? When to Call Your Doctor

If you are concerned that your baby has a speech delay, talk with your doctor about it—without delay. If something is wrong, resources are available to help. If nothing is wrong, the conversation will put your mind at ease.

my girls that she had memorized in her life. My girls loved to listen to my mom, and for a while my older daughter even picked up a British accent!

Talking didn't come as easily to my son. At age two, he wasn't talking at all. He would look at me and say, "Dada." That was all he could say, but I could tell that he actually thought he was talking. My husband and I were concerned, so we took our son to the doctor, who promptly told me, "Why should he talk? He has two big sisters to talk for him."

On my own, I took my son to a speech therapist, who made the diagnosis of verbal apraxia. With patience and speech therapy, he did fine, on his own timetable. The lesson here: Trust yourself as well as your doctor. Having the speech evaluation done gave me peace of mind, and affirmed my intuition. It never hurts to have another opinion.

—*Lesley Burton-Iwinski, MD*

A mother will speak to her child all day long—in words, through touch, or with a look. She doesn't have to give a single thought to "teaching" her child to talk, or "encouraging" her child to talk, or "supporting" her child in talking. A mother will express her love in her own unique way. The loving attention and fascination that a mother and her baby have for one another will, without much thought, create a relationship in which the child speaks—through a look, with a touch, and eventually with words. Children learn to talk as a result of being involved in intimate human relationships. The wellspring of child development is inside the child, and only needs the parents' joy (and safety) to unfold.

—*Elizabeth Berger, MD, a mom of a 28-year-old son and a 26-year-old daughter, a child psychiatrist, and the author of* Raising Kids with Character, *in New York City*

Switching to Organics

It's kind of funny that buying organic food seems "new." Before pesticides were introduced in the 1930s, everything was organic!

Organic foods are grown without the use of pesticides, synthetic fertilizers, sewage sludge, genetically modified organisms, or ionizing radiation. (Yes, you read that right, sewage sludge. Ick.) Animals that produce organic meat, poultry, eggs, and dairy products are not given any antibiotics or growth hormones.

To buy organic food, look for the green-and-white USDA Organic seal. That seal is a promise that the food is organic. Fresh organic produce in stores will be indicated by signs, or look on the foods sticker for a code beginning with 9.

When you buy organic food, it supports the farmers who *grow* organic food. That means fewer pesticides and chemicals are released into our air, water, soil, and bodies. Studies show that infants are exposed to hundreds of harmful chemicals before they are even born. According to the National Academy of Science, "Neurologic and behavioral effects may result from low-level exposure to pesticides."

It just makes common sense: If a chemical was developed to kill an insect, how on earth could it be healthful for your baby?

I try to buy organic foods whenever I can. A generation ago, people smoked because they didn't know how bad it was. Now we know. Along the same lines, I believe that we might not yet know how bad conventionally grown foods are, but someday we will.

The one thing I always buy organic is milk. There's a dramatic price difference between conventional milk and organic, but I think organic milk is well worth the extra cost. Milk is a huge staple of my son's diet, and it's one thing I can't wash.

For fruits and vegetables, I try to buy organic when I can. When I can't buy organic, I wash the fruits and vegetables three times in cold water, very vigorously.

—*Wendy Sue Swanson, MD, FAAP, a mom of four- and two-year-old sons, a board-certified pediatrician, and a blogger for Seattle Children's Hospital, in Washington*

When my older son was a baby, there wasn't much organic baby food available except what we could grow ourselves. But as soon as I was able to get a hold of organic foods, I shifted over to an almost all organic diet. Today, about 90 percent of the food that we eat is organic. We belong to an organic cooperative, and I buy almost all locally grown organic vegetables, meats, and poultry.

People often say organic foods are too expensive, but actually I think that the opposite is true. Because organic foods are more nutritious than highly processed or simple carbohydrate foods, you eat less. Plus, you can pay a lot for packaging in all of those processed foods. Farmers' markets are good places to buy organic food less expensively.

—*Michelle Storms, MD, a mom of 24- and 20-year-old sons and a 21-year-old daughter, the assistant director of the Marquette Family Medicine Residency Program, in Marquette, MI, and a member of the health professionals board for Intact America*

∽

When I buy food and other items for my daughter, I always try to choose the most natural products I can, organic if possible. For example, I didn't buy the baby mattress with antibacterial agents. But the organic mattress cost $500, so I didn't buy that one either. Instead, I bought a regular mattress, and I've been very comfortable with that decision.

Along the same lines, I don't buy toys or baby products with antibacterial chemicals in them. We don't know enough about those chemicals to know that they are safe. My daughter received a doll one year for Christmas that had a bad petrochemical smell to it. Two years later, it still smells! That's the type of thing I wouldn't put in my daughter's play area, especially since she's mouthing everything in sight!

—*Katja Rowell, MD*

∽

My older son ate a fair amount of organic baby food. It wasn't necessarily because I believe organics are better than conventionally grown foods, but because an organic baby food company kept sending me samples.

—Carrie Brown, MD, a mom of seven- and five-year-old sons and a general pediatrician who treats medically complex children and specializes in palliative care at Arkansas Children's Hospital, in Little Rock

I would like to buy more organics, but it just is not a huge priority for us. As long as my kids eat, I'm fine with that!

—Jennifer Gilbert, DO

I think buying organic food is a fad and unnecessary. Is buying organics really going to grow healthier kids or save the world? I don't think so.

—Melanie Bone, MD

Chapter 11
11th Month

Your Baby This Month

YOUR BABY'S DEVELOPMENT

As your baby grows, he experiments with all of his senses. These days, your baby is likely very interested in different scents. The delicious smells of baking cookies, a spritz of Daddy's cologne, or the salt in the air by the sea are all bound to grab your baby's interest.

Around this time, your baby might start standing alone for a few moments. He might even take a few tentative baby steps. Most babies take their first steps on their tiptoes, with their toes turned outward. Most children don't walk with a mature stride, with their toes pointed ahead and their heels striking the ground, until they are around three years old.

Along the same lines, most babies learning to walk also instinctively bend their arms, as if they're carrying a tower of books. As your baby gains confidence walking, his arms will straighten, and he'll look much more relaxed.

These days, though, your baby is still probably mostly cruising from furniture to furniture, holding onto the couch, coffee table, or dog for dear life. Soon your baby will be able to stand alone, for a few uncertain moments, before plopping back down. It's ironic that standing is so much easier than sitting, and getting started is so much easier than stopping. Lots of bumps and bruises are in your baby's future. If you consider buying your little adventurer a crash helmet, rest assured you won't be the first parent to think of it!

If you have stairs, it's a good bet your baby is doing his best to scale them. Babies learn to climb stairs long before they learn to descend them. This is why wall-mounted safety gates are critical at the top *and* bottom of every staircase.

At this time, babies start to refine their pincer grasp. It becomes more precise, and it changes from an assisted pincer, where a baby rests his wrist on a surface for support, to a "neat" pincer. Your baby will start to pick up objects with his thumb and forefinger, without any help from his wrist. As your baby's pincer grasp develops, he'll be better at picking up and manipulating small objects.

Most things your baby picks up still go into his mouth, and anything in his grasp will be taste-tested. That's because babies even at this age still explore their world with their fingers and their mouths.

At 11 months, some babies can say "DaDa" and "MaMa" discriminately, on purpose and correctly. Some babies can say another word or two as well. Most babies understand the word "no" by this stage.

Babies this age delight in games that involve picking things up and dropping them. Your baby is also probably practicing using his motor skills, delighting in that all-time favorite baby game "knocking stuff down."

Taking Care of You
Sign up for a class to learn something new. Why should your baby be the only one learning and growing?

Justification for a Celebration
You're in the homestretch of your baby's first year!

Taking a Vacation

Is a vacation with a baby a vacation at all? It can be, with the right planning and preparation.

A topic that's been in the news lately is the U.S. Transportation Security Administration's rules on traveling with breast milk, formula, and juice. These rules change, but currently, mothers flying both with and without their babies are permitted to bring breast milk, formula, or juice in amounts greater than three ounces. Moms are encouraged to bring only as much of these liquids as needed until they reach their destinations.

The liquid must be separate from any other liquids, gels, and aerosols, which are to be placed in a quart-size zip-top bag. It must be presented for inspection, even possibly opening, by the security officers.

You would never hold your baby while driving down the highway in a car at 65 miles per hour. Why would you hold her on your lap when you're hurtling through the air at *500* miles per hour? Your arms aren't strong enough to hold your baby securely in the event of turbulence, especially if it's sudden and unexpected.

Babies should have their own seats on the plane. If you're flying, check for a discount when making reservations. Many airlines offer discounts of up to 50 percent for babies younger than two.

The Federal Aviation Administration strongly urges parents to buckle children into approved child restraint systems when flying. You can ask if the airline has a child restraint system for you to use, but more likely you'll have to bring your own. Check your baby's car seat label to make sure it says, "This restraint is certified for use in motor vehicles and aircraft." Otherwise, you might have to check it with your luggage.

Child restraint systems can only be used in window seats on airplanes so that they don't impede anyone's escape path in an emergency.

Of course, not everyone flies to their vacation destination.

See "Keeping Your Baby Happy and Safe in the Car" on page 76 for information on car safety.

∽

When we traveled, we were sure to pack lots of snacks. Dried fruit and whole wheat crackers were always easy choices because they wouldn't spoil.

—*Ari Brown, MD, a mom of two, a pediatrician with Capital Pediatric Group, and the author of* Baby 411, *in Austin, TX*

∽

Even when my daughter was a baby, we traveled a lot. I became an expert at packing for and traveling with a baby. Collapsible baby bottle inserts were invaluable. They packed well, and they didn't need to be sterilized.

I always took along a collapsible stroller. I could fold it up and stow it in the overhead bin of the airplane, and then we'd have our stroller with us when we got off the plane.

Our fellow passengers would look at us when we got on the plane, worried that our daughter was going to cry the entire flight. But she didn't. I think because we took her with us from a very early age, she was accustomed to it. Plus, I always packed plenty of games to keep her busy, and I made up stories to keep her entertained.

—*Debra Jaliman, MD, a mom of a 19-year-old daughter, a dermatologist in private practice, and an assistant professor of dermatology at Mt. Sinai School of Medicine, in New York City*

∽

We traveled right away with our son. Both of our boys were born in the summer, and we always spend two weeks at the shore. I probably overpacked, but I wanted to be prepared.

One thing that was very handy was a travel bassinet. It folded up into the size of a booster seat, and then my husband and I set it up in the middle of our bed, so the baby slept between us. You have to be very careful about cribs at hotels. Before you use one of those cribs, inspect it closely to make sure you can't fit a soda can between the slats and that all of the hardware is tightened very well.

With that said, I think it's a lot easier to travel with a baby than a toddler. With a baby, pretty much all you need are diapers and one-sies. You can contain a baby in the car seat. Once babies hit that stage where they can walk, but they can't talk, traveling with them is very difficult.

I remember being with my older son when he was a baby, on an airplane doing a sticker book for hours. It's all about knowing your baby and being prepared with a bag of tricks to keep him busy.

—Heather Orman-Lubell, MD, a mom of 10- and six-year-old sons and a pediatrician in private practice at Yardley Pediatrics of St. Christopher's Hospital for Children, in Pennsylvania

When my girls were five and three years old, and our youngest was less than a year old, my husband and I decided to take them to San Diego for a week. Packing for that trip was like moving our entire house to the hotel.

Mommy MD Guides-Recommended Product
Go-Go Kidz Travelmate

"For travel, I love the Go-Go Kidz Travelmate. You strap your baby's car seat to it, put the baby in the car seat, pull out the handle, and away you go," says Lennox McNeary, MD, a mom of a two-year-old son, a specialist in physical medicine and rehabilitation at Carilion Clinic, and a cofounder of the Mommy Doctors Bakery (makers of Milkin' Cookies), in Roanoke, VA.

"It's wonderful to have at the airport because you don't have to take a stroller. Use it to transport your baby and car seat right to the gate, then check the Travelmate and the car seat at the gate. This made going to the airport with our baby so much easier."

Go-Go Kidz Travelmates cost around $80, and you can buy them online.

We had luggage, car seats, strollers, and even a hot plate so I could boil the water to heat my son's bottles. At one point, we had to cross a busy, divided highway to get from the parking lot to our hotel, carrying all of our stuff and three kids, all of whom were young enough to be runaway threats.

My husband and I looked at each other, dismayed.

"I'll take care of the kids; you bring the stuff," I said.

Midway across the street, while we were standing on the median, my younger daughter proclaimed that she had to go to the bathroom!

When we got home after that vacation, we were exhausted. For the next few years after that, we only went to local hotels. That way if we needed something, I could run home and get it, rather than bringing everything!

—*Lisa Dado, MD, a mom of three children, ages 21 to 16, a pediatric anesthesiologist with Valley Anesthesiology Consultants, and a cofounder and CEO of the Center for Human Living, which teaches life skills and martial arts training, in Phoenix, AZ*

Traveling with a baby is a challenge, and traveling with twins is even more so. When we flew with our babies, we held them on our laps on the airplane. We fly Southwest Airlines because it's easiest. We get into line early so we can pick good seats.

The first time we flew with the twins, my husband and I got all settled into our seats next to each other. Then the flight attendant came by and told us that one of us had to move because they only permit one lap child per row in each section! Now we sit across the aisle from each other, and we can still pass things back and forth.

Bringing a DVD player with Dora DVDs and packing some small new toys, which we gave to our children on the plane, made things much easier.

—*Brooke Jackson, MD, a mom of 3½-year-old twin girls and a 14-month-old son and a dermatologist and medical director of the Skin Wellness Center of Chicago, in Illinois*

RALLIE'S TIP

Years ago, my sister and I started a tradition of going to the beach with our husbands and children every summer. When we were younger, it was the only way we could afford to take a vacation. We'd scrimp and save and pool our resources and split the cost of just about everything.

My sister and I had our first babies around the same time, and this made things really fun! Our children had a great time playing with each other on the beach during the day, and in the evenings, we'd take turns babysitting. While my sister and her husband went out to eat, my husband and I would watch the children. The next night, we'd switch. I felt totally comfortable leaving my baby with my sister and her husband for a few hours, so I was really able to enjoy myself—and my husband's company.

My husband and I are very lucky that we're able to travel and expose our kids to many different cultures. I think it was ideal to start this even before they turned a year old.

Sure, it's a little scary to be far from home with a baby. When our youngest baby was only four months old, we took her to New Orleans for my best friend's wedding. All of the ladies there told me, "Your baby's out in the wind; she's going to catch a cold." Sure enough, she did. But more likely she caught it from the recirculated air on the plane than the wind at the wedding!

Despite all of that, I think it's valuable to take kids places early in life. It gives you more flexibility later on down the road.

—Nancy Rappaport, MD, a mom of 21- and 16-year-old daughters and an 18-year-old son, an assistant professor of psychiatry at Harvard Medical School, an attending child and adolescent psychiatrist in the Cambridge, MA, public schools, and the author of In Her Wake: A Child Psychiatrist Explores the Mystery of Her Mother's Suicide

My daughter has asthma, and new environments sometimes triggered her asthma attacks. I sometimes travel for work, and I enjoyed taking her along if possible. But I had to weigh the pros and cons of that carefully.

Once we were in Philadelphia, and my baby had a sudden, violent asthma attack. Fortunately, I was familiar with the city, and I knew that Jefferson Hospital was only a few blocks from our hotel.

Rather than getting into the car, I ran with my daughter down to the front desk, asked them to point me in the direction of the hospital, and I sprinted with her to the ER. After being treated, my daughter was fine.

Take a MOMcation

Back in 2009, Fawn Rechkemmer started taking weekend vacations by herself to get some much-needed relaxation and quiet time. She found that these "retreats" helped her repair herself mentally and physically from the wear and tear of mothering two toddlers. Fawn also found that other mothers craved such an escape but didn't have the resources to get away on their own. So Fawn, along with a committee of volunteer moms, created MOMcation.

A MOMcation is a vacation for Mom, away from the kids, with the goal of relaxing, renewing, and repairing Mom so she can be an even greater mom when she returns home.

MOMcation retreats feature opportunities to connect with and learn from other moms as well as spend some quiet time alone in self-reflection. The retreats are organized by moms who realize the importance of taking a break from it all to refresh and revive your spirit and connect with who you are, aside from being a mom.

Attendees are encouraged to participate in events throughout the weekend such as a welcome party, hayride, karaoke, and hikes. But the organizers emphasize that "all activities are optional. You choose where your retreat takes you."

MOMcations are held from Friday to Sunday, and they cost between $80 and $180. The cost includes all meals, lodging, and activities. Relaxation, renewing, and repairing are all included too! Visit **MOMCATION.ORG** to learn more or to register.

Generally, it was wonderful to have my babies with me on trips, but sometimes if there was a concern about them getting sick, it was less stressful to leave them at home. It's no fun being in a hotel room with a sick baby!

I enjoy traveling with my family, and here are a few tips I found to be invaluable during my babies' first years, which you can read more about on my blog WaterWineTravel.com.

• Always have a change of clothing (including undies) for yourself and your kids in your carry-on bag. My kids have had unexpected bouts of diarrhea and vomiting both on car and plane trips.

• The lips and skin can get dry during air travel, so keep some lip balm and lotion (no more than three ounces) in your carry-on bag.

• Hotel rooms can be close quarters for families. We usually rent a home when we travel. The benefits include spacious quarters for two or more families, a full kitchen (which reduces our meal costs), a laundry room, and often a pool and/or hot tub.

• Consider renting car seats, a Pack 'n Play, and strollers at your destination. Baby equipment rental is a popular service in many resort areas that cater to families. In addition, some hotels and vacation homes can provide this service.

—*Ann V. Arthur, MD, a mom of a nine-year-old daughter and a seven-year-old son, a pediatric ophthalmologist in private practice at Park Slope Eye Care Associates, and a blogger at WaterWineTravel.com, in New York City*

Learning to Walk

As far as milestones go, learning to walk is one of the biggest. It's truly amazing to watch a baby develop from pulling himself up to taking those first baby steps.

∽

My older son crawled at eight months and walked very early. But he didn't talk! My younger son didn't walk until he was over a year old, but he talked a lot. I figure they can only focus on one thing at a time.

—*Sandra Carson, MD, a mom of two grown sons and the director of the Center for Reproduction and Infertility of Women and Infants Hospital, in Providence, RI*

❧

All kids reach milestones like learning to walk in their own time. My son was the kind of kid who did things slower. He crawled until he was almost 2½, and then he ran!

—*Nancy Rappaport, MD*

❧

I loved seeing my son crawl for the first time and pull up to stand for the first time. He crawled at eight months and pulled to stand at nine months. He cruised up till 12 months, then let go and stood for minutes. He didn't walk without help until 14 months because he was afraid of moving, and then he ran at about 16 months.

—*Sonia Ng, MD, a mom of seven- and two-year-old sons, a pediatrician, and a sedation attending physician at the Children's Hospital of Philadelphia Pediatric Care and the University Medical Center at Princeton in Princeton, NJ, and the Pediatric Imaging Center in King of Prussia, PA*

❧

My daughter was a very chubby baby. She didn't roll over for a long time. But suddenly, at eight months, she started to walk, without any crawling in between.

Watching my daughter learn to walk was nerve-wracking. She was very little and quite round. She didn't seem to have any clear direction of where she was going; she just walked around randomly. Things like the edge of the rug were constantly tripping her, and she'd fall down.

We actually put a bicycle helmet on her to try to protect her head. But that threw her balance off completely, and she fell down even more! So we gave up and tried to steer her onto soft surfaces.

—*Penny Noyce, MD, a mom of 23- and 21-year-old daughters, two 21-year-old sons, and a 13-year-old son, the author of the preteen novel* Lost in Lexicon, *and an internal medicine specialist, in Weston, MA*

My son was born prematurely, and he's been a little slow reaching physical milestones like crawling and walking. I've been keeping a close eye on that.

When my son started to walk, I noticed that he was having trouble with his right leg. I talked with his pediatrician, and he dismissed my concerns.

"Kids develop at different times," he insisted.

I felt that it wasn't a delay in development; something looked wrong to me. I talked with my friend Cheri Wiggins, MD, who is also a specialist in physical medicine and rehabilitation. She agreed and also suspected that my son had mild cerebral palsy and encouraged me to take him to physical therapy. My husband and I have taken him to the park every day, and we encourage him to run on uneven ground. He's done very well so far, and I'm glad that I didn't ignore my gut.

Trust your mom instinct! You know your child. Don't worry about being the "difficult parent." It's your job to advocate for your child.

—*Lennox McNeary, MD, a mom of a two-year-old son, a specialist in physical medicine and rehabilitation at Carilion Clinic, and a cofounder of the Mommy Doctors Bakery (makers of Milkin' Cookies), in Roanoke, VA*

Saving Money on Baby Things

The adage that the most expensive gifts come in the smallest packages sure does hold true for babies. According to the U.S. Department of Agriculture (USDA), it will cost a middle class U.S. family about $222,360 to raise a baby born in 2009 to adulthood. A family earning more than $98,120 can expect to spend $369,360.

According to the USDA, the cost to raise a child varies by location, location, location. Expenses are the highest for families living in the urban Northeast, followed by the urban West and urban Midwest. Families living in the urban South and rural areas have the lowest child-rearing expenses.

According to the USDA's report, costs for food, shelter, and other child-raising necessities total from $11,650 to $13,530 per year, depending on the age of the child. Housing costs are the single largest expenditure on a child, averaging $70,020 or 31 percent of the total cost over 17 years. Child care, education, and food are other large expenses.

You can visit the USDA's online cost-of-raising-a-child calculator at cnpp.usda.gov/calculatorintro.htm. This handy calculator will help you estimate how much it will cost annually to raise a child. This could help you to plan better for overall expenses, including food, or to purchase adequate life insurance.

Fortunately, there are lots of ways to save money, even on baby things.

෴

If you sign up on baby product manufacturers' websites, often they send you coupons and samples. I received a lot of samples of organic baby food.

—*Carrie Brown, MD, a mom of seven- and five-year-old sons and a general pediatrician who treats medically complex children and specializes in palliative care at Arkansas Children's Hospital, in Little Rock*

෴

I bought my older son a bunch of educational toys. That was a total waste of money. He was totally happy playing with anything that made noise or that he could chew on. By the time my second son was born, all of those educational toys had fallen by the wayside.

--*Sandra Carson, MD*

෴

Rather than buying expensive prepared baby foods, my husband and I mainly made our own baby food. We simply mashed up what we ate! It's far less expensive to do it that way. Plus, who knows what's in that prepared food!

—*Susan Besser, MD, a mom of six grown children, ages 26, 24, 22, 21, 19, and 17, a grandmom of one, a family physician, and the medical director of Doctors Express-Memphis, in Tennessee*

෴

Thinking of buying a video monitor? Save your money. I really loved my sound-only baby monitor. It gave me the freedom to move around my house without being at my baby's bedside and still know she was okay. I don't have a video monitor, though. I thought that was a little too much hovering. You can easily go overboard with all the new "gadgets" out there to entice/guilt the new parents. I feel that I really don't need to be watching my babies every single second of their existence. As long as I can hear them, that's fine with me.

—*Sadaf T. Bhutta, MD, a mom of a five-year-old daughter and three-year-old triplets and an assistant professor and the fellowship director of pediatric radiology at the University of Arkansas for Medical Sciences and Arkansas Children's Hospital, both in Little Rock*

Often friends' recommendations are helpful, but you really do have to consider your own lifestyle. A friend of mine recommended a Snap and Go stroller, which is a frame that you put the baby car seat into. I bought one, then ended up only using it twice.

—*Rebecca Reamy, MD, a mom of six- and one-year-old sons and a pediatrician in emergency medicine at Children's Healthcare of Atlanta, in Georgia*

One thing we saved a lot of money on was our double jogging stroller. We bought a used one from a bike-and-stroller store, and it worked out just fine.

—*Alanna Kramer, MD, a mom of an eight-year-old son and a six-year-old daughter and a pediatrician with St. Christopher's Hospital for Children, in Philadelphia, PA*

With six kids, clothing got passed from kid to kid. That saved a lot on the clothing bills! But not all of my kids have the same body type. Some are tall and thin, and others are short and chunky. So not every outfit worked for all of the kids. Also, by the time my sixth baby was born, some of the clothes were simply worn out.

Another thing that saved a lot of money was buying durable brands, even if they cost a little more initially. I loved Osh Kosh, but I noticed that by the time my sixth baby was born, the brand wasn't quite as durable anymore.

—*Susan Besser, MD*

One of my hobbies is clipping and using coupons. I like to save money! I started clipping coupons when I first opened my medical practice and I was six months pregnant. I didn't have many patients those first few months, and so at times I sat at my desk clipping coupons while I waited for my patients to arrive.

Today I keep a basket full of coupons for baby items such as diapers and baby food in my waiting room for moms to take.

—*Charlene Brock, MD, a mom of 28-, 25-, and 23-year-old sons and an 18-year-old daughter and a pediatrician with St. Chris Care at Falls Center, in Philadelphia, PA*

RALLIE'S TIP

When my first son was born, I wasn't just on a budget. I was too poor to even have a budget. I never shopped at an upscale baby store, but I was able to find everything my baby needed—and lots of stuff he didn't! On Saturday mornings, my friend Joy and I would load our babies in the car and head out to the yard sales. We'd buy clothes and toys and strollers and swings for next to nothing. Some of those items had been very expensive the first time around, and there's no way I could have afforded them brand-new.

Buying most baby items secondhand is an excellent way to save money without scrimping. Babies grow so fast that they might only wear an outfit once or twice, or they might play with a certain toy for only a week or two before they lose interest in it. Joy and I had a great time shopping those yard sales. It was like going on a treasure hunt!

I found that a good financial strategy was to do my research and invest money in baby products that I would be using a lot. Then I saved money on things I wouldn't be using as often.

I learned this the hard way, though. We bought four baby carriers before we finally spent the big money to get a decent one! I spent more on the first four than I would have spent if I had gotten the good one right from the start.

Most of our baby clothes are hand-me-downs, and we often bought onesies and Carter's rompers from a used-clothing store.

I made the art for my daughter's room, which was fun and personal *and* saved money. We hung her grandfather's childhood quilt on the wall for another decoration. Ikea has been another great resource for baby bedding and other products we use day-to-day.

—*Katja Rowell, MD, a mom of a five-year-old daughter, a family physician, and a childhood feeding specialist with FamilyFeedingDynamics.com, in St. Paul, MN*

This isn't so much about saving money, but about *making* money. I've sold some of my kids' baby clothes on Craig's list or places like that.

—*Kristie McNealy, MD, a mom of eight- and five-year-old daughters and three- and one-year-old sons and a blogger at KristieMcNealy.com, in Denver, CO*

Keeping Fears and Worries in Check

The fact that it will cost more than $222,360 to raise your little one to adulthood aside, worries come with the parenting territory. When you were pregnant, you likely worried about your baby almost nonstop: *I can't see him, so how do I know he's okay?* Now that your baby is born, you might have a new worry: *Now that he's out in the world, how can I keep him okay?*

There's so much for moms to worry about. Will someone abuse my baby? Will he be run over by a car? Will someone feed him peanuts and he'll have an allergic reaction?

Parents can become so fearful that it affects the children. Bad things can happen if we are there or not, so we need to learn to let go. Most of us make it to adulthood. I can only suggest that you do the best you can and have faith.

—*Melanie Bone, MD, a mom of four, ages 16, 15, 14, and 13, a grandmom of one grandson, a gynecologist, the founder of the Cancer Sensibility Foundation, and the author of the syndicated column* Surviving Life *and the book* Cancer, What's Next?, *in West Palm Beach, FL*

When my third son was a baby, he was up every few hours to breast-feed. One night, he slept a lot longer than usual. I had to wake him up, and he wasn't interested in nursing. I was concerned that he might have a serious infection. I made an appointment to see his pediatrician, and sure enough, by the time we got to the office, my son looked fine.

As a physician, you know what all of the worst cases could be. So it's very easy to get worried as a new parent. As time went on, I probably went to the opposite extreme. My kids had to prove to me they were really sick before I'd believe them!

—*Charlene Brock, MD*

MomMy TIME — Keep a Journal

Often when we worry, our minds get stuck in a continuous loop. *What if? What if? What if?*

An effective way to get your brain off of worry mode is to write down your thoughts. You're not likely to write down the same thing over and over again, and so writing helps you to unstick your stuck thoughts. Journaling can help you to work out problems, learn about yourself, clarify your thoughts and feelings, and reduce stress.

If you begin to journal, you join a long, storied history of journalers that dates to at least 10th-century Japan. Many famous and successful people kept journals, including Anne Frank, Lewis Carroll, Virginia Woolf, George Washington, Thomas Jefferson, and Harry S. Truman.

To make journaling more appealing, buy a journal that you will want to use, preferably one with lines, and find a pen that you like to write with. Keep the journal and the pen handy, but consider keeping them in a private place so you don't feel you have to censor your thoughts.

So that journaling doesn't add to your stress, don't pressure yourself. Write what you want, when you want.

Once you have a baby, I think he's first and foremost in your mind, and you're always thinking about him on some level—a psychological parent. That clicks in as soon as the baby is born, and it never goes away. When your "baby" turns 16 and gets his driver's license, that worry is still there; it's just different. I think that you can mitigate these fears some by choosing the best child care that you can find.

—*Sandra Carson, MD*

Before our daughter was born, I told my husband that I didn't think I had any maternal instincts, and I didn't know how I would do as a mom. My baby's first few days, I was so paranoid about her. I worried, *Is she going to develop this problem? That problem? Some other problem?* I was thinking too much, and those worries were always swirling around in the back of my head.

I kept telling myself, *You've got to get through this. She's eating, she's growing. Everything is going to be okay.*

—*Jennifer Bacani McKenney, MD, a mom of a two-month-old daughter and a family physician, in Fredonia, KS*

When you have children, maternal worries come to the forefront. This is true for physicians as well. When my children are sick, what I learned in medical school becomes a blur.

It's our nature as moms to think the worst—to exaggerate and overconcern ourselves. That's been a continuing challenge for me. I try to keep my head and not worry that every cough is pneumonia or every blemish is a viral rash.

What I do is use my husband as my touchstone. He's there to tell me a cold is just a cold. He's able to view things more rationally than me.

—*Silvana Ribaudo, MD, a mom of a five-year-old son and a two-year-old daughter and an assistant clinical professor at the Columbia University Medical Center, College of Physicians and Surgeons, and at ColumbiaDoctors Eastside, both in New York City*

During your baby's first year, you can anticipate that *something* bad is going to happen. One time, my husband was watching our two oldest kids. He had one baby in a backpack on his back, and he had the other in a backpack that was sitting on the ground. All of a sudden, the backpack toppled over, and our baby hit his head on the ground! Thank goodness, he was fine, but it was very scary.

After that, my husband and I had a lot of discussions about blame. He had correctly sensed that my attitude was, "If something happens on your watch, you're screwed. I will never forgive you because these are my most precious kids."

My husband explained that this attitude added an extra burden for him: the fear that I would never forgive him if something happened and the added pressure of losing me too if something happened.

It really is by the grace of God that kids don't do something to hurt themselves regularly. Babies are a huge responsibility. I completed a pediatrics internship, and so I saw the worst-case scenarios. My imagination was always fairly active. One of the many challenges of being a new parent is not to overexaggerate the risks.

—*Nancy Rappaport, MD*

Socializing with Family and Friends

"To have a friend and be a friend is what makes life worthwhile."
—Unknown

Friends are one of life's greatest gifts. With a new baby, it's easy to get stuck in your own life—in your own *house*—and miss time with friends. But showing your baby how to make friends, how to *be* a friend, and the value of friendship is a terrific lesson. And when those friends are also *family*, it's a wonderful thing.

☙

I enjoy spending time with my friends from church. We get together for Bible study, prayer, and encouragement. We share any concerns we have, and we pray for each other.

—*Charlene Brock, MD*

When you have a baby, you get a whole new lifestyle. You have to get home at a certain hour, and you can't leave in the morning before a certain hour. There are also questions as to which events you're going to take the baby. For me, having a baby ruled out certain activities that I had done prior. I chose to forgo activities rather than be away from my baby.

—*Sandra Carson, MD*

Instead of having large parties during my baby's first year, I enjoyed small gatherings with close family and friends. I think that large productions take away from the pleasure of the experience.

I especially enjoyed spending time with my friends who also had babies, many of whom I met in my prenatal yoga classes. I enjoyed that intimacy of womanhood and motherhood.

Consider Mothers of Preschoolers (MOPS)

In Wheat Ridge, CO, in 1973, eight moms met for lunch. Little did they know they were starting an organization that would grow to more than 102,000 members, in 4,052 groups, across 30 countries.

Mothers of Preschoolers (MOPS) is an organization of local MOPS groups where moms—of children from conception through kindergarten—meet to build friendships, receive encouragement, gain hope, and grow as leaders while their children attend a MOP-PETS program, which is a preschool-like setting.

MOPS groups vary in size, from 10 to 200 women. Some groups meet once a week; others meet once a month. Some groups meet during the school year; others meet year-round. Groups meet during the day, in the evenings, or on weekends.

Each year, MOPS holds a convention, with speakers and other fun activities. To learn more about MOPS or to find—or start—a group near you, visit **MOPS.ORG**.

—Lauren Feder, MD, a mom of 17- and 13-year-old sons, a nationally recognized physician who specializes in homeopathic medicine, and the author of Natural Baby and Childcare *and* The Parents' Concise Guide to Childhood Vaccinations, *in Los Angeles, CA*

∾

It's hard to get out with a baby, so we tried to invite people over as much as possible. During my baby's first summer, we held a huge Fourth of July barbecue and invited all of our friends and neighbors. We asked people to bring their kids' favorite toys, and we sectioned off an area of our yard for the "crawlers" with safe toys just for them.

—Jeannette Gonzalez Simon, MD, a mom of a two-year-old daughter who's expecting another baby and a pediatric gastroenterologist in private practice, in Staten Island, NY

∾

I think it is possible and also helpful for children to be made part of some adult social experiences from early infancy. Then the child learns to participate in the ebb and flow of conversation, and that attention is sometimes directed at the child and sometimes directed at other matters. A child who is among grown-ups (who are right there, when he needs them) but who is also allowed to think his own thoughts, to play with a carrot or pretzel, or to nibble on the edge of a cloth napkin is enriched by the experience.

Of course, parents have a need to get away from the baby at times and enjoy some adult conversation without tending to an infant. But in many cultures, babies hang out with the grown-ups much more of the time than they do in ours. And, interestingly, in many cultures, babies are given a variety of grown-up food pretty much as soon as they can manage it.

—Elizabeth Berger, MD, a mom of a 28-year-old son and a 26-year-old daughter, a child psychiatrist, and the author of Raising Kids with Character, *in New York City*

Preventing and Treating Constipation

Because we moms are right there at so many of our babies' diaper changes, it's easy to get a little obsessed with our babies' "bathroom" habits. When a baby is first born, the stool is thick, tarry, sticky meconium. It's made up of the baby's old skin cells that are shed and then swallowed in the womb before the baby is born.

During the first weeks, a breastfed baby's stools are usually soft and yellow, around eight to 10 of them each day. These stools actually change over time because breast milk changes over time, adapting to the baby's growth. Most breastfed babies drop to about four stools per day by the time they're four weeks old.

Formula-fed babies' stools are often tan or yellow and firm. They don't change over time, unless you change formula. Formula-fed babies generally have fewer bowel movements per day than breastfed babies. By around eight weeks old, both breastfed and formula-fed babies have a bowel movement about once a day.

Constipation generally isn't common in babies, but it can occur, especially during transitions such as from breast milk to formula or baby food to table food.

If your baby is straining to move his bowels, it might be helpful to let gravity work in his favor: Pick him up. Hold his knees against his chest. Don't use laxatives, mineral oil, or enemas to treat a baby's constipation.

～

When my daughter got a little constipated, I just gave her a little apple juice. As long as she had about four ounces of apple juice a day, she was usually regular.

—*Jeannette Gonzalez Simon, MD*

When my babies were breastfeeding, they didn't seem to poop that often. I think it was because breast milk is so well digested. But the truth is, a breastfed baby can poop seven times a day or once every seven days and either extreme is still normal. The key is to watch your baby for patterns and whether or not she's comfortable.

If your baby isn't pooping but she's not uncomfortable, count your blessings—and all of the money you're saving on diapers!

—*Amy Baxter, MD, a mom of 13- and 10-year-old sons and an 8-year-old daughter, the CEO of MMJ Labs, and the director of emergency research of Children's Healthcare of Atlanta at Scottish Rite, in Atlanta, GA*

My son has regular bowel movements, but when he was around a year old, he got terribly constipated. He was screaming and crying. I bought some baby glycerin suppositories. My mom was visiting, and she helped me administer them. They gave us the results we were looking for. After that, I was careful to give my son more to drink. He didn't have a problem again after that. (Talk with your doctor before giving your baby this or any medication.)

—*Michelle Hephner, DO, a mom of a two-year-old son and eight-month-old daughter and a family physician in private practice with Central DuPage Physician Group, in Winfield, IL*

Newborns are almost never constipated. Even if they're grunting and pushing, those are generally normal sounds that we all make on the toilet. We just don't share them with the world!

One of my favorite mentors, who is a poop specialist (a gastroenterologist really), says your poop is normal as long as you have a poop anywhere between seven times per day or once every seven days. It's not so much how often your baby poops to watch for, but what the poop looks like. Constipated poop is scribolous, little tiny balls of poop stuck together.

Sometimes when moms are mixing formula, they won't add as much water as they should, and that can constipate a baby. Also, a 12-month-old who is eating a lot of table food without a lot of fiber or without enough liquid could become constipated. Ninety-nine percent of the time when a baby is constipated, it's diet related. Give the baby more liquid to drink and more fiber-rich foods to eat, such as fruits, vegetables, and grains.

—*Hana R. Solomon, MD, a mom of four, ages 35 to 19, a board-certified pediatrician, and the author of* Clearing the Air One Nose at a Time: Caring for Your Personal Filter, *in Columbia, MO*

My second son only pooped once a week, which is completely okay for a breastfed baby. From the time my son was around eight weeks old until he was five months old, he only pooped on Wednesdays before 10:30 a.m. I am not kidding.

Because my son pooped so infrequently, when he did poop, it went everywhere. It ran down his legs, and he'd be sitting in a soppy mess in his bouncy seat. Every poop was a have-to-wash-everything event.

My husband was a stay-at-home dad at the time. Early on, he decided that Wednesday mornings would be a great time to have a babysitter. I think the babysitter probably assumed that our baby pooped like that all of the time, and that it was just bad luck it happened while she was there. She didn't know that we set her up.

—*Carrie Brown, MD*

Watching Out for Teeth Grinding

Parents aren't generally surprised by most of their babies' sounds: soft coos, cheerful giggles, even piercing shrieks. One sound parents don't expect to hear is the gnashing of teeth! Yet a surprising percentage of babies, almost a third of them, do grind their teeth.

Teeth grinding is also called bruxism. No one knows why people, let alone babies, grind their teeth. They might do it in response to pain, such as an earache. Or they might do it because their teeth aren't aligned properly.

Teeth grinding can actually cause babies to chip their teeth or cause jaw pain. But generally kids outgrow it, sometimes when they lose their baby teeth or later, when they become teens—and they have a whole new repertoire of ways to drive their parents crazy!

RALLIE'S TIP

My middle son started grinding his teeth when he was around a year old. The first time I heard him doing it in the middle of the night, I had no idea what that noise was or where it was coming from. When I followed the sound all the way to my son's crib, I couldn't believe that his little teeth could make such a racket. I had never heard anything quite like it. When I asked his pediatrician about it, the doctor reassured me that it was very common for babies to grind away during teething, and that it would likely resolve on its own. He was right! The teeth grinding stopped in a couple of months.

? When to Call Your Doctor

If you hear your baby grinding his teeth, talk with his dentist, who will examine the teeth for chips and wear and tear. The dentist might be able to come up with the cause of teeth grinding and offer some solutions.

I don't recall my babies grinding their teeth at all. It wasn't a problem, and I wasn't worried about it.

—*Ann Kulze, MD, a mom of 22- and 15-year-old daughters and 20- and 19-year-old sons; a nationally recognized nutrition expert, motivational speaker, and family physician; and the author of the best-selling book* Eat Right for Life, *in Charleston, SC*

Teaching Your Baby Values

It might be hard to imagine, but even in your baby's first year, he is learning values, just by watching every move you make, every step you take, and every rule you break. That's a lot of pressure!

The fundamental value is the love that the parent has for the child. That's the child's first value. It's something that the child experiences. It's the sum of everything that the parent is.

—*Elizabeth Berger, MD*

Be an active part of raising your children to be adults with character and good hearts because they all start out as blank slates. You are their most influential teacher.

—*Ann Contrucci, MD, a mom of 12-year-old boy-girl twins who works as a pediatric emergency physician, in Atlanta, GA*

It's so important to be part of a community that shares similar values to yours so that your children are exposed to that. I'm sure that much of what our children learned was from the families of their friends. Our community came from our religious and school affiliations.

—*Cathie Lippman, MD, a mom of 30- and 28-year-old sons and a physician who specializes in environmental and preventive medicine at the Lippman Center for Optimal Health, in Beverly Hills, CA*

Our Christian faith is a priority to my husband and me. One thing that is important to us is going to church. I tell new parents not to take their babies out in crowds until they're around three weeks old. However, in thinking back, I remember that my babies were in church at a week of age. We sat in the back, so I could take them out or nurse them if need be. Our church has a nursery, but at that age, I felt it was better to keep my babies with me.

—*Charlene Brock, MD*

I try to make dinnertime fun. It's one of my favorite times of the day because we're all together, and I want my sons to learn to enjoy this time too. We all talk about our favorite events of that day, and even my middle son will ask me, "How was your day?" At the end of dinner, we sing songs or do other fun things to make staying at the dinner table enjoyable. It's a great way to connect with each other. I hope that because I've made it fun, my boys will still enjoy eating dinner with us when they're teenagers.

—*Amy Thompson, MD, a mom of four- and two-year-old and nine-month-old sons and an ob-gyn at the University of Cincinnati College of Medicine, in Ohio*

RALLIE'S TIP

When my sons were babies, I was always amazed by the reactions they drew from adults. In stores and restaurants, total strangers would stand over them, smiling and cooing at them. As a new mother with my first child, this type of behavior worried me a bit. By the time my third son was born, I was used to it, and I even enjoyed watching the joyful interaction between my child and another adult.

As moms, we want to protect our babies, and older children definitely need to learn about "stranger danger." But not when they're babies. The smiles and coos from other adults are a critical part of a baby's socialization. Allowing your baby to interact with other adults lets your baby know that the world is a good place to be, and that he is an important and welcome person in our society.

Chapter 12
12th Month

Your Baby This Month

YOUR BABY'S DEVELOPMENT

By your baby's first birthday, she has likely tripled her birth weight and grown 10 inches! A baby's head also grows four to five inches in circumference during her first year.

A baby's fontanels—those soft spots on her head—usually close before she turns one year, or at the latest, by 18 months.

Although your baby is still a bit nearsighted, she can see pretty much just like you can. She also probably hears well, and she should immediately and predictably turn toward sounds.

You probably notice your baby's drooling less and less. That's because she's developing more and more motor control of her mouth.

Most babies near their first birthdays sleep for just 2½ hours during the day, possibly even at only one nap. With a little luck, your baby sleeps around 11½ hours each night.

Some babies can drink from a cup at this age, though many can't do this until 16 months. Even though your baby is used to being fed by a spoon, she's probably not very good at using one herself yet. Most babies can't feed themselves with spoons until they're around 15 months old.

Around this time, your baby is probably pretty good at cruising. She might be able to stand all alone for a few wobbly moments. Your baby might take her first steps. Interestingly, while half of babies are walking tall by their first birthdays, the other half aren't. One in ten babies won't take his or her first steps until they're 15 to 18 months old. All in good time.

Some babies can now roll a ball back to you. More than half of one-year-olds can imitate activities. They love to comb their hair, brush their teeth, and wash their faces—just like you do!

Babies this age often shift from play using their fine motor skills to exercising their large muscles. Your little one might love pushing, throwing, and knocking things down. By this age, most babies are able to actually initiate games such as peek-a-boo.

Just when you thought it was over, separation anxiety often makes a return at this stage. It interestingly often coincides with a baby's learning to walk. Many babies have fears of strangers long past their first birthdays.

By the time your baby is a year old, her laugh has changed from a high-pitched squeaking sound to a sound more like your own laughter. She can understand many simple words and phrases. Although many babies don't say their first words until 14 months or later, some babies can say "DaDa," "MaMa," and even another word or two by now—though you and your family might be the only ones who can understand them. Your baby can likely respond to simple instructions, like "Wave bye" or "Blow out the candles on your birthday cake!"

TAKING CARE OF YOU
Have a massage and/or spa day!

JUSTIFICATION FOR A CELEBRATION
You made it through your baby's first year! Happy MomDay!

Transitioning to a Sippy Cup

A search on Amazon.com for "sippy cup" nets 2,097 results! So if you try one type of sippy cup and your baby doesn't like it, simply try another one. Eventually, you'll find one your baby likes. Most doctors agree that babies should stop drinking from bottles by their first birthdays. Also at around a year, most babies are ready to make the leap from formula to cow's milk. Even if you're still breastfeeding, your baby should start to drink cow's milk, juice, or water from a cup.

 ❧

Before the end of the first year, it's important to introduce a sippy cup. After a year, a baby shouldn't be drinking from a bottle anymore because it's risky for her baby teeth. Also it's important for a baby to learn to drink from a cup because it improves her language skills.

—*Amy Baxter, MD, a mom of 13- and 10-year-old sons and an 8-year-old daughter, the CEO of MMJ Labs, and the director of emergency research of Children's Healthcare of Atlanta at Scottish Rite, in Atlanta, GA*

 ❧

It can be hard to transition a baby to a sippy cup from a bottle. Babies work hard to train their parents not to do this. I helped my daughter make the transition by giving her a bottle with nothing in it. Then I'd put her juice or formula into a sippy cup. It was so funny to watch her process this, *Well, I want this bottle here, but the juice I want is in that cup over there.* It wasn't too long before she started to drink from the sippy cup.

—*Christy Valentine, MD, a mom of a five-year-old daughter, a specialist in pediatrics and internal medicine, and the founder of the Valentine Medical Center, in Gretna, LA*

 ❧

My older daughter drank from a sippy cup. I bought the Gerber sippy cups, which had valves that you could remove and wash separately. Another brand had a valve that didn't come out, and those things can get really grody.

My younger daughter skipped over the sippy cup step. She

wanted to drink from an open cup right away. I didn't worry about the mess too much because I only gave her water to drink in it.

—*Robyn Liu, MD, a mom of seven- and four-year-old daughters and a family physician with Greeley County Health Services, in Tribune, KS*

Introducing Finger Foods

A baby's first year features so many firsts, and first finger foods are especially fun. It's wonderful to watch a baby learning to feed herself. Some babies are ready for this around nine months, others later. Offer your baby soft, small pieces of food. You might also want to try dry cereals and crackers, cooked pasta, and shredded cheese.

Always be 100 percent present with your baby when she is eating. Be sure to avoid the following foods, which can be choking hazards.

- Pieces of raw vegetables or hard fruits
- Raisins
- Whole grapes (peel and quarter them)

- Cherry tomatoes (peel and quarter them)
- Whole or sliced hot dogs and kiddie sausages (peel and cut into very small pieces)
- White bread (which can squish into little round balls)
- Pieces of hard cheese

∽

Three finger foods my son really enjoyed are Goldfish crackers, Cheerios, and Gerber Puffs. What is it about Goldfish crackers kids love so much?

—*Lennox McNeary, MD, a mom of a two-year-old son, a specialist in physical medicine and rehabilitation at Carilion Clinic, and a cofounder of the Mommy Doctors Bakery (makers of Milkin' Cookies), in Roanoke, VA*

∽

Cheerios are absolutely wonderful! Every one of my kids loved them. They practically melt in your mouth, so you don't have to worry so much about the baby choking. They were great to help my kids learn hand-to-mouth dexterity. They're fun to play with and portable. Give a kid a bag of Cheerios, and you have an instantly happy kid.

—*Susan Besser, MD, a mom of six grown children, ages 26, 24, 22, 21, 19, and 17, a grandmom of one, a family physician, and the medical director of Doctors Express-Memphis, in Tennessee*

∽

My daughters loved sweet potatoes when they were babies. I'd cook a sweet potato in the microwave, and then smash it up with a little breast milk. Sometimes I'd add very finely chopped spinach. Then I'd roll the mixture into raisin-size pellets, and my daughters would just gobble them up.

—*Robyn Liu, MD*

∽

One food that I loved to feed my babies is avocado. It's the perfect baby food! Avocados have the right balance of protein, monounsaturated fat, and carbs, plus a bunch of vitamins. And they have a bland taste that most babies tolerate well.

—*Michelle Storms, MD, a mom of 24- and 20-year-old sons and a 21-year-old daughter, the assistant director of the Marquette*

Family Medicine Residency Program, in Marquette, MI, and a member of the health professionals board for Intact America

⊘

My daughter was always happy to have finger foods, but she mostly made a mess with them before she was 12 months old. She loved soft, crumbly crackers, bananas, plums and apricots with the pits and skin removed, and muffins.

— Stuart Jeanne Bramhall, MD, a mom of a 30-year-old daughter and a child and adolescent psychiatrist, in New Plymouth, New Zealand

⊘

My son loves the Gerber Puffs sweet potato flavor. He now likes chili from Wendy's, potato smilers, spinach, soft carrots, noodles, and rice. Scrambled eggs and pancakes are his favorite. He loves maple syrup. He'll rub his face with the drippings when he thinks I'm not looking. He gets bathed often for stickiness.

—Sonia Ng, MD, a mom of seven- and two-year-old sons, a pediatrician, and a sedation attending physician at the Children's Hospital of Philadelphia Pediatric Care and the University Medical Center at Princeton in Princeton, NJ, and the Pediatric Imaging Center in King of Prussia, PA

It really helps kids to eat better if you make eating healthy foods fun. I have a very creative husband.

Once my daughter was eating a baby carrot, and it fell into her milk.

"Oh, that's great! I love my carrots dipped in milk!" my husband said.

And so my daughter gobbled it up.

—*Charlene Brock, MD, a mom of 28-, 25-, and 23-year-old sons and an 18-year-old daughter and a pediatrician with St. Chris Care at Falls Center, in Philadelphia, PA*

As my babies were beginning to eat more foods, I found it helpful to keep in mind that the food, and food combinations, that I found pleasing might not necessarily be what my kids would eat. My daughter, for instance, ate her pancakes with ketchup.

Plus, I found that my babies ate much more varied foods than I expected. I'll never forget one Easter, when we took our family to brunch at a resort. My son was eight months old at the time, and he ate an entire shrimp cocktail with spicy sauce. He was just chowing down! Give kids a chance to try something new.

—*Lisa Dado, MD, a mom of three children, ages 21 to 16, a pediatric anesthesiologist with Valley Anesthesiology Consultants, and a cofounder and CEO of the Center for Human Living, which teaches life skills and martial arts training, in Phoenix, AZ*

RALLIE'S TIP

I was determined not to introduce chicken nuggets and French fries to my children until they had sampled every fruit and vegetable under the sun. One of the physicians in my residency program had started feeding her daughter chicken nuggets when she was just a baby, and that child didn't want to eat anything else. If she couldn't have those chicken nuggets, she'd clamp her jaws shut, and then she would refuse to eat whatever she was offered.

I figured that if babies found chicken nuggets and French fries that addictive, I'd just bypass them altogether. I started feeding my boys tiny pieces of bananas and grapes and other fruits, and then moved on to bits of cheese, meat, and cut-up vegetables. Fortunately, none of my boys ever developed a serious addiction to chicken nuggets or French fries.

∽

With my twins, I was very careful about what foods I gave them. They ate no foods with added sugar for the entire first year!

That's a tougher act to follow with another baby. Although my third baby was on breast milk exclusively her entire first year, when she was nine months old, I took my twins to an ice cream store. While I was figuring out how to hold my ice cream cone, hold my baby, and pay the cashier, my baby lapped up about half of my ice cream cone—with no adverse results.

—*Lillian Schapiro, MD, a mom of 14-year-old twin girls and an eight-year-old daughter and an ob-gyn with Peachtree Women's Specialists, in Atlanta, GA*

∽

? When to Call Your Doctor

As you introduce each new food to your baby, keep an eye out for allergies. Signs and symptoms include a rash, diarrhea, or vomiting. If any of these occur, call your baby's doctor the next business day.

If your baby has trouble breathing, it could signal a severe allergy. If that happens, call 9-1-1.

As I introduced my babies to finger foods, I offered them a variety of healthy food, especially Eastern foods. People in those countries have healthier diets overall than we do because their baseline foods are healthier.

For example, my family loves chickpeas. Another favorite is dahl, which are lentils that come in many different types and are a great source of protein and fiber. When my sons were babies, I'd mix dahl and rice and mash them together for a tasty, delicious treat. We also enjoy pita bread and naan.

Dosa is a South Indian dish similar to crepes, which are made from flour and water. We stuff them with spiced potatoes or lentils and cut them into fours. They're great for kids to pick up and eat. You can buy dosa batter at any Indian store and make it yourself, like a pancake or a crepe.

—*Mona Gohara, MD, a mom of four- and two-year-old sons, a dermatologist in private practice, an assistant clinical professor in the department of dermatology at Yale University, and a cofounder of K&J Sunprotective Clothing, in Danbury, CT*

⁓

As my kids began eating more table food, I put a few choices in front of them. My attitude was matter-of-fact: This is the meal. If they don't like it, they can figure out what to make to eat. I am not a short-order cook! Don't turn it into a power struggle.

—*Ann Contrucci, MD, a mom of 12-year-old boy-girl twins who works as a pediatric emergency physician, in Atlanta, GA*

⁓

From the very beginning, I have pretty much let my kids eat all foods, in moderation. I believe if you're too restrictive, your kids will rebel. I saw that firsthand: Children who weren't allowed to eat candy at home loved to come to the Bone house for a forbidden snack! To this day, we all love chocolate and eat it almost every day, but we also eat salad and protein and whole grains as well.

—*Melanie Bone, MD, a mom of four, ages 16, 15, 14, and 13, a grandmom of one grandson, a gynecologist, the founder of the Cancer Sensibility Foundation, and the author of the syndicated column* Surviving Life *and the book* Cancer, What's Next?, *in West Palm Beach, FL*

⁓

One thing I was very concerned about during my son's first years was choking. I'm certified in advanced lifesaving and basic CPR, and I trained everyone else in our house too. As a precaution, I always made sure my son was sitting down when he was eating.

Two things that people might not realize are that experts don't recommend doing the finger sweep of the mouth anymore to clear the airway if someone is choking because it can push the item in further.

Also, if someone is coughing to get something out, you shouldn't give them water to suppress the cough. The cough is your body's mechanism for getting it out.

—*Sharon Giese, MD, a mom of a two-year-old son and a cosmetic plastic surgeon in private practice, in New York City*

Transitioning to a Convertible Car Seat

It can be nerve-wracking driving with your baby facing backward. Some babies hate it and cry. But experts recommend keeping infants in the back seat, in rear-facing child safety seats, as long as possible within the limits of the car seat. So that means you should keep your baby rear-facing until she reaches the maximum height or weight for the seat she rides in. All infants should ride rear-facing until they are one year old and weigh 20 pounds. The American Academy of Pediatrics just released new guidelines that say toddlers should ride rear-facing until age two.

Once it is time to switch your baby from an infant car seat to a convertible car seat, the National Highway Traffic Safety Administration offers this advice: The best car seat is the one that fits your child properly, is easy to use, and fits your vehicle correctly. Be sure that the seat is installed properly and use it every single time your baby is in the car.

It's a great idea to have a certified Child Passenger Safety (CPS) technician look over your car seat to ensure that it is properly installed. You can find lists of certified CPS technicians and Child Seat Fitting Stations on NHTSA.gov and SeatCheck.org or by calling 888-327-4236 or 866-SEATCHECK (866-732-8243).

‿〜◦

I'm a huge proponent for extended rear-facing car seats. We didn't turn my daughter's car seat around to forward-facing until she was almost three and hit the upper weight limit for rear-facing in her car seat.

—*Cheri Wiggins, MD, a mom of four- and two-year-old daughters, a specialist in physical medicine and rehabilitation at St. Luke's Magic Valley, and a cofounder of the Mommy Doctors Bakery (makers of Milkin' Cookies), in Twin Falls, ID*

We switched to a convertible car seat when our twins were about nine months old. Before I bought the car seats, I consulted all of my Facebook friends. The consensus was that the best seat was the Britax Marathon. It's definitely pricey, especially when you have to buy two. But it is wonderful. We only have car seats in my husband's car, and whenever we go anywhere with the kids, that's what we drive.

—*Jennifer Gilbert, DO, a mom of 18-month-old twins and an ob-gyn at Paoli Hospital, in Pennsylvania*

Carrying Your Heavier Baby without Injuring Yourself

Even though most babies weigh three times as much on their first birthdays as they did when they were born, that doesn't mean they want to be carried any less! It's important to protect yourself from injury as much as you protect your baby from injury. Parenting is a marathon, not a sprint.

RALLIE'S TIP

I never hurt myself carrying one of my children in my arms or on my hip, but carrying my baby in one of those gigantic, awkward baby carriers was a different story! Is there any way to comfortably carry a baby carrier? The best thing I could come up with was having my husband wrestle with the baby carrier while I carried the baby in my arms.

I think I probably carried my babies around a bit excessively. They all loved to be held, and I loved to hold them. My children were born before it became fashionable to wear one's babies, so I never used a baby sling or accessorized with my children in any way. When my boys were tiny newborns, I just carried them in my arms, snuggled against my chest. When they got big enough to help support themselves, I'd just nestle them on one hip or the other. When I got too tired or too hot lugging around one of those chunky babies, I'd just pop him in an umbrella stroller or hand him off to my husband. When my boys got too big for me to carry without risking bodily injury to one or both of us, I used the stroller to transport them. If one of my boys needed to be held, I'd sit down, take him out of the stroller, and hold him on my lap. Holding and carrying your baby is one of the greatest joys of motherhood, and it's one of the things that I miss the most.

I see a lot of problems in pregnant and new mothers in my practice. Carpal tunnel syndrome and de Quervain's tenosynovitis are super common. New mommies also get *a lot* of neck and back pain, shoulder pain, and elbow pain (tennis elbow), and many still suffer from lower-extremity joint pains because of the pregnancy hormones.

I try to rest my daughter's head on a pillow or the armrest of our rocker instead of in my hand so that I am not stressing the tendons around my wrist. I also try to notice when I am holding, changing, or bathing my baby in a position that is horribly uncomfortable for me and then adjust my position. I try to hold my daughter close to my body so that I am lifting her with my biceps (upper arm) muscles rather than my forearm muscles, because this is a big cause of tennis elbow.

My husband carries our baby in the car seat whenever possible because the combination of a heavy baby, a heavy car seat, and a seat designed to keep baby (not your arms and neck) safe is rough.

Mommy MD Guides-Recommended Product
Playtex Hip Hammock

Many baby front carriers max out at around 22 pounds. So as your baby gets bigger, you can't use them anymore. A product that makes it easier to carry a heavier baby is the Playtex Hip Hammock, which is designed for babies who weigh between 15 and 35 pounds.

Because you wear your baby on your hip, it's easier to walk or do chores without your baby blocking your reach. You can wear your baby on either hip. One of your hands will naturally curl around your baby, while the other will be totally free. The Hip Hammock has a toy hook that can hold a toy, and you can clip your keys to the key chain on the waist strap.

Hip Hammocks roll neatly and compactly, so they're easy to pack. You can buy Playtex Hip Hammocks online and in stores for around $50.

I started wearing wrist splints at night to rest my wrists while I sleep. I also have an "I-Need" neck massager from Brookstone (about $100) that just pummels the knots in the upper back muscles. Who has time for a massage appointment?!

—Rachel S. Rohde, MD, a mom of a five-month-old daughter, an assistant professor of orthopaedic surgery at the Oakland University William Beaumont School of Medicine, and an orthopaedic upper-extremity surgeon with Michigan Orthopaedic Institute, P.C., in Southfield, MI

I returned to work approximately two months after having my second son. When he was five months old, I developed this *terrible* pain between my right thumb and wrist. It was particularly bad at night. I tried wearing a splint and taking nonsteroidal anti-inflammatory medications, to no avail. It also became a serious problem for my work as a gastroenterologist, because I needed that hand to do colonoscopies and endoscopies.

I consulted with one of the rheumatologists at the hospital, and he diagnosed me with de Quervain's tenosynovitis, after doing a Finkelstein's test. For the Finkelstein's test, you make a fist with the thumb inside the fingers, and then the doctor pushes the wrist toward the outside (the pinkie), and that should reproduce the pain. I guess de Quervain's tenosynovitis is also called "baby wrist" because it can occur in postpartum mothers. It's thought to be due to carrying large, heavy babies with the wrist flexed. The rheumatologist who treated me injected the area with steroids and advised me to wear a wrist splint for about a week. The problem never came back.

To prevent this condition from occurring, I would make several suggestions. First, try to shift your baby from one side of your body to the other. Also, keep all the muscles you use to carry your baby in a "neutral position," particularly the muscles of the spine and wrist. Finally, try to keep the baby at the center of your body.

—Stacey Weiland, MD, a mom of a 12-year-old daughter and 7- and 5-year-old sons and an internist/gastroenterologist, in Denver, CO

Preventing and Treating Other Conditions

Babies change and grow so much during their first years, and unexpected things sometimes happen. Be on the lookout for changes and concerns, knowing that help from your doctor is only a phone call away.

❧

My younger son got conjunctivitis as a baby. He had very red, goopy eyes. Rather than being caused by a virus or bacteria, it was a sensitivity issue in his case. I tried numerous treatments, and they worked for a while, but the condition came back.

We were living in a house with old carpeting, and when we had the carpeting taken out, the conjunctivitis stopped. I think there was so much mold and dust in the carpet that he was reacting to that.

—Cathie Lippman, MD, a mom of 30- and 28-year-old sons and a physician who specializes in environmental and preventive medicine at the Lippman Center for Optimal Health, in Beverly Hills, CA

❧

My first child was born with a tethered frenulum, which is sometimes called "tongue tied." It was easy to spot; I noticed it immediately, as we were trying to figure out nursing together.

The medical literature at the time was very ambiguous about whether or not to have it clipped. It made sense to me to have it clipped right away. We had it done at an ear, nose, and throat specialist who was recommended by my son's pediatrician. I think that having the frenulum clipped definitely helped my son to breastfeed better.

—Amy Baxter, MD

❧

When my son was born, he was tongue tied. We didn't do anything, just watched it carefully. It didn't cause a problem with him breast-feeding or eating. I think it just stretched out in time.

My daughter had blocked tear ducts on both sides. She would develop green-yellow goop in her eyes. I used warm compresses to soften it up so I could clean it away. When she was about three months old, one of her tear ducts got infected. It was very red, goopy, and swollen. I took her to an urgent care center, and the doctor prescribed her an antibiotic. The infection cleared up just fine, and we haven't had any problems with her tear ducts since.

—Michelle Hephner, DO, a mom of a two-year-old son and eight-month-old daughter and a family physician in private practice with Central DuPage Physician Group, in Winfield, IL

At first, I thought my husband was crazy when he ordered a Hisense Monitor. The sensor is placed below the crib mattress and, when on, senses when there is a lack of motion in the crib. It's sensitive enough to sense the movement of breathing; when there is no movement, an alarm sounds.

During the first few weeks, we had some false alarms because our daughter was so mobile that she would roll to the side of the crib not fully sensed by the monitor. Now that she is bigger, it is great. If she stops breathing, we would rather know immediately so that we can do something about it. It's worth the false alarms.

—Rachel S. Rohde, MD

When my older daughter was a few weeks old, I noticed that she was using her right hand more than her left hand. I mentioned it to her pediatrician, thinking perhaps she was going to be right-handed. It turned out it was actually a symptom of a much larger problem. My daughter was diagnosed with cerebral palsy.

My husband and I had just recently moved to Florida. I was working in a brand-new job, and we didn't know a soul here. It was very tough to cope. Our family flew in for support, and I walked every day with a friend who also had a new baby. Talking was a big part of the healing process for me. Even though my days were filled with anxiety and worry, my beautiful daughter brought a lot of sunshine into my life. Part of me wishes I could go back now and tell my younger self that it would get better—in time.

—Eva Ritvo, MD, a mom of 20- and 15-year-old daughters, a psychiatrist, and a coauthor of The Beauty Prescription, *in Miami Beach, FL*

Coping with Tantrums

Oh, the whining, crying, fussing, yelling—and that's just us moms. Around their first birthdays, some babies start to throw temper tantrums. They're equally common in girls and boys, and they usually occur between ages one and three, especially during the second year of life.

Temper tantrums are like an emotional storm. A baby is frustrated, tired, hungry, or uncomfortable, and she has no way to express that, other than with kicking-and-screaming chaos. Just as kids vary, so do temper tantrums. Some kids have them regularly; others very rarely. Temper tantrums are very normal, and they usually diminish on their own in time. As your baby matures and develops better communication skills as well as a better understanding of her world, she'll be less frustrated and feel more in control, and the emotional "weather" should improve. Our prediction: Clear skies ahead.

You have to pick your battles and decide what is really important for your children to do. You also need to give them choices as much as possible. For example, I'll tell my son, "You can wear this pair of pajamas, or that pair. Which do you want?" That way, he gets to choose, but I still get him to put on pajamas. By giving children a choice, you're less likely to trigger a tantrum. We try to ignore tantrums, although it is hard. If we pay attention to the behavior, they learn that it achieves something, and this is not good in the long run.

—Amy Thompson, MD, a mom of four- and two-year-old and nine-month-old sons and an ob-gyn at the University of Cincinnati College of Medicine, in Ohio

My oldest son was—and still is—very strong willed. Sometimes when he didn't get his way, he would get himself all worked up. If I couldn't distract him or redirect him early enough, he would end up having a full-blown temper tantrum. It seemed as if it always happened at the most inconvenient times or in the places I'd be most embarrassed, like right in the middle of a church service or in the mall parking lot. Whenever my son was in full meltdown mode, there was no stopping him. No matter what I tried, it just seemed to make matters worse.

I'd just move my son's writhing little body to a safe place and let him get it all out. I really think those temper tantrums were the only way he knew to release his frustrations. Afterward, he'd go back to being his old sweet self. I think he outgrew them by the time he was about three years old, and as far as I know, he hasn't had one since!

When my daughters have tantrums, I try to remain patient and calm and follow the rules. For example, if one of my daughters wants to watch TV, she might cry and scream and leave the room. I kindly tell her that it is not time to watch TV. I say it only one time in a calm voice. (If you get angry, you lose.) For example, "Sweetheart, it is not time for TV; it is time for dinner." A little while later, she'll come back and say, "I love you, Mommy."

If you follow the rules, don't let yourself feel guilty, act naturally, and continue doing what you are doing, they notice you are just not going to pay attention to the tantrum. It all works out.

—*Gabriella Cardone, MD, a mom of five-, three-, and one-year-old daughters and a pediatric emergency physician at Texas Children's Hospital, in Houston*

In parenting, you need to be 100 percent consistent. But not a lot of people realize that, with kids, it's perfectly okay to call a do-over! And then you restart the consistency.

Simply sit down with your child and say, "Okay, we have a new thing going into effect from now on." You can actually do this several times, as long as you make it seem like a new plan each time. I've found this to be a great way to introduce new patterns or fix bad habits or behavior such as tantrums. It's even better if you build it up for a few days: "Starting Saturday . . ." If you've been inconsistent for a while, you need to start fresh with consistency.

Kids are never too young for natural consequences. Instead of saying, "From now on, we're not going to throw your doll into the toilet," the natural consequence is "You can't have the doll until it's been run through the dishwasher." When a toy is the subject of a dispute, sometimes I'll put the *toy* in time-out. I tried the Solomon solution, but our kids would have let me cut a disputed toy in half rather than give in.
—*Amy Baxter, MD*

⌒

I found that it's best to avoid the tantrum to start with, by steering the overall situation so that the child's frustration does not become too much for her to manage. Of course, for some children under some circumstances, it is impossible to always succeed with this goal. If a tantrum can't be avoided, the best thing to do is to lay aside all other agendas for the moment and work on soothing the child so that the tantrum ends.

The best way to achieve this is sometimes tricky. Some children need to be in your lap, while others need to be quietly near you. Other children need an interesting distraction. The basic cause of a tantrum is that the child cannot manage the level of stimulation and has just "gone to pieces." Worrying about "giving in" to the child is usually irrelevant—unless, of course, it is an issue of safety. The child who has gone to pieces isn't manipulating you, bullying you, or trying to get the better of you. Children who have gone to pieces need a lap so they can pull themselves together again, or they need to get out of the busy store, or they need something that feels secure and comforting. The parent's goal is to deliver that thing.
—*Elizabeth Berger, MD, a mom of a 28-year-old son and a 26-year-old daughter, a child psychiatrist, and the author of* Raising Kids with Character, *in New York City*

There are few things more distressing than a tantrum, especially in public. The best advice I can give is to find a way to make a graceful exit, and ignore the stares of the judging public. Usually, tantrums occur because a child is tired, hungry, sick, uncomfortable, or feeling overwhelmed or discouraged. Occasionally, tantrums are a learned response that a child uses as a way to get something.

Use each tantrum as a learning opportunity. Ask, "What did I learn?" and "What will I do differently next time to prevent this from happening?" Meet the child's need, whatever it is. If your child is sleepy, give her a nap. If she's hungry, give her something to eat. If her shirt tag is bothering her, cut it out. Once the child has calmed down, you can move forward. If the child was feeling powerless, you can give her some choices so that she doesn't feel as helpless. If she was feeling frustrated and discouraged, you can find a way to break a task or activity into smaller, more manageable pieces. If you think your child is having a tantrum to get her way, offer empathy but hold firm to your limits. To do otherwise is to perpetuate the problem.

Every child (and adult, for that matter) should have a special place where they go to feel better. This is not "time-out" in the traditional sense. Help them create a "self-calming area," either in a special place or use a basket that is portable. What goes in this area is different for each child. One might like to listen to music. Another might like to look at a picture book. Some like Play-Doh, or rubbing a silky cloth, or snuggling with a favorite stuffed animal. When they have calmed down, then they are ready to come out. Problem solving and planning "for the next time" is much more possible when everyone is in a quiet frame of mind. Once they know how to do it, kids are usually better at this than grown-ups! World peace will be built on the foundation of that sort of learning.

—*Lesley Burton-Iwinski, MD, a mom of 20- and 18-year-old daughters and a 14-year-old son, a retired family physician, and a parent and teacher educator with Growing Peaceful Families, in Lexington, KY*

Considering Weaning

By age one, some babies have long been weaned from the breast. Others still nurse for nourishment, comfort, or both. The American Academy of Pediatrics (AAP) recommends that a combination of solid foods and breast milk be given until a baby is one year old. After that, the AAP recommends continued breastfeeding beyond the first birthday as long as mutually desired by mother and child. So if Mom is ready to stop, or if Baby is ready to stop, then it's time to stop. Around one, most babies are becoming more and more interested in drinking from a cup and eating solid foods, so this might be an easy transition time.

⌒⌒

I breastfed all three of my kids. It was difficult with my first baby because the nurses had given him a bottle before bringing him to me. When my second son turned 5½ months old, he suddenly decided that he didn't want to nurse anymore. That was it. To this day, he doesn't drink milk! My daughter would have breastfed forever, but I weaned her when she was seven months old because of work issues. I wish I hadn't. Breastfeeding really helped me to lose weight and feel connected to my daughter. It also was so much easier to breastfeed than to use formula.
  —*Michelle Storms, MD*

⌒⌒

I breastfed my daughter until she was 10 months old. My daughter self-weaned at that point. She totally lost interest.
  —*Stuart Jeanne Bramhall, MD*

⌒⌒

By the time my daughter was a year old, I expected her to lose interest in breastfeeding. But she didn't! I didn't have a plan to wean her, but a few months later I didn't want to nurse anymore. She didn't respond to weaning well, but she got over it.
  —*Dina Strachan, MD, a mom of a five-year-old daughter, a dermatologist and director of Aglow Dermatology, and an assistant clinical professor in the department of dermatology at Columbia University College of Physicians and Surgeons, in New York City*

My oldest and youngest babies became very interested in food when they were five months old. They practically stalked it! So when we started them on solid food at six months, they were ready to go, and at that point they weren't interested in breastfeeding anymore.

My middle child, on the other hand, would have breastfed until college if I would have let him.

—Amy Baxter, MD

RALLIE'S TIP

I had planned to stop breastfeeding my youngest son when he was seven months old because I was getting ready to start a critical care rotation at a hospital that was nearly an hour away from my home. I wanted him to be comfortable taking a bottle from my husband or the babysitter in the evenings. On the weekend that I had planned to stop nursing, my son got a cold, and he was so miserable that I couldn't bear to take away his greatest source of comfort right then.

Weaning can be stressful for babies—not to mention their mothers—so it's important for babies to be as healthy and happy as possible before the big transition. I put off weaning my son for what turned out to be another three months. By then, he was really ready to be done with nursing, and I couldn't wait another minute to have my body all to myself again!

⌢

I breastfed my first son until he was one. I plan on doing the same for my second child. Weaning was tough for both my first child and for me. I stopped nursing him during my lunch break initially and then I stopped the nighttime feeds. I am still nursing my second child. I anticipate that weaning him will be even tougher.

—Bola Oyeyipo, MD, a mom of three-year-old and six-month-old sons, a family physician in private practice, and the owner of SlimyBookWorm.com, in Highland, CA

⌢

My son is 25 months old, and he's still breastfeeding. He developed Kawasaki's disease at a year of age and had a very small aneurysm, and so I rarely let him cry. He also has speech delay and looks like he doesn't understand me yet, so I don't want to cut him off until he can understand that I'm taking it away because he's too old rather than I'm taking it away because I'm being mean to him.

—*Sonia Ng, MD*

Thinking about Another Baby

Where does the time go? It probably feels like yesterday that you were thinking about having this baby. Could it be time to think about another?

One thing to consider, whether or not you considered it with your first baby, is banking your baby's cord blood. Deciding whether or not to bank your baby's umbilical cord blood is a very personal decision. Because you have only one opportunity to bank your baby's blood, on the day she's born, it can also be a very difficult decision to make. The blood in the umbilical cord contains stem cells, which have the potential to treat leukemia and some inherited disorders now and have the possibility of treating more diseases in the future.

When the baby is born, the doctor or midwife collects the cord blood from the part of the umbilical cord that is attached to the placenta. Normally, this blood would be disposed of as medical waste. The blood is placed into bags or syringes and carried by courier to a cord blood bank. There it's given an identifying number and frozen in liquid nitrogen. Theoretically, the stem cells in the sample can last forever if stored properly. But because the research only began in the 1970s, no one knows for sure how long they'll last.

Cord blood banking comes with a cost, around $2,000 for the initial collection and processing and an annual storage fee of around $125. You can donate your baby's cord blood to a public bank for free, but it is not reserved for your family's use.

∽

I waited until late in life to have kids, and now I look back and think, *If I'd have known how much fun kids are, I'd have started earlier and had more of them.*

—*Rebecca Reamy, MD, a mom of six- and one-year-old sons and a pediatrician in emergency medicine at Children's Healthcare of Atlanta, in Georgia*

Our son was very challenging for his first seven weeks, and my husband was threatening he might be an only child. But things quickly got easier.

My husband and I knew that we wanted to have at least two kids. When my son was around a year old, I was in my thirties, and we didn't want to wait too long. We had wanted our kids to be close in age. We didn't know how long it would take to get pregnant, and so we started trying, and it happened right away. It has been much easier to adjust to a second child; I think that having a little experience made the transition easier.

—*Michelle Hephner, DO*

My husband and I adopted twins, and when we were thinking about adopting a third baby, we realized you really have to rethink everything. Going from a family of four to a family of five can be challenging logistically. We have an SUV, and the middle row is all car seats! A

Mommy MD Guides-Recommended Product
Cord Blood Registry

Of the many cord blood banks in the United States, Cord Blood Registry (CBR) is the world's largest and most experienced, entrusted with storing more than 350,000 cord blood collections for individuals and their families.

CBR's laboratory storage facility in Tucson, AZ, was the first family cord blood stem cell bank in the world. Inside, the lab is an amazingly high-tech facility. But outside, the building is nondescript, in an almost secret location, for security purposes.

In its 20-year history, CBR also helped more clients use their cord blood stem cells for lifesaving transplants and experimental regenerative medicine therapies than any other family bank.

Visit **CordBlood.com** to learn more about cord blood banking.

vehicle that should fit seven adults only fits two adults plus three kids in car seats.

Parenting our son is a piece of cake. With the younger child, you learn to relax all of your paranoias. You have to let all of that go. Having kids has helped me to delegate more, and roll with the punches better. That's all that you can do!

—*Brooke Jackson, MD, a mom of 3½-year-old twin girls and a 14-month-old son and a dermatologist and medical director of the Skin Wellness Center of Chicago, in Illinois*

When we were thinking about having another baby, I found it helpful to read books with my older child that explained what was going to happen. Some books focus only on the positive aspects of having a baby sibling. I recommend also reading books about the not-so-great things—books that talk about angry feelings and how tough it can be to share your mom and dad.

One book I really like is *Julius, Baby of the World*, by Kevin Henkes. It tells the story of a big sister who at first thought it would be great to have a new baby in the family, but she later embarks on a rejection campaign. My older child laughed so hard when I read that book to her because she could really identify with the feelings he described.

—*Michelle Paley, MD, PA, a mom of two and a psychiatrist and psychotherapist in private practice, in Miami Beach, FL*

I'm currently pregnant, so I'm thinking a lot about having another baby! I'm a proponent of cord blood banking. I banked my daughter's cord blood, and I intend to bank my next child's cord blood also. There are so many possibilities that scientists are working on regarding cord blood research. Who knows what diseases they will be able to cure with cord blood in the future? For me, the expense of banking cord blood is well worth the risk of hopefully never needing to use it.

The advice that I received from my ob in choosing a cord blood banking company was to choose one of the larger companies that have been around for a while versus one of the many new start-up companies. If the new ones close down, what happens to your baby's cord blood?

—Jeannette Gonzalez Simon, MD, a mom of a two-year-old daughter who's expecting another baby and a pediatric gastroenterologist in private practice, in Staten Island, NY

When I was thinking about having another baby, it was important to me to bank the baby's cord blood. It wasn't readily available yet when my twins were born, and the technology had come very far in those six years.

When I was pregnant with my youngest daughter, the decision to bank her cord blood was a no-brainer. I have a younger sister who was born with brain damage. If she had been able to have her stem cells given back to her as a young child, it might have made all of the difference.

The other reason I wanted to bank my baby's cord blood is because it can be used to treat a lot of conditions that don't run in families. You can't predict things like cerebral palsy, leukemia, and lymphoma. But if you have banked your baby's cord blood, you can treat them.

—Lillian Schapiro, MD

RALLIE'S TIP

Cord blood banking wasn't an option when I was pregnant, but if it had been, I definitely would have taken advantage of it. Umbilical cord blood is a rich source of stem cells, which are considered to be the master cells of the body, and they've been used to successfully treat more than 80 serious diseases, including leukemia and other cancers and blood disorders. In the future, it's likely that doctors will use stem cells from banked cord blood to repair damaged or diseased tissues and organs.

Cord blood collection is safe and simple for moms and babies. In the moments after your baby is born, the doctor or midwife simply collects blood from the part of the umbilical cord that is attached to the placenta. If this blood isn't collected, it will end up being discarded as medical waste. Some families want to allow the cord blood to continue to pulse to the baby after delivery, and that is perfectly acceptable. Once the doctor or midwife has collected the blood, it's placed into bags or syringes and delivered to a cord blood bank, where it is given an identifying number and frozen in liquid nitrogen. Theoretically, the stem cells can last indefinitely if stored properly. Hopefully, your child will never have to use them, but you can take comfort in knowing that they're available if you ever need them.

Celebrating Your Baby's First Birthday!

People might think of a baby's first birthday as a milestone for her, but it's also a huge milestone for *you*. You've been a mom for an entire year! Happy MomDay!

꩜

My husband and I didn't make a big deal of our babies' first birthdays. The best I remember was giving them a big chocolate muffin or a Dove chocolate bar and watching them smear chocolate all over their faces. When our kids got older, we had birthday parties with the neighborhood kids.

—*Michelle Storms, MD*

꩜

For our babies' first birthdays, we had pretty low-key celebrations, with a few gifts and a cake. The babies really didn't get it at all. In general, we try to have home birthday parties, rather than going out. Also I try to make sure there are at least two other adults there to help out. Birthday parties can get quite chaotic!

—*Lesley Burton-Iwinski, MD*

꩜

We had two parties for my son's first birthday: one for my folks and another for my in-laws. My son touched his cake and then cried hysterically because he had icing all over his fingers. He didn't know to simply lick it off!

—*Michelle Hephner, DO*

꩜

I remember all of my babies' first birthdays, especially the chocolate cakes and the mess that went along with that.

My oldest son loves chocolate, but even as a baby, he was a neat freak. He couldn't stand to have food on his hands. So at his birthday party, he'd take a bite and then wave his hands in the air for them to be wiped. Then he'd take another bite.

—*Susan Besser, MD*

For my younger daughter's first birthday party, I made teddy bear–shaped, carrot, sugar-free cakes, with M&M's for the eyes. All anybody ate were the eyes. My twins were seven years old and horrified that I'd serve anybody such disgusting cake. Even the one-year-old babies who were there quickly figured out that sugar-free cake is not a winning concept.

—*Lillian Schapiro, MD*

To celebrate my younger daughter's first birthday, I planned a big family party at our house, and it was mayhem. Our house was filled with people, and our new Great Dane puppy was wreaking havoc, including chewing on all four legs of my dining room table.

Our older daughter had her first loose tooth at the time. Just after I had cleaned up the dinner dishes and was getting out the cake, my dad, who was a dentist, thought it would be a great idea to pull my daughter's loose tooth out! She started running around the house, crying hysterically with blood running out of her mouth because the tooth was pulled too soon. It was a nightmare! My perfect moment of my daughter's first birthday photo op was ruined. Just goes to show, you can plan and prepare as much as possible, but things often don't go as you hope. This all is remembered as a memory never to forget. So make it okay for things not to go perfectly and laugh at these precious moments when they don't.

—*Lisa Dado, MD*

RALLIE'S TIP

When my oldest son turned a year old, I was at a really low point in my life. I was 22 years old, and my husband and I were separated. We had gotten married when we were both really young, and neither of us had a clue about what it took to make a marriage work. I got pregnant right away, and the stress of having a new baby was just too much for our relationship.

I dropped out of college to work full-time so that I could support my son and myself, but it was nearly impossible to make ends meet with my minimum wage job. We were living well below the poverty level, and there was never enough money for food or rent, much less a nice party and presents to celebrate my son's first birthday! I felt like a complete failure. Earning a college degree had been my dream, but I had almost given up on it. How could I work, raise my son, and go to school at the same time?

On my son's first birthday, I remember dressing him in a little sailor suit that I bought for a dollar at a yard sale and promising him that his next birthday would be better. I would find a way to get back in school and earn my degree. Of course my son couldn't have cared less whether his mother had a college education, and he didn't realize that we were poor. As long as he felt safe and loved, he was the happiest baby in the world. I should have followed his example! Instead, I practically killed myself trying to do it all. Three years later, I graduated from college with a bachelor's degree, and ultimately I ended up graduating from medical school.

I know now that when our children are young, they need our love and attention more than anything. If I had known this on my son's first birthday, I would have enjoyed his little celebration as much as he did!

What I wish I had known on my son's first birthday is that it would all work out, and there was no need to beat myself up about the past, or to worry so much about the future. Life is full of second chances, and there is always more than one path that can lead us to our dreams.

Index

Note: Underlined references indicate boxed text.

BRAT diet, 250

Breast abscess, 17

Breast enlargement, in newborns, 3

Breastfeeding. *See also* Breast milk
  acid reflux and, 168, 169
  baby's bowel movements and,
      432, <u>432</u>, 433, 434
  baby's growth and, 339
  benefits of, 12–13, 14, 19, 21, 289
  birth control and, 108, 109
  challenges of, 15–19, 20, 21–24,
      25, 26–27, 27–28, 29,
      30–31, 34
  clipping baby's nails during, 259
  colic and, 160–61
  considering weaning from, 457–
      59
  for dehydration prevention, 250
  depression and, 180, 181
  elimination diet and, 378
  frequency of, 99
  help with (*see* Lactation
      consultants)
  introducing other liquids with,
      440
  introducing solid foods and, 207,
      314, 405
  isolation with, 322–23
  jaundice and, 46, 47
  leaking urine and, 155
  Mommy MD Guides–
      Recommended Products
      for, <u>13</u>, <u>16</u>, <u>23</u>
  nighttime, 95, 98, 99, 104
  nutrition required for, 298
  pacifier use and, 42–43
  in public, 270

  after returning to work, 122–23,
      124, 125, 126, 184
  sleep location for baby and, 95,
      96
  sleep loss with, 321
  as special experience, 14, 21, 25,
      277
  statistics on, 12
  supplementing with formula,
      103–4, 340
  twins, 15, 147
  during visits from family and
      friends, 37
  When to Call Your Doctor
      about, <u>18</u>

Breast milk
  air travel rules about, 414
  allergy to, 158, 160–61
  increasing production of, <u>13</u>, 16
  leakage of, 22–23, 125
  nutrients in, 260
  as primary beverage, 293, 295,
      296
  pumping, 15, 16, 22, 24, 26,
      27–28, 30, 31, 34, 103, 121–
      26
  storing, 121–22, 125

Breast pain, from breastfeeding, 17,
      18–19, <u>18</u>, 20, 21, 22, 24, 52.
      See also Mastitis

Breast pumps, 121, 122–24, <u>122</u>,
      125, 126

Breast shields, 16

Breathing, of newborns, 3

Breathing difficulty
  from allergy, <u>317</u>, <u>376</u>
  from asthma, 253–55, <u>255</u>

Cerebral palsy, <u>46</u>, 422, 452–53, 462

Cetaphil products, 128, 134

Chamomile packs, for breast pain, 21

Cheerios, 442

Child care. *See* Babysitters; Day care; Nannies

Child Passenger Safety (CPS) technician, for checking car seat installation, 79, 447

Child-rearing expenses, saving money on, 422–26

Child restraint systems. *See also* Car seat
for air travel, 414

Choking, 228, 230, 441–42, 446–47

Circumcision, 4, 65, 66
When to Call Your Doctor about, <u>67</u>

Cleaning house. *See* Housework, keeping up with

Cleaning products, nontoxic, 247

Clean Shopper, <u>269</u>

Clenched fists, of baby, 3, 110

Clipping fingernails and toenails, 258–60

Clothing
carrying change of, 75
dressing baby in, 80–81
hand-me-down, 424, 425
organizing, 343–46
reselling, 426
secondhand, 425
stain removal for, 223–24
for sun protection, 140–41, <u>142</u>, 143

taking pictures of, 367

washing, 82–83

weather-appropriate, 330–32

Clutter, 228, 249

Cocoa butter, as moisturizer, 130

Cold air, for croup, 403, 404

Cold flashes, after delivery, 53

Cold medications, 287, 290, 291

Colds, 285–91, 370, 373
When to Call Your Doctor about, <u>286</u>

Colic, 156–62, 267, 377, 378
When to Call Your Doctor about, <u>160</u>

College, saving for, 382–83

Comfort items, attachment to, 390

Comfort Silkie, <u>405</u>

Communication methods, of baby, 5, 111, 148, 149, 150, 305, 361, 390–91, 413, 439

Condoms, 108, <u>189</u>

Congestion. *See also* Colds
in newborns, 3

Conjunctivitis, 451

Connecting with your partner, 235–37

Constipation, 53, 431–34
When to Call Your Doctor about, <u>432</u>

Contraception, resuming, 108–9

Contrucci, Ann, 15, 35–36, 40–41, 56–57, 73–74, 84, 94–95, 106–7, 120, 147, 157, 163, 251, 281–82, 321, 333, 339, 436, 446

Convertible car seat, 447–48

Cooking safety, 225, 226

Friends
 introducing baby to, 35–39
 for overcoming isolation, 322,
  324
 socializing with, 429–31
Fruits, 295, 312–19, 409, 444
Furniture, babyproofing, 227, 228,
 229

G

Games, 305, 335, 361, 391, 413,
 439
Garcia, Joseph, 399
Gastroenteritis, 249–50
Gates, safety, 229, 309, 310, 312,
 348, 350, 393, 413
Gatten, Mike, 103
Gatten, Mindi, 103
Gaynor-Krupnick, Darlene, 19, 28,
 113, 123, 189, 190, 235–36,
 272–73, 290, 373–74
gDiapers, 61
Genitals, of newborns, 4
Gentle Naturals Cradle Cap Care,
 133
Gerber 100% Organic Apple Juice,
 295
Gerber Puffs, 442, 443, 443
Germs, fear of, 252
Giese, Sharon, 26–27, 38, 68, 228,
 252, 299, 306, 365, 376,
 446–47
Gilbert, Jennifer, 32, 76, 80, 98,
 176–77, 229–30, 241–42,
 258, 259, 261, 267–68, 342,
 343, 369, 394, 411, 448
Girlfriends' Guide to Pregnancy, 275

Go-Go Kidz Travelmate, 416
Gohara, Mona, 142, 144–45, 147, 151,
 211, 284–85, 287, 445–46
Grocery cart covers, 268, 269
Grocery shopping, 248, 267–70
Growth of baby
 by first birthday, 438
 tracking, 338–40
Guardian, appointing, 92, 93
Guilt, 175, 186, 241, 242, 246, 317,
 381, 386
Gums, cleaning, 257, 258
Gymboree, 113

H

Haircuts, 176–78
Hair growth, of baby, 2
Hair loss
 of baby, 2, 134
 of mother, after delivery, 53
Hands of baby
 for communication, 265
 control of, 149, 195, 239, 265,
  304, 334–35, 390
 as entertainment, 265
Hand washing, 37, 287, 373
Happiest Baby on the Block, The, 101,
 105
Hats
 for sun protection, 141, 143, 144
 for warmth, 50, 332
Head circumference, 10, 338, 438
Head control, of baby, 4–5, 111,
 149, 195, 238
Head injuries, 347
Health insurance, adding baby to,
 92–93

J

Jackson, Brooke, 32–33, 104, 147, 163, 167, 182, 240, 251–52, 271–72, 281, 290, 338, 417, 460–61

Jaliman, Debra, 126, 184, 234, 295, 316, 348, 415

Jaundice, 30, 45–49
    When to Call Your Doctor about, 46

Jogging stroller, 205, 234, 296, 297, 384, 424

Johnson & Johnson's baby wash, 90

Journaling, 427

Juice, 293–96, 327, 414, 432, 440

Julius, Baby of the World, 461

K

K&J Sunprotective Clothing, 142

Kangaroo care, for premature babies, 34–35

Kegel exercises, 156

Kickboxing, as exercise, 234–35

Kitchen, babyproofing, 225–26, 309

Knifty Knitter, 342

Koala Bibs, 369

Kosher baby foods, 318

Kramer, Alanna, 9, 25, 51, 78, 80–81, 97, 105, 115, 141, 200, 291–92, 322, 328, 424

Kulze, Ann, 33, 158–59, 218, 256–57, 261, 267, 277, 296, 300–301, 308, 310–11, 315, 333, 339–40, 362, 370, 397, 435

K-Y Jelly, 190

L

Lactation consultants, 15, 16, 17, 19–20, 21, 22, 23, 27, 30, 34, 88

Lactation cookies, 13

Lansinoh nipple cream, 24

Lansky, Vicki, 356

Laufer-Cahana, Ayala, 186, 301

Laughter, of baby, 5, 57, 148, 149, 195, 196, 439

Laundry, 82–83, 249

Laundry detergent. *See* Detergent

Leaking urine. *See* Urinary incontinence

Leash, baby, 310, 311

Legs
    baby bearing weight on, 238, 265
    of newborns, 4

Levenstein, JJ, 186–87

Life insurance, adjusting, 92, 93

Light reflex test, 12

Light treatment, for jaundice, 46, 47, 48–49

Lil' Dressers Drawer Labels, 344

Lippman, Cathie, 14, 82, 87–88, 153, 162, 240, 247, 260, 291, 377, 436, 451

Liu, Robyn, 101, 119, 171, 176, 216, 220, 224, 237, 253, 258, 261, 295, 299, 300, 313, 320, 368, 377, 440–41, 442

Living room, babyproofing, 226–27

Lumbar puncture, 137

Lyle, Kristin C., 16–17

M

Maclaren Volo stroller, <u>203</u>

Magnesium, in Natural Calm, <u>164</u>

Mailing labels, for birth announcements, 91

Malone, Mary Ann, <u>204</u>

Manicure, <u>258</u>, 361

Marriage, nurturing, 235–37, 300–301

Mastitis, <u>18</u>, 23, 24

McAllister, Rallie

  on asking for help, 85

  on baby as car passenger, 79–80

  on baby shoes, 364–65

  on baby's sleep location, 96

  on bathing, 130

  on bellyaches, 252–53

  on breastfeeding, 22–23, 26

  on carrying heavier baby, 448

  on celebrating baby's first birthday, 464–65

  on changing diapers, 59, 329–30

  on changing doctors, 396

  on clipping fingernails and toenails, 259

  on colic, 159

  on cord blood banking, 462–63

  on corralling toys, 393

  on cradle cap, 132–33

  on croup, 403

  on date nights, 237

  on diaper rash, 173–74, 175

  on diapers, 59, 329

  on ear infections, 371–72

  on enjoying sex, 190–91

  on exercising, 234

  on family traditions, 397–98

  on foods, 444–45

  on getting back into shape, 297–98

  on going back to work, 184–85

  on hiring a nanny, 274–75

  on housework, 248–49

  on introducing juice, 294

  on keeping baby happy and safe in car, 79–80

  on leaking urine, 155–56

  on making time for yourself, 386

  on napping, 322

  on organizing baby's clothing, 345–46

  on pet safety, 352

  on placing baby on tummy, 218–19

  on playdates, 241

  on playing with baby, 114–15, 359

  on preserving memories, 367–68

  on reading to baby, 152

  on recovering from birth, 56

  on resuming birth control, 109

  on saving for college, 383

  on saving money on baby things, 425

  on skin care products, 135

  on sleep location for baby, 96

  on stressing less, 165, 382

  on sun protection, 143

  on tantrums, 454

  on teaching values, 437

  on teeth grinding, 435

  on transitioning to stroller, 206

  on umbilical cord stump care, 65

  on vacations, 418

  on weaning, 458

About the Authors

RALLIE MCALLISTER, MD, MPH, MSEH

Dr. McAllister is a nationally recognized health expert. Dr. McAllister is the cofounder of Momosa Publishing LLC. She is the coauthor of *The Mommy MD Guide to Pregnancy and Birth*. Dr. McAllister's tips, articles, and blog are featured on **MOMMYMD GUIDES.COM**.

Her nationally syndicated newspaper column, Your Health, appeared in more than 30 newspapers in the United States and Canada. It was read by more than a million people each week.

Dr. McAllister has been the featured medical expert on more than 100 radio and television shows. She has appeared on *Good Morning America Health* and *Fox News*. She's the former host of *Rallie on Health*, a weekly regional health magazine on WJHL News Channel 11 with over one million viewers in a five-state area, and *No Bones about It*, a weekly radio talk show.

Dr. McAllister's healthy-eating tips and interviews have been featured in dozens of popular publications, including *USA Today, Women's Day, Better Homes and Gardens, Redbook, Family Circle, Parenting, Prevention, Men's Health, Women's World, Cosmopolitan, Glamour, Health Magazine, Energy Times, Arthritis Today*, and dozens of other newspapers.

Dr. McAllister has authored hundreds of health articles, with millions of additional readers, on dozens of health-related websites, including WebMD.com, LifetimeTV.com, iVillage.com, ParentsMagazine.com, msn.com, ParentingBookmark.com, FamilyResource.com, ChristianMommies.com, WomenOf.com, and BabyCenter.com.

She is the author of several books, including *Healthy Lunchbox: The Working Mom's Guide to Keeping You and Your Kids Trim*.

Dr. McAllister is a mom of three sons and a grandmom of one granddaughter.

JENNIFER BRIGHT REICH

Jennifer is a writer and editor with more than 15 years of publishing experience. Jennifer is the cofounder of Momosa Publishing LLC. She is the coauthor of *The Mommy MD Guide to Pregnancy and Birth*. Jennifer's tips, articles, and blog are featured on **MOMMYMDGUIDES.COM**. She has contributed to more than 150 books and published more than 100 magazine and newspaper articles. She's the author of *The Babyproofing Bible*.

Jennifer proudly served as a Lieutenant in the U.S. Army for four years, including one year working directly for the three Commanding Generals of I Corps at Fort Lewis, WA.

After that, Jennifer worked for seven years on staff at Rodale before launching her own editorial services business, Bright Communications LLC, in 2004.

Jennifer lives in Allentown, PA, with her husband and their two sons.

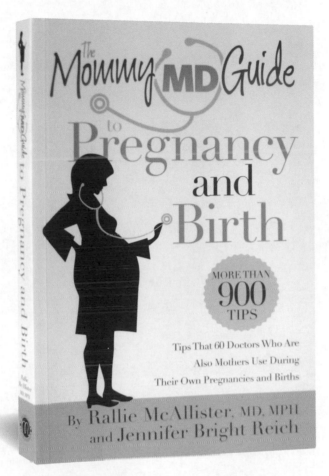